What constitutes a traumatic event? How and why does trauma affect people differently and what is a normal response? These are important questions asked by mental health professionals, counsellors, lawyers and primary care physicians on a daily basis. This concise yet comprehensive guidebook critically evaluates the evidence for causation and aetiology of post-trauma mental distress. It provides an accessible and highly referenced resource of practical advice and information which will be welcomed by a wide range of professionals, trainees and other interested readers. Dr O'Brien's coverage ranges from a brief historical perspective on post-traumatic illness and its prevalence right through to the present-day legal implications. We are reminded that post-traumatic stress disorder is by no means the only possible response to trauma and a helpful chapter is also devoted to the definition of a normal response. A broad range of theoretical and practical viewpoints is closely examined, including an evaluation of management approaches, possibilities for prevention and future research.

TRAUMATIC EVENTS
AND
MENTAL HEALTH

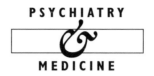

PSYCHIATRY

MEDICINE

Over recent years, the extent of psychiatric morbidity among patients seen in general hospital practice and primary care has been well established. Physicians and surgeons are becoming increasingly aware of the importance of recognizing and treating the psychiatric problems that their patients experience, and consultation–liaison psychiatry has become a distinct field for research and clinical practice. In the context of general medicine and its specialties, psychiatric morbidity may coexist with definite organic pathology or present largely with somatic symptoms in the absence of organic disease. This area is receiving more attention in postgraduate and undergraduate teaching, but there are few specialist textbooks which cover the topic.

This series reviews particular areas of medicine in which psychological factors and psychiatric morbidity are especially significant. Each book is written or edited by a clinician with extensive experience in the area, and combines clinical insight with a discussion of relevant research. The series is aimed at senior clinicians and trainees, particularly in psychiatry, internal medicine and general practice, and individual volumes will interest a wider audience in the health professions.

TRAUMATIC EVENTS
AND
MENTAL HEALTH

L. STEPHEN O'BRIEN

Aintree Hospitals NHS Trust,
Liverpool, UK

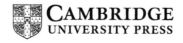

CAMBRIDGE
UNIVERSITY PRESS

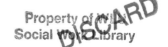

PUBLISHED BY THE PRESS SYNDICATE OF THE UNIVERSITY OF CAMBRIDGE
The Pitt Building, Trumpington Street, Cambridge CB2 1RP, United Kingdom

CAMBRIDGE UNIVERSITY PRESS
The Edinburgh Building, Cambridge CB2 2RU, United Kingdom
40 West 20th Street, New York, NY 10011-4211, USA
10 Stamford Road, Oakleigh, Melbourne 3166, Australia

© L. Stephen O'Brien 1998

First published 1998

Printed in the United Kingdom at the University Press, Cambridge

Typeset in Monotype Garamond 10/13 [SE]

A catalogue record for this book is available from the British Library

Library of Congress cataloguing in publication data

O'Brien, L. Stephen, 1956–
Traumatic events and mental health / L. Stephen O'Brien.
p. cm. – (Psychiatry and medicine)
Includes index.
ISBN 0 521 57027 1 (hc). – ISBN 0 521 57886 8 (pbk.)
1. Post-traumatic stress disorder. I. Title. II. Series.
RC552.P67027 1998
616.85′21–dc21 97-22865 CIP

ISBN 0 521 57027 1 hardback
ISBN 0 521 57886 8 paperback

CONTENTS

FOREWORD

Post-traumatic stress disorder is nowadays widely known (usually by its acronym PTSD), although it is also widely misunderstood, as is often the case with matters which attract considerable media interest. Hence, facts and fantasies are often mixed in accounts and reports of PTSD. Post-traumatic stress disorder is not a new problem, but one which has long been acknowledged, particularly in military contexts, at least by commanders and others with 'eyes to see' and 'ears to hear'.

Stephen O'Brien has military and civilian experience which, allied to academic discipline and a capacity for lucid writing, make this book an authoritative account of PTSD. Useful details are given of the history of this disorder and its relationship to other post-traumatic states is discussed. Clinical manifestations and treatment approaches are also dealt with, completing a text suitable for all who seek a balanced and authoritative view of this most important and potentially very disabling condition.

J.P. Watson MD, FRCP, FRCPsych

Professor of Psychiatry, United Medical and Dental Schools
Guy's Hospital, London
Honorary Civilian Consultant in Psychiatry to the Army

CHAPTER 1

INTRODUCTION AND HISTORICAL PERSPECTIVE

This book is intended to be a brief but comprehensive textbook of the mental disorders or difficulties which can follow trauma and traumatic events. It is hard to argue with the suggestion that disasters, catastrophes, violence and traumatic incidents are all too common in modern society. Nobody would seriously suggest that previous centuries were idyllic peaceful times; natural disasters have always occurred. However, the sheer scale of the efforts which we have made to kill and maim each other this century has far outclassed the equally brutal but probably far less efficient activities of our forebears. Increased speed has its effect. Not only do we move around at greater and greater speeds, with the results of accidents being more horrific, but information moves around the world at faster and faster rates so that communication may be almost instantaneous. Some of the particular problems associated with the impact of trauma on the psyche could not have happened until the last decade. Only now can a mother sit at home and watch live footage of a shipwreck in which she believes that her son has drowned.

The frequency and diversity of traumatic events which may affect one person or thousands are such that the consequences of trauma will probably impinge upon all of us at some time. They will certainly impact upon the work of health and other service workers in general and mental health and social work professionals in particular. There is a need for a relatively brief text on the problems, their background, diagnosis and management. In addition, this book is meant to act as a source of relatively detailed information as well as a resource book pointing to relevant data and references. Hopefully this may be of value for those researching or teaching the topic, and for those who have to plan, purchase or provide services.

It is no accident that the title does not mention post-traumatic stress disorder (PTSD). While it is recognised that PTSD is a very important topic and the major focus of research into the psychological consequences of extreme stressors, it is not the whole story of post-traumatic illness (PTI) and by no means explains all the possible reactions to various traumatic events. How people react to trauma is influenced by a whole range of factors including the nature, severity and meaning of the traumatic event, and factors in the individual such as his or her personality, previous history, experience, support and subsequent experience. Not only is PTSD not a universal response to trauma, but it is not the only response.

Most people adjust satisfactorily following exposure to even the most traumatic of events. Almost all are affected in some way by their experience and many suffer distress in the immediate aftermath, but most recover well. Of those who do develop significant mental disorders, not all suffer from PTSD, but many develop one or more of a wide range of post traumatic illnesses similar to the illnesses occurring in other situations. The evidence is that many of those who do develop PTSD also suffer from some other mental disorder in addition.

In the context of this book, PTI is taken to mean a recognisable mental disorder other than PTSD which follows a traumatic event and which is postulated to have been caused or precipitated by it. Possible PTIs commonly include other anxiety disorders, affective disorders, adjustment reactions, substance abuse disorders, and a range of other axis 1 disorders.

This first chapter is intended to give a brief overview and introduction to the purpose of the book, skating over some of the arguments and issues dealt with in the other chapters. It will also address two particular questions in some detail: questions concerning the history of PTI, and the validity and applicability of the concept. These seem to be fundamental questions which must be addressed first if we are going to be able seriously to consider the effects of trauma upon mental health. The second part of the chapter will review much more briefly the other issues and questions which will be discussed in the later chapters in an attempt to orient the reader to some of what is going to be said about this, surely the most popular diagnosis or diagnostic area in psychiatry today. It seems that PTSD is about the only psychiatric diagnosis that people do not object to being given.

Why is PTSD such a popular subject?

It has been recognised for many years that there can be psychological as well as physical consequences of trauma. The association between physical and mental health is generally accepted, both in terms of physical illness having an adverse effect upon mental state, and of mental illness aggravating or prolonging phys-ical problems. There is also a long history of recognition, at least anecdotally, that survivors may also suffer mental health difficulties, even if they have not sustained physical injury. There was relatively little medical research into this aspect of trauma until the large numbers of cases produced by war in this century. Indeed, interest has waxed and waned as wars have come and gone. Time and again it has been noted that lessons in the management of mental health problems in battle have had to be relearned with each new conflict. Nowadays there is enormous interest in the psychological consequences of trauma. It is a sort of psychiatric 'dish of the day' which is comprehensible and accessible for mass media and adds 'human interest' to disasters. Every time there is some form of individual or collective tragedy in the UK today we are told by radio, television, and newspapers that trained counsellors are being deployed to help the survivors come to terms with the trauma. The fiftieth anniversary of the end of World War II brought stories about the still-suffering veterans and about the potential trauma caused by reminders.

It is as if PTSD in particular is an acceptable face of mental illness, more understandable than schizophrenia and easier to associate with. There is an acceptance that it could happen to 'anyone, even to a member of my family'.

This media interest is partly because PTSD is 'a good story', but also partly because the media played a part in the synthesis of this disorder in a way in which they have not for any other. Newspaper and magazine articles, popular books and films, television documentaries, all played a part in bringing the plight of Vietnam veterans to the attention of America.

The increasing general interest also reflects a development in professional interest in PTI. The PILOTS database contains over 9000 references on the subject and includes book chapters as well as a wide range of author submitted papers. A recent search of major international on-line data services found over 5000 indexed references. The vast majority of these papers are recent and it seems clear that the growth of interest in matters post-traumatic has been reflected in a very rapid expansion in production of papers in recent years. A team from the American National Center for PTSD investigated this percep-tion and confirmed that there was a major increase in production of papers around and after the description of PTSD in 1980 (Blake, Albano and Keane 1992). Most of these articles were initially written about either war or sexual violence, with considerably more of the former. It seems that PTI is inevitably linked to warfare. In a review article in the *British Journal of Psychiatry*, Gersons and Carlier (1992) looked at the history of PTSD and said that 'the "introduction" of the new diagnosis of PTSD was seen and felt to be a recognition of the psychic consequences of war, especially as experienced by Vietnam veterans'.

If the media has been interested in PTI and PTSD in recent years, the law has had such an interest for a rather longer period. One of the criticisms, as well as the commendations, of PTSD is that it is a way to facilitate compensation claims for psychic injury. It appears clear that English law began to recognise the ability to gain relief for 'nervous shock' in the absence of physical injury in the nineteenth century. Interestingly, then as now, much of the reluctance and resistance to accept this concept was based on the 'flood gates' argument that says that if you grant relief for nervous shock then there will be an unstoppable tide of cases, including spurious ones. Legal papers on the subject have also increased rapidly in recent years, and there has been a recent Law Commission consultation paper on Liability for Psychiatric Illness (Law Commission, 1995). While there may continue to be debate about how often PTI may gain relief at law, there does not seem to be any argument in legal circles or elsewhere that it does not exist. Gersons' paper notes that when PTSD was formally described, 'another important aspect of the new diagnostic category was that it facilitated compensation claims'.

Gersons and Carlier went on to note that 'the emphasis of this side effect implied that it was considered a normal human reaction to an extremely unpleasant event.' This has been an important feature of the perception of PTI, and of PTSD in particular, as people debate whether such responses are normal or pathological. Paradoxically, although Gersons and Carlier see the facilitation of compensation as 'normalising' the reactions, the law is clear that normal responses and normal shock cannot lead to compensation. This demand that PTI is a normal reaction has been used by some to attract sufferers into help-seeking, although it may also take management of such difficulties out of health care hands or even make sufferers refuse treatment on the grounds that their suffering is normal.

Today consideration of traumatic events and mental health inevitably focuses on PTSD even though this is not the only response to traumatic events. As response to trauma becomes more acceptable and more respectable, it is easy to forget that most people survive traumatic events without developing significant mental health problems. Although some studies have shown extremely high rates of PTI, the majority have not. If we look at survivors of trauma who recognise the need for, or seek, help, then rates are lower still. Although almost everybody who is exposed to a major traumatic event is affected in some way, the majority adjust effectively and continue to function well.

In addition, not everybody who develops PTI suffers from PTSD. A range of mental health problems can present for the first time after trauma. They may or may not be associated with the event. Even if they are, the range of clinical presentations is wide and to label them all as PTSD is not only inaccurate but is likely to be unhelpful. It may help people gain compensation, but it may make them less likely to get appropriate treatment for the cause of their disability. For the purposes of this book, PTSD will be considered as one type or presentation of PTI. Although there will be considerable emphasis on PTSD as perhaps a paradigm of PTI, other conditions which can follow trauma will also be considered, as will the range of normal responses to traumata.

Is PTSD a new condition?

The first question addresses the history of PTSD, and particularly where PTSD comes from. It was only defined in 1980. Is it new?

The idea that PTI, or more specifically PTSD is not a new concept is widely championed. Many papers tell us that PTSD is merely the renaming or the synthesis of an age-old condition. This attitude has generally been accepted, but what is the evidence?

Most authors cite anecdotal papers or present the simple statement that PTSD is the same as soldier's heart, railway spine, battle shock etc. This may well be the case, but it is worthwhile considering these assertions critically rather than accepting them at face value. In fact, there is a great list of synonyms for 'traumatic neurosis' that have been used in litigation and in clinical situations (Table 1.1). It can be seen that the more pejorative have tended to be used where legal or compensation issues are to the fore.

There are powerful reasons for wanting PTSD not to be a new condition. The formulation of PTSD in the *Diagnostic and Statistical Manual of Mental Disorders*, third edition (DSM-III) was met with some scepticism. One of the major complaints was that there was no justification or explanation of the development of a 'new condition'. It is difficult for professionals or the public to accept that a condition such as PTSD can be new. It is, by definition, a response to events which may be more frequent today but which are not unique to the latter half of the twentieth century. Therefore it must have existed before. By the same token it is probably unacceptable, at least to professionals, that there was no knowledge or recognition of the existence of the PTSD syndrome before its definition. It therefore becomes essential that the definition of PTSD comprises the redefinition and recategorisation of a pre-existing

Table 1.1. *Terms used to describe PTI in litigation and in clinical practice*

Accident aboulia	Neurotic neurosis
Accident neurosis	Nostalgia
Accident victim syndrome	Physioneurosis
Aftermath neurosis	Post accident anxiety syndrome
American disease	Post traumatic stress syndrome
Attitudinal pathosis	Post traumatic syndrome
Battle shock	Post Vietnam syndrome
Combat fatigue	Profit neurosis
Combat stress neurosis	Railway brain
Commotio cerebri	Railway spine
Compensation hysteria	Rape trauma syndrome
Compensationitis	Secondary gain syndrome
Compensation neurosis	Shell shock
Da Costa's syndrome	Soldier's heart
Entitlement neurosis	Syndrome of disproportionate disability
Erichsen's disease	Traumatic hysteria
Functional overlay	Traumatic neurasthenia
Fright neurosis	Traumatic neurosis
Gas hysteria	Triggered neurosis
Greek disease	Unconscious malingering
Greenback neurosis	Vertebral neurosis
Justice neurosis	War neurosis
Litigation neurosis	Wharfie's back
Mediterranean back	Whiplash neurosis
Mediterranean disease	

syndrome which was known under other names, rather than the description of a new phenomenon.

What, then is the background to PTI and PTSD?

The history of PTI

Various authors vie to come up with the earliest record of PTI, citing cases going back thousands of years. In general, the older the references, the less empirical they are, the less detailed the description of symptoms, and the more likely it is that case studies are autobiographical. However, like that other 'twentieth century' mental illness, anorexia nervosa, there are some very old possible cases recorded.

Earliest reports

It is suggested that the Romans, in their Lex Talionis or Law of Retaliation, were codifying a phenomenon accepted in Old Testament times that immediate retribution for trauma may be an automatic response which is outwith a victim's control and was therefore socially sanctioned.

The author's favourite early case is the description in the seventh century Welsh legends surrounding King Arthur, the man who was provided with a round table and a brotherhood of knights some five hundred years later. It is said in the original stories that Merlin, or Lailoken, was a wild man who went away to live alone in the woods for some years as he was affected by the sounds and sights of terrible battle. He avoided people and lived as a hermit for several years, only to return refreshed and with his special powers. The comparison with PTSD here is that he appears to have suffered from intrusive memories and perhaps flashbacks, as well as subsequent social isolation and loss of former interests.

Seventeenth century

The first scientific description of actual symptoms as a consequence of 'violent commotion of the mind or strong emotions' may be credited to the seventeenth-century physician Sydenham (Mendelson, 1987).

Samuel Pepys' diary is said to contain descriptions of symptoms indicative of PTSD following the Fire of London. In his paper, one of the earliest to address the new American diagnosis of PTSD in the UK press, Daly (Daly, 1983) gives a detailed account of Pepys' response to the Fire of London of 1666, using descriptions taken from his diaries. It seems that Pepys was not under direct physical threat from the fire but managed to get his family and possessions out of the way. However, he did spend a significant amount of time in the vicinity of the fire, initially as a bystander and then in an official capacity. There is record of a psychological reaction to the event. He notes being 'much terrified in the nights nowadays with dreams of fire and falling down of houses'. There is evidence of arousal at reminders, and perhaps of irritability, although it is not clear that the latter is associated with the fire. It is perhaps significant that there is no evidence of dysfunction, no good evidence of avoidance behaviour, and a good outcome.

Eighteenth century

A single paper (Parry-Jones and Parry-Jones, 1994) purports to show supportive evidence for the concept of PTSD from an eighteenth-century natural disaster. It is based on study of three contemporary sources, including detailed
medical records. The essence of the traumatic event was that three female
members of the same family were confined for 37 days in a space six feet by four
feet by two and a half feet after the barn they were sheltering in was buried by
an avalanche. They were eventually rescued and all survived. They had lived on
snow mixed with milk from the two goats trapped with them. They had wisely
decided not to eat the putrefying chickens raw. Their physical problems are
described, as are very clear-cut, acute psychological reactions. The descriptions
recorded would not be considered diagnostic of PTSD but do confirm recognition of a psychological reaction to trauma at that time. Interestingly, they not
only sought and received compensation for their plight from the sovereign, but
also went on at least two of what might be described as lecture tours, and 'by the
piteous recital of their long and great suffering, excited so much compassion,
that they were everywhere met with a charitable reception, and plentiful relief'.

Nineteenth century

In the nineteenth century the arrival of the railways heralded a new form of
trauma with the development of 'railway spine' (Trimble 1981). Fatalities from
train accidents started on the first day of the commercial service. In addition to
physical injuries there is very good evidence of PTI, and of the pursuit of
compensation. It was in association with the problem of illness induced by the
great fear caused by a near miss from a train that the concept of nervous shock
came to be developed. It appears that accidents involving trains were not
uncommon. Indeed Charles Dickens was in a train crash in which ten were
killed and 49 wounded. He subsequently described symptoms which would not
fulfil DSM-IV criteria for PTSD (American Psychiatric Association, 1994), but
which certainly represent a PTI. He wrote of feeling weak, of being able to eat
and sleep well, but being unable to concentrate on his writing because of feeling
'faint and sick', and of anxiety on exposure.

At this time there was, as later, a debate as to whether the cause was physical
or psychological. Erichsen believed the symptoms to be due to 'molecular
degeneration' of the nervous system, while Page disagreed and saw a psychological cause. Psychological explanations centred around new studies and
definitions of hysteria.

In the American Civil War, soldiers are said to have developed symptoms of lethargy and withdrawal, sometimes called nostalgia as it was thought to be related to a profound distress at being away from home. Later there were descriptions of soldier's heart or irritable heart, conditions which appeared clearly to have more to do with 'heartache' and psychological distress than with heart disease. There was a series of personal accounts of the distress of this war. There seems no doubt that there were significant numbers of cases of PTI, but none of the accounts really seems to describe PTSD. The war was also of interest because, like Vietnam, it was a controversial war in which there was not general acceptance of the motives of those involved, or of the conduct of the conflict.

First World War

The first large-scale groups of cases to be documented in detail occurred in the First World War. Large numbers of troops became unable to fight and presented with an array of symptoms including conversion hysteria, apparent stupor, and overarousal. Initially they were evacuated to hospital in England, where many did not recover. First studies were done by neurologists, who thought the condition to be due to pressure or chemical effects upon the brain of close or prolonged exposure to the forces associated with explosions (Mott, 1917). However, failure to recover and the growing scale of the problem led to the involvement of psychiatrists and the establishment of NYD-P (not yet diagnosed-psychiatric) units.

Presentations were well documented both by a number of professionals and by contemporary novelists and poets. There were whole units presenting with classical conversion hysteria, with well-documented accounts of lines of soldiers marching miles for treatment of dyspnoea, confusion and light-headedness thought to be attributable to poison gas to which, in fact, they had not been exposed (Mareth and Brooker, 1985). Others had apparent organic confusional states. By 1917 there were 40 000 (20% of the total) war pensioners with psychiatric disabilities (Salmon, 1917).

In 1920, Rivers (Rivers, 1920) confirmed that the presentations were similar to those of neurotic illness in peacetime. This is of particular interest as it was a view that predominated for many years. It was generally accepted that trauma precipitated recognised psychiatric illnesses, usually in those more than normally susceptible. Rivers, like others, did not propose that there was a specific post-traumatic illness. The Shell Shock Enquiry supported this view and therefore recommended that the term shell shock be abandoned (Report of the War

Office Committee of Enquiry on Shell Shock, 1922). At this time the received wisdom was that trauma precipitated a variety of mental illnesses which usually resolved unless they solidified into a chronic case of one of the recognised neuroses or psychoses. It was not felt that trauma produced a single durable clinical presentation.

Second World War

During the Second World War there was again ample evidence that trauma could be followed by mental illness. In fact Cline (Cline and Rath, 1982) has suggested that in 1940 the French Army itself became a psychiatric casualty, despite having had lower rates of chronic PTI and higher rates of recovery in World War One due to treatment close to the trauma (near the front line). General Beaufre said of the advancing German army 'two guns and a hundred men could have held them up for half a day. . . . But how could people get a grip of themselves in the midst of this general chaos?'. Whole units fled in disarray without even engaging the enemy.

Several discoveries important to the future of PTI were made during this conflict. It was noted that the rate of PTI appeared to be proportionate to the severity of the traumatic stress. Rates of casualties went up with intensity of battle, number of physical casualties, poor preparation of the troops, and physical tiredness or deprivation.

In 1942, Rado (Rado, 1942) produced a detailed description of traumatic neurosis. He described conversion hysteria symptoms, marked trembling and impotence. However, he also described hyperarousal, sleep disturbance with vivid nightmares, and irritability with self-pampering behaviour, and marked sensitiveness. These latter symptoms are closely related to those of PTSD and this gives weight to the idea that at least some of the neuroses seen in World War Two were PTSD.

Following the Coconut Grove nightclub fire in which 500 people died, Lindemann (Choy and de Bosset, 1992) produced a very detailed account of the symptomatology of acute grief. The descriptions were of an acute PTI, a severe form of grief, but the symptoms as reported could not be said to be definitely equivalent to PTSD.

Pre-Vietnam

DSM I (American Psychiatric Association, 1952) did not include a condition equivalent to PTSD. It did recognise that extreme stressors could be followed by mental health problems in that it included the diagnostic category of gross stress reaction. However, this was seen as a self-limiting condition. It was felt that chronic problems only occurred in those with severe premorbid personality disturbance. In such cases, the condition solidified into a recognisable psychiatric disorder.

In 1968 DSM-II (American Psychiatric Association 1968) moved away from gross stress but still focused on previous vulnerability in that it included 'transient situational disturbance of adult life' which should again be considered as transitory, with persisting symptoms being rediagnosed in accordance with one of the existing diagnostic categories. In the same year Keiser (1968) expressed an opposite view in his book *The Traumatic Neurosis*, clearly describing a specific problem following trauma. Many papers cite this monograph as proof of the existence of the clinical syndrome of PTSD prior to Vietnam.

Vietnam

The history of PTSD, and therefore to a great extent the history of PTI, does, inevitably, tend to centre around Vietnam. Nobody can seriously doubt that despite the ongoing background interest in PTI, it was not a particularly popular topic before Vietnam. There was some interest in the effects of the Holocaust and of violent sexual crime against women, but it was essentially consideration of the fate of Vietnam veterans which led to the development of the diagnosis of PTSD. Indeed, part of the brief of the research committee which came up with the diagnosis was to consider the possible validity of a 'post-Vietnam syndrome'.

What was different about Vietnam as compared with other conflicts that led to the concept of PTSD being formulated? The number of casualties and the extent and intensity of the war were less than in World War II, yet after the dust of that war had settled there was relatively little interest in chronic PTI until after Vietnam and PTSD. The exception was, of course, the Holocaust, which led to a constant background level of interest and research. Indeed, there was a reasonable amount of research on chronic disability in concentration camp survivors and other victims of the Nazis, but it is important to note that there was no assumption that such information could be generalised to other situations. The Holocaust was seen as something different, something unique. In 1991 Weisaeth and Eitinger (1991) reminded us that post-war interest in post-traumatic mental health problems in Europe was dictated by the form of involvement in the war. He states 'occupied countries suffered forms of civilian casualties above and beyond those caused by bombings or the ordinary stresses of war . . . these varied traumatic stress experiences led to intensive research'. It was only after Vietnam that the 'ordinary' casualties of World War II were studied in any detail.

Vietnam is said to have been different from other wars. It was an unpopular, prolonged, relatively low intensity, distant, guerrilla conflict which did not involve the majority of the people, and was lost by the Americans. Returning Vietnam veterans were not welcomed as heroes. At best they were ignored and at worst they were vilified for the part that they had played in an unpopular war. Initially they were not thought of as being victims but as deserving any problems that they had because they should not have been there in the first place. Gradually, however, there developed a database of information which was mostly in the public domain. Scientific studies were initially small scale and perhaps less than wholly unbiased. The information broadcast by the popular press was certainly not unbiased. The plight of suffering veterans was highlighted, usually focusing on single cases. Vietnam began to be associated with social problems, poor integration in society, criminal behaviour, and mental health problems. There were widely publicised dramatic criminal cases in which post-Vietnam problems were successfully argued as the cause of the criminal behaviour. Films and books began to feed a national guilt at how the veterans had been treated and there was a growing demand that they receive some form of specific help or treatment.

Congress finally agreed in 1979 (Kelly, 1985) to funding for 'shop-front' services for Vietnam veterans with readjustment problems. These readjustment problems were described as 'a low-grade motivational or behavioural impairment which interferes with a victim's overall ability to cope reasonably effectively with his or her daily life problems. A readjustment problem does not usually amount to a definable psychiatric illness'. Previous requests for such services had been turned down by Congress for the preceding six years because it was not accepted that Vietnam veterans had needs different from those of veterans of other wars, or that there was any specific need. It was an acceptance that Vietnam was different which led to this intervention.

It had been increasingly obvious, and increasingly difficult to ignore, that many veterans of Vietnam had not settled and reassimilated into life in the same way that other veterans of foreign wars had done. Although Borus' paper on the incidence of maladjustment in Vietnam veterans actually stated that the rate of problems was not higher than in other veterans and strongly criticised other papers as being biased and unselected (Borus, 1974), this was clearly a minority view. Much attention was being paid by those promoting the concept of problems following Vietnam, to a 'post-Vietnam syndrome', and to problems specific to Vietnam veterans as differentiated from other veterans (Friedman, 1981; Walker 1981; Stuart 1982).

A paper by Fleming (1985) is of interest in this regard because a Vietnam veteran and associate professor of psychology actually had the audacity to question the uniqueness of Vietnam. For one thing he noted that it was not only after Vietnam that there was a shortage of home-coming parades. There were indeed many victory parades and great welcomes for veterans after the First World War, but the way in which troops were returned to the USA after the Second World War contributed to the fact that there was only one official heroes welcome parade in the whole country. He said that Vietnam was not different from all previous wars. He compared it with the Indian wars and the Philippine insurrection, saying that each of these was as brutal as Vietnam. He noted that these too were guerrilla wars, that there were demonstrations against the Philippine insurrection intervention, and that the average age of combatants in the American Civil War was 18 compared with 19 in Vietnam. He says that the system of fixed-term rotation of individual soldiers rather than whole units started in Korea rather than Vietnam, and that the practice of having pools of men to replace wounded individuals in units rather than replacing the units themselves had started in World War II.

Later studies suggested that 300 000 to 700 000 or more of the 3 000 000 who served in Vietnam had PTSD. These studies were specifically designed to measure the size of the problem after its nature had been accepted. They were prompted by the less acceptable presentations of PTSD which were capturing public attention. There was a series of books, films, television programmes and newspaper articles which emphasised the plight of veterans and fuelled the national and executive guilt for the way in which these people had been treated by society. Veterans were seen as being marginalised and significantly socially handicapped. They apparently had much higher rates of criminal behaviour, of divorce, and of substance abuse. They were said to be more likely to be unemployed, and to feel that they had been rejected by their country. This contrasted with previous veterans (and also subsequently with Gulf and Panama veterans) who had been lionised and treated as heroes on their return. Investigation showed a consistent pattern of symptomatology in sufferers which was defined in DSM III as PTSD.

There was a further contrast with previous wars. In the First World War there had been very large numbers of acute casualties and large numbers of chronic casualties. Initially great store was laid in the fact that Vietnam had low rates of psychiatric casualties (Jones, 1967). The rapid growth in incidence during later years was mostly due to substance abuse rather than the more usual forms of

PTI. Nevertheless, despite the much lower rates of acute illness, there were apparently much higher rates of chronic illness as PTSD in veterans after they had left the army. This is surprising and gave further fuel for the debate as to whether there was something specific about Vietnam that made it different from other traumatic events.

Post-Vietnam

The definition of PTSD sparked a further frenzy of research and interest in the problem area. Initially most of the work continued to focus on Vietnam and it is true that even today this has been the primary source of data. A search of the PILOTS database held at Dartmouth College shows that references concerning Vietnam outnumber those referring to all other wars by a factor of three.

However, there was some research done into PTI outwith the stress of war before Vietnam, and rather more afterwards.

New areas of interest grew rapidly. Papers started to be published noting PTSD in groups of people other than Vietnam veterans. Prevalence rates varied widely. In female survivors of sexual abuse, rape and physical abuse, rates varied from 4% (Greenwald and Leitenberg, 1990) to 81% (Kemp *et al.*, 1995) . Post traumatic stress disorder was reported in patients with physical illness without external trauma, and even after childbirth (Ballard, Stanley and Brockington, 1995). For example, rates of 15% in those with unexplained temporo-mandibular joint pain (Aghabeigi, Feinmann and Harris, 1992), 25% following heart attack (Kutz *et al.*, 1994), and 46% in people with a psychotic illness (McGorry *et al.*, 1991) were all reported. Traumatic physical injuries were also studied, with rates varying from less than 1% following accidental injury (Malt, 1988) to 45% in burn victims (Tarrier, 1995) . Rates for those exposed to natural disasters had been reported varying from 5% in children who survived a hurricane (Shannon *et al.*, 1994) to 60% in survivors of a tornado (Madakasira and O'Brien, 1987) . The nature of qualifying stressors and the importance or otherwise of the stressor criterion in PTI will be discussed in Chapter 5.

Studies were also done on veterans of other wars, particularly World War II. Elderly veterans rates varied from 0% to 12% (Spiro, Schnurr and Aldwin, 1994) for 'ordinary' veterans depending upon the extent and the intensity of their combat exposure, to 56–67% in ex-prisoners of war (Muse, 1986; Zeiss and Dickman, 1989).

There is clear evidence that some sort of PTI has been recognisable, no matter how frequently, for many hundreds of years. There are similarities between historical accounts of these problems and recent descriptions of

PTSD. However, the accounts over the centuries are not unequivocally co-terminous with current descriptions of PTSD. This may be a problem of recording and of interpretation over time. However, it is probably not safe simply to assume that all previous PTI is the same as PTSD.

Is PTI a valid concept?

The second question in this chapter concerns the validity of the concept of post-traumatic illness. Is there any evidence that such disorders exist?

Validity is an interesting concept in itself. Dictionary definitions describe valid as meaning well-founded, of a robust argument. In scientific practice we commonly talk of different forms of validity. For example, Horowitz, Weiss and Marmar, (1987) in a commentary on the validity of the diagnosis of PTSD consider four necessary types of validity:

- face validity
- descriptive validity
- predictive validity
- construct validity.

We will consider the validity of PTSD specifically, rather than that of PTI in general.

Face validity

A concept has face validity if it seems well-founded; if it makes sense. Both a priori reasoning and the lessons of history indicate that there is face validity for the concept of mental disorder following traumatic events or stressors. The section on the history and development of the concepts of PTI and PTSD strongly supports the face validity of PTI as it has consistently been recognised for hundreds, if not thousands, of years that in a significant number of cases mental distress or disorder follows events that are generally recognised as being traumatic. More recent work supports the concept of PTSD itself as a recognisable response to trauma.

Descriptive validity

A concept has descriptive validity if it allows the content to be described in such a way that it is possible to group the instances together and also to separate them from what does not belong. For example, to define PTI as a consequence of trauma is sufficient to include all cases of PTI, but could also include orthopaedic injuries or homelessness. To define it as mental distress occurring after trauma would again include all cases but would also include normal reactions and unrelated mental disorders occurring in anyone who has suffered a traumatic event. In fact this is a particular danger in work with PTI. There is a common human drive to seek meanings or explanations of events and as a consequence there is a temptation to ascribe everything that follows a traumatic event to that event, even when no causal relationship exists.

If we use PTSD as the paradigm for PTI, then it does appear to have descriptive validity as the definition includes the traumatic event, a temporal relationship to that event, a required duration of difficulties and demonstrable disability, and a specific symptom pattern with content related to the event. Thus it attempts to include like events and to separate them from both normal responses and unconnected mental and physical disorders. There is evidence that the syndrome is stable and relevant, with all criteria being to a greater or lesser degree associated with trauma as represented by exposure to a range of particularly stressful events including combat, crime and natural disasters. Factor analytic research has also supported the concept of the three symptom groups – intrusive, avoidant and arousal (Silver and Iacono, 1984) – as used in DSM.

Predictive validity

If the concept of PTI or PTSD is valid, then we will be able to predict certain things from the diagnosis. We will be able to predict that it will only follow traumatic events, that it will generally respond in a particular way to treatment, and that it will generally have a predictable course or range of courses. In general, this seems to be the case and PTSD is a valid concept in terms of predicting its occurrence and choosing appropriate therapy. There are, however, questions raised. Scott (Scott and Stradling, 1994) has raised a question as to whether or not PTSD has predictive validity in this way. He describes a number of cases in which the symptom criteria for PTSD have occurred in cases in which the stressor would not be considered to be a qualifying one which was likely to result in PTSD. He argues for the abolition of the stressor criterion as it has been defined in the various editions of DSM or suggests an alternative diagnosis in addition to PTSD, of 'prolonged duress stress disorder' in which all the criteria other than the stressor would be similar to those in PTSD except that they would not be related to a single stressful event. He is not alone in raising questions about the importance of the stressor criterion, which will be discussed later.

Construct validity

To have construct validity, PTSD must give support to theoretical models explaining the signs and symptoms said to comprise the syndrome. There are a

16

number of studies in various areas which appear to give external validity to the concept of PTSD as a syndromal presentation of specific neurobiological consequences of stress.

It has been shown that video films of relevant stressors not only result in more intrusive symptomatology and experienced affect than do neutral stimuli, but are also related to states of increased physiological arousal not observed in control subjects or in subjects with other mental disorders. These findings have been replicated and can be seen as external validators of the concept of an abnormality of arousal and stress response in PTSD. They will be discussed further in Chapter 4 with regard to aetiology, and in connection with assessment in Chapter 7.

Diagnostic validity

Wolfe and Keane have reviewed the diagnostic validity of PTSD (Wolfe and Keane, 1990). They recognise that the face validity has been generally accepted, and describe four routes by which attempts have been made to validate the diagnosis:

- assessment efforts in diagnosis, including a 'comprehensive, structured assessment battery' to increase diagnostic accuracy by using multiple overlapping or concordant measures
- the establishment of models to explain the observed phenomena
- the search for biological changes or markers
- epidemiological study.

In each of these areas there has been support for the validity of the diagnosis of PTSD. A wide range of diagnostic instruments (which are described in some detail in Chapter 7) has been shown to have convergent validity as well as reliability. Models to explain PTSD centre around an interaction between neurobiology and psychosocial processes rather than the original psychoanalytic theories of Freud and others, and there is increasing support for such models from animal, in-vitro and in-vivo experiments. In association with this there are increasingly reproducible biochemical, physiological and hormonal changes seen in PTSD. Epidemiological studies have shown the occurrence of PTSD and PTI in widely differing samples, both after a variety of traumatic incidents, and in the general population.

PTSD certainly seems to be a valid concept which has considerable empirical support for face, construct, descriptive and predictive validity.

Nosological considerations

Several investigators have considered the nosology of PTI or PTSD in particular (Davidson and Foa, 1991; O'Donohue and Elliott, 1992). Classification is an important issue in mental health. Before discussing classification methods it is important to consider the reasons for using any classificatory system.

O'Donohue and Elliot describe three main groups of purposes or functions for classification. The first are meta-scientific functions in that classification provides the ontology, defines what is said to exist and defines order in systems. The scientific functions allow description in defining what is similar and what is different or outside the group. They predict both antecedents and future behaviour, and they allow explanation and understanding of the objects under investigation. The third group of functions are pragmatic. Principally they include facilitation of communication and of data storage and retrieval. Classification provides a sort of shorthand which allows professionals and others to talk about cases which are similar, in language which has the same meaning for both parties.

Davidson and Foa describe the four classificatory systems generally used in medicine. These are, in increasing levels of importance or robustness:

- symptomatological or syndromal
- anatomical
- pathogenetic
- aetiological.

In mental health, most disorders are classified according to symptoms. In DSM-IV a small number of groups of conditions are defined aetiologically. These are the organic brain syndromes and substance abuse disorders. PTSD is also defined aetiologically, but it is included in the group of anxiety disorders, the other members of which are defined symptomatically. This is anomalous and is one of the reasons why the position of PTSD in the classification system has been questioned.

There is considerable argument about where PTSD should be placed in the classification system. In both revisions of DSM-III, and in DSM-IV, PTSD is consistently placed amongst the anxiety disorders. Is this appropriate?

Brett (1993) has discussed four possible nosological positions of PTSD.

PTSD as an anxiety disorder
This is the current position. There is some support for the theory that PTSD is an anxiety disorder. Comorbidity studies have shown a somewhat stronger

link with anxiety disorders than with other disorders. Investigations of family history in sufferers have been less than dramatic in their findings, but there is a stronger family history of anxiety disorders than of affective disorders in PTSD sufferers.

There is rather stronger support for PTSD as an anxiety disorder in consideration of symptomatology and of physiological responses. PTSD shares symptomatology with panic disorder, phobic anxiety, generalised anxiety disorder, and obsessive compulsive disorder, although none of these diagnoses covers the whole of the PTSD syndrome. Not only the symptomatology, but also physiological assessment indicates that PTSD, like anxiety disorders, involves an increase, or at least an abnormality, in sympathetic nervous system activity.

PTSD as a dissociative disorder

Hypnotisability has been used in a number of studies as a measure of dissociation (Stutman and Bliss, 1985; Spiegel, Hunt and Dondershine, 1988). It has been shown that levels of hypnotisability in patients with PTSD are higher than those in patients suffering from a range of other mental health problems. In particular they were found to be twice that generally found in cases of generalised anxiety disorder.

Another observation which is believed to be associated with dissociative disorders is that of an analgesia on exposure to stressful events which is reversible with naloxone. In Vietnam veteran patients with PTSD, this naloxone-reversible analgesia has been found on exposure to films of combat but not to neutral films or films of unrelated stressors (Pitman *et al.*, 1990).

However, dissociative symptoms such as flashbacks and amnesia, unlike anxiety symptoms, are by no means universally present in PTSD. Dissociative phenomena, including marked behavioural disorganisation, are relatively common in the immediate aftermath of trauma, but tend to reduce with time.

PTSD in a broad group of stress response syndromes

An alternative classificatory group which has been suggested for PTSD is that of a group of stress response disorders. This was one of the options considered by the DSM-IV task force on PTSD. If this were adopted, PTSD would be placed in an aetiologically defined group of disorders which follow various stressful events. It is placed in such a group in ICD-10. Suggested members of such a group would be:

- acute stress disorder
- PTSD

- pathological grief reactions
- bereavement
- adjustment disorders.

There is doubt about the inclusion of adjustment reactions which, to a great extent, are seen as a sort of container for all problems which do not really fit diagnostic criteria for any other Axis-I disorder and are considered to be short lived and mild.

In addition, bereavement responses have been carefully excluded from the diagnostic classification and are seen as conditions which do not amount to a mental disorder but may be a focus of medical attention.

PTSD in a narrow group of DESNOS

The other suggested new classification system was intended to avoid inclusion of questionable or particularly minor conditions and not to dilute the importance of PTI. Suggested members were:

- acute stress disorder
- PTSD
- disorders of extreme stress not otherwise specified (DESNOS).

This last has been suggested as a new diagnosis but not accepted by the American Psychiatric Association. It was intended to recognise the frequent presentation of patients who have clearly suffered significant disability following traumatic events, but who did not fulfil diagnostic criteria for PTSD either because of the nature of the stressor criterion or because of the symptom profile.

PTSD in DSM-IV and ICD-10

In fact, DSM-IV did not change the nosological position of PTSD. It and a new PTI, acute stress disorder, were firmly included in the anxiety disorders section. DESNOS was not accepted but will be further studied, and bereavement is still considered to be a normal process although it may be a focus of medical attention. Adjustment disorders remain in a separate category as a catch-all at the end of Axis-I.

ICD-10 is the first edition specifically to include PTI as PTSD. It has also included acute stress disorder. The previous edition was produced before PTSD was defined in DSM-III. In ICD-10, the nosological situation of these PTI disorders is somewhat different as there is a group of stress-related disorders unlike DSM-IV. Here too bereavement is not seen as a disorder or disease. Again, adjustment disorders comprise a separate group at the very end of Axis-I.

The status of PTSD and PTI as illness

The question is often asked as to whether PTSD is a mental disorder or a normal reaction. The point is of more than academic interest. In the provision of mental health care in today's National Health Service in particular, there is increasing pressure to 'target' services on the mentally ill, and specifically on the severely mentally ill. Other life difficulties or problems cannot be afforded attention by health professionals. It is therefore difficult to obtain resources for the provision of treatment for PTSD sufferers. If it were thought that it was not a true mental illness, then it would not be seen as a suitable area for assessment or intervention at all.

This question of whether or not PTSD is an illness will be explored in great detail in the next chapter. Suffice it to say that there has been great pressure both for PTSD to be accepted as a genuine illness, and for it to be accepted as a normal response to an abnormal situation.

There is a downside to the successful campaign for the recognition and acceptance of PTSD. It has become so much of an accepted concept that a backlash is perhaps beginning to develop against sufferers, particularly in the area of compensation and litigation. A trend can be seen to consider that people today are less sturdy or robust than their forebears and that they are unable to cope with stresses that they should take in their stride. This is particularly so in those who have been traditionally considered to be strong, 'macho' representatives of the public, such as the police and army. A number of newspapers have run articles indicating disappointment at the perceived readiness of such people to seek compensation and to be unable to cope with the stresses of their job. Examples of such articles include 'Hillsborough Officers Lose Trauma Claim in Hillsborough Football Disaster' (1995), and headlines like 'The Cap Badge says Death or Glory, Not "Or Compensation"' (1994), and 'Hillsborough Police Claims Repugnant' (1995). There seems a real danger that the promotion of PTSD and PTI as an acceptable and 'normal' response which is different from the general run of psychiatric illnesses has led to a trivialisation of the concept and a perception, shared to some extent by the courts, that it is only a means of gaining compensation.

How common is PTI?

The structured research has been focused upon PTSD rather than upon other illnesses following traumatic stress. While a range of the latter is recognised, particularly anxiety disorders, depression and substance abuse, much of the focus has been upon the question of whether other disorders should be seen as evidence of comorbidity, rather than on studying the other disorders as separate entities. The importance of the recognition of the existence of forms of PTI other than PTSD will be dealt with in Chapter 6.

It is worth remembering that it is not only mental disorders which have been linked to stress. As early as 1927, Bram reported that 85% of 3000 cases of thyrotoxicosis gave a history of some traumatic or stressful event in the period leading up to the onset of the illness. Clearly this does not prove that the one caused the other. They may be of quite separate causation or may both indirectly be caused by a third factor. However, there is considerable evidence to link the onset or exacerbation of physical illnesses to traumatic events.

Most of the studies of prevalence of PTSD have been based on groups at particular risk because they are known to have been exposed to traumatic events. Investigators have studied rates of PTSD in subgroups exposed to the same stressors at different intensities and duration, or have looked at the rates of PTSD following a wide range of different stressors. Incidences and prevalences vary markedly from stressor to stressor, and to a lesser extent from study to study. Rates appear to be uniformly high following certain stressors such as rape, much more variable following combat in general, and comparatively low following medical problems or road traffic accidents.

There have been some community studies of prevalence of PTSD in representative samples of the general population not at particular risk. These will be discussed further in Chapter 3, but it is worth noting that the better studies are fairly consistent in producing lifetime rates of 1% or 1.3% and current rates a little below half that. While a lifetime prevalence rate of about 1% appears to represent an uncommon problem, it is of the same order as schizophrenia. This suggests that at any one time there should be about 250 000 active cases of PTSD in the United Kingdom.

Does PTI occur in isolation?

One of the most consistent findings in studies of PTSD or PTI is that the great majority of sufferers fulfil the diagnostic criteria for other disorders in addition to those for PTSD. This question of comorbidity is of considerable importance in consideration of both the validity of the concept of PTI and of the causes or underlying pathology. On average studies have shown that 80% of PTSD sufferers also fulfil diagnostic criteria for at least one other condition (Sierles *et al.*, 1983, 1986; McFarlane and Papay, 1992), and that a significant number could actually be diagnosed as having three or more current Axis-I diagnoses. Some association has been found with almost all disorders. Comorbidity is discussed in Chapter 6.

What causes PTI?

Superficially this appears a perfectly simple question. By definition, PTI must be caused by trauma. However, the situation is far from being that simple. If PTI was simply a consequence of trauma then there would be a clear and simple relationship between trauma and its occurrence. For example, one of two situations might exist. There might be a level of trauma below which people did not get PTI and above which almost everybody did so. More credibly, there would be a direct relationship between trauma and incidence of PTI so that it would be possible to forecast that a certain trauma would result in, say, 50% of those exposed developing PTI.

Clearly this is not the case. There are two very obvious problems. One lies in the differences between people, and the other in measurement of traumatic stress. Why is it that two apparently very similar people can be standing next to each other in the same trench when an attack occurs yet one develops PTI and one does not? How does one measure and compare stresses or traumata? It is very difficult to rank order, being wounded in battle, being shot at in battle, shooting a criminal in the course of duty, attending a multiple road traffic accident as a rescuer, watching helplessly as a stranger is killed, watching a relative be killed, being raped, being held hostage, and suffering severe accidental injury. There is a real temptation to order them by post hoc reasoning, counting the most traumatic as that producing the highest rate of PTI. However, this may be fallacious as it is not measuring intensity of trauma, but is assuming that rate of PTI measures intensity of trauma and ignoring the possibility that trauma may not be uni-dimensional, but there may be differences in quality and in meaning as well as in intensity.

In fact, the two questions of individual response and extent of trauma are not at all clearly separated. DSM-IIIR recognised in the text of the manual, and DSM-IV recognised in the actual diagnostic criteria, that a victim's perception of a traumatic event is of major importance. While it is clear that some events such as rape are universally negative, the impact may vary from person to person. Some other events may simply not be traumatic for some. One man's trauma may be another's hard day's work or even an exciting and exhilarating event.

The question of aetiology of PTI will be addressed in detail in Chapter 4.

How do we know who has PTI?

In theory, the diagnosis of PTI is simple: patients who present with symptoms and a history of exposure to traumatic events in circumstances in which it seems likely that the symptoms constitute an illness that would not have occurred if it were not for the traumatic event have a PTI. In practice, of course, things are not nearly so simple.

PTI patients do not always complain

Much has been made of the importance of avoidance symptoms and their effect upon help-seeking behaviour (Veale, 1991). Kolb in particular has emphasised the view that sufferers are reluctant to seek help, that when they do seek help they do not mention the trauma, that when the trauma is mentioned they avoid talking about it and do not present it as a focus on their problems, and that health care providers may often collude in this denial of the problem, so that many cases are missed (Kolb, 1989).

In fact, there is very little empirical as opposed to anecdotal evidence that sufferers with severe disability associated with PTI fail to seek help because of the effect of their severe PTI symptoms. One study showed that increased symptomatology soon after the trauma was associated with help-seeking (Yule and Udwin, 1991). There is some evidence of delay in help-seeking. Israeli attempts to study the phenomenon of delayed onset PTSD found that only 10% of cases were of true delayed onset, while most represented delayed help-seeking (Solomon, et al., 1989). In one of the very few, if not the only, study directly to investigate help-seeking versus none help-seeking behaviour in PTI, the Israelis (Solomon, 1989) discovered that help-seeking was related to symptom severity, to self efficacy, and to the experience of negative life events. In essence, those who did not seek help had less severe symptoms and had more personal resources to cope with their symptoms. This contradicts the idea that the most severe cases do not seek help.

There is no single diagnostic test for PTI or PTSD

PTIs other than PTSD do not have specific symptomatology which sets them apart from other general psychiatric illness. The presentation of depression after a traumatic event is similar to that when the depression has no known origin. Only the relationship in time, the course, and perhaps the symptom content can help make the diagnosis.

For PTSD there is a specific symptom cluster which is used to define the diagnosis. This makes the diagnosis apparently simple if the patient seeks help. Trauma plus the symptoms of PTSD plus disability equals PTSD. However, while there is clearly a need for a high index of suspicion of PTSD and for systematic routine enquiry about trauma, it must also be remembered that at clinical interview there is no objective test for PTSD. This can cause problems when there is financial or other gain associated with the diagnosis of PTSD. Litigation, worker's compensation, criminal responsibility, or pension issues may be involved. In addition, there is the powerful need of sufferers to seek meaning for their situation.

Failure to diagnose PTI will lead to a failure to provide treatment which may significantly reduce disability, and may also lead to a failure of the sufferer to gain recompense to which he is entitled. On the other hand, inappropriate diagnosis may lead to inappropriate treatment, unfulfillable expectations, and also to a shift of responsibility for self and adoption of a victim role which robs the sufferer of the ability to cope.

Diagnostic methods

There is a need in the clinical mental health and trauma settings always to be aware of the possibility of PTI and to enquire systematically about traumatic events. At the same time there is a need for caution and to resist the temptation automatically to make the equation:

$$history\ of\ trauma + mental\ illness = PTI$$

Diagnosis in the clinical setting should use one of the structured interviews which have been well validated. Psychometric tests can be supportive in diagnosis and may be more robust than interview, although many are quite transparent. It should be noted that none of them was designed and validated in an adversarial or forensic situation. Further robust support for the diagnosis may be gained from physiological testing, from prolonged observation, and from information from neutral informants.

What is the management of PTI?

If it had been shown that there was a single, simple, effective treatment programme for PTSD and other PTI, then Chapter 8 on management and outcome would be very brief. Unfortunately, this is not the case. Amongst the thousands of papers on PTSD and PTI there have been surprisingly few controlled trials of treatment and outcome. The results are far from clear, although there is some evidence that both behavioural approaches and medication have some effect. Some centres focus on psychotherapeutic approaches, individually, in group therapy, or in 'rap groups'. Others have a problem-centred or 'package' approach, with a number of different treatment modalities used either in a formalised treatment programme or as modules specific for a patient's needs.

The various forms of management and the evidence or otherwise for their efficacy will be considered in detail. It is worth noting that ICD-10 says of PTSD that 'the course is fluctuating but recovery can be expected in the majority of cases'. This may be at variance with the experience of those who spend a significant amount of time treating patients with PTSD. However, it is certainly possible that the process of selection which leads to patients coming to those with a particular interest in PTI means that only the worst prognosis cases are seen. What evidence there is consistently shows that symptoms generally decrease in intensity with time.

Success has been claimed for a wide range of treatments including psychotherapy (Horowitz, 1973; Brom, Kleber and Defares, 1989), group therapy (Besyner, 1985), individual and group therapy (Brende, 1981), behavioural therapy (Foa and Rothbaum, 1989), rewind technique (Muss, 1991), saccadic eye movement desensitisation (Shapiro, 1989), mono-amine oxidase inhibitors and tricyclic antidepressants (Frank *et al.*, 1988), selective serotonin re-uptake inhibitors (Davidson, Roth and Newman, 1991), and buspirone (Duffy and Malloy, 1994), to name but a few.

Is PTI only related to compensation cases?

The answer here is an almost unqualified no. There is clear evidence that only a small proportion of the total numbers of Vietnam veterans said to suffer from PTSD have sought compensation. The Israeli experience is that compensation-seeking behaviour is associated with severity of exposure to combat, and of reported disability and symptomatology (Solomon *et al.*, 1994). There is considerable evidence that the course of illness is not affected by the presence or otherwise of compensation claims, and that resolution of litigation does not produce recovery (Braverman, 1977; Mendelson, 1982; Burstein, 1986a, 1986b). The impression that PTI is only associated with compensation can be gained by looking at a number of papers which have only considered compensation seekers (Bell *et al.*, 1988; Brooks and McKinlay, 1992).

There has been some considerable concern in the civil legal field that plaintiff lawyers and experts will come together to construct arguments for PTI in every case without consideration of the validity of the case (Law Commission, 1995). There is very little evidence for this and it seems that the Law Commission is, in its consultation paper on 'Liability for psychiatric illness', playing devil's advocate to provoke further consideration of the topic.

There have been occasional dissenting voices. There has been a suggestion that the Veterans Administration system in the US (Mossman, 1994) encourages illness and personal incapacity through the process of funding and rewarding illness. There was also an article in which it was suggested that PTI was a condition caused or perpetuated by the law and in which well-meaning professionals damage their patients or clients in the process of trying to obtain financial compensation for them (Tyndel and Tyndel, 1984). These are minority views.

While those practising in a medico-legal setting will see many plaintiffs seeking compensation, those working in a clinical setting will see many who have no recourse to compensation or have not chosen to seek it, or have had their compensation claim settled.

Is PTI related to criminal behaviour?

Forensic issues and PTI is a vexed topic. One of the earliest observations about Vietnam veterans and PTI was the apparently high prevalence of criminal behaviour and especially violence in sufferers. The evidence is perhaps less clear cut than the early reports suggested.

Headlines such as 'Paying the price for Vietnam: PTSD and criminal behaviour' (Erlinder, 1984) contrast with 'The "Vietnam syndrome" defense: a "G.I. bill of criminal rights"?' (Menefee, 1985) to show the opposing extremes of the public perception. The former suggests that criminal behaviour by Vietnam veterans with PTI is an inevitable consequence of Vietnam, while the latter suggests that Vietnam is simply being used to explain away criminal behaviour and to absolve veterans of responsibility for their actions.

There has been suggestion of a specific connection between Vietnam veteran status and criminal behaviour in that a study in 1979 (Beckerman and Fontana, 1989) showed that 15% of prison inmates were Vietnam veterans while 10% were veterans of other wars. However, neither this study nor the one which showed that 25% of Vietnam veterans had had serious legal difficulties (Marciniak, 1986) connected criminal behaviour with PTSD or PTI per se rather than with simple Vietnam veteran status.

A comparison of Vietnam veterans who were inmates with those in the community showed that criminal behaviour was related to pre-military behaviour and that rates of PTSD were equivalent (Shaw *et al.*, 1987). A study of cases in which a plea of not guilty by reason of insanity was entered showed that less than half of one percent of cases used a diagnosis of PTSD (Appelbaum *et al.*, 1993).

More recently authors have stressed the dangers of inappropriate use of PTSD as a defence in the courts. It has been suggested (Packer, 1983) that PTSD is seldom the cause of offences, and that criminal behaviour generally bears little relationship to traumatic experience (Bisson, 1993).

Almost all of the work associating PTSD sufferers with crime as opposed to the production of PTSD by violent crime, has been in the area of Vietnam and PTSD. This is because of the major political connotations of this connection. That Vietnam veterans have a higher rate of principally non-violent crime seems proven. That this crime is associated with PTI is not proven. There is considerable scepticism as there have been widely publicised controversial cases and as PTSD has been used to explain everything from murder to drug dealing and tax evasion. It is important to emphasise that there is no evidence that these results can be generalised from Vietnam to Vietnam-related PTSD or other sources of PTSD. Nor can they be generalised from PTSD to other types of PTI.

The various medicolegal aspects of PTI will be addressed in more detail in Chapter 9.

Is it possible to prevent PTI?

There are different approaches to prevention.

Traditionally armies, and latterly other organisations whose members may be exposed to traumatic events in the course of their duties, have trained personnel in order to enhance their ability to withstand stressors. Over the years there have been attempts to select out those who are most susceptible to the adverse effects of traumatic events. These have generally had limited success. All organisations have some degree of selection and there is also self-selection in the people who apply to be members of such organisations. Probably the largest experiments in selection were carried out by the Americans in the Second World War. They had the highest ever rejection rate of recruits for psychological reasons but failed to lower the rate of psychological casualties significantly. Attempts to define selection procedures and pick those who are most suited to the job as well as least likely to develop PTI continue. There may, however, be conflicts if those who are most likely to be effective at the task in hand are also most likely to expose themselves to the stressor and therefore most likely to develop PTI.

Most recent interest in the subject of prevention has been in secondary prevention. It seems to be received wisdom that early intervention can prevent PTI. This would appear to be a logical position and is one which is supported by a number of authors, although the empirical evidence is far from clear (Brom and Kleber, 1989; Armfield, 1994; Lundin, 1994). Indeed, Bisson and Deahl (1994) have pointed out that there is no good empirical evidence of the value of debriefing as an early intervention in preventing PTI.

Chapter 10 looks in detail at methods used to prevent PTI, at the evidence for their efficacy, and particularly at the very fashionable use of debriefing techniques in the early aftermath of a traumatic event.

What is the future?

There is a great deal that is still not known about PTI.

- Little is known about PTI other than PTSD. We need to understand its course and response to treatment as well as its relationship to the same conditions occurring other than in the aftermath of trauma.
- The relative roles of trauma and pre-existing factors are still not clearly understood.
- Response to treatment and logical treatment choice are still major issues and there is a need for large-scale outcome studies.
- The role of selection in prevention needs further study.
- The question as to whether or not debriefing is preventive needs to be answered.
- There is a need for a method of assessing trauma and its effect on an individual.
- More robust diagnostic methods are still required, specifically ones which are not transparent and not readily open to a charge of falsification.
- There is a need for courts to come to some clear understanding of the position of PTI, both in criminal responsibility issues and in the area of what sort of PTI in what sort of situation is to be afforded relief at law.
- It needs to be recognised that PTI is not the inevitable consequence of trauma and that not all PTI is PTSD.
- The predictive value of symptomatology in the immediate aftermath needs further exploration to help in the targeting of resources.

References

Aghabeigi, B., Feinmann, C. and Harris, M. (1992). Prevalence of posttraumatic stress disorder in patients with chronic idiopathic facial pain. *British Journal of Oral Maxillofacial Surgery*, 30, 6: 360–4.

American Psychiatric Association (1952). *Diagnostic and Statistical Manual of Mental Disorders*, 1st edition. Washington: APA.

American Psychiatric Association (1968). *Diagnostic and Statistical Manual of Mental Disorders*, 2nd edition. Washington: APA.

American Psychiatric Association (1994). *Diagnostic and Statistical Manual of Mental Disorders*, 4th edition. Washington: APA.

Appelbaum, P.S., Jick, R.Z., Grisso, T. and Givelber, D. (1993). Use of posttraumatic stress disorder to support an insanity defense. *American Journal of Psychiatry*. **150**, 2: 229–34.

Armfield, F. (1994). Preventing post traumatic stress disorder resulting from military operations. *Military Medicine*, **159**, 12: 739–46.

Ballard, C.G., Stanley, A.K. and Brockington, I.F. (1995). Post traumatic stress disorder (PTSD) after childbirth. *British Journal of Psychiatry*, **166**: 525–8.

Beckerman, A. and Fontana, L. (1989). Vietnam veterans and the criminal justice system: A selected review. *Criminal Justice and Behavior*, **16**, 4: 412–28.

Bell, P., Kee, M., Loughrey, G.C., Roddy, R.J. and Curran, P.S. (1988). Post-traumatic stress in Northern Ireland. *Acta Psychiatrica Scandinavica*. **77**, 2: 166–9.

Besyner, J.K. (1985). Multimodal inpatient treatment of Vietnam combat veterans with post-traumatic stress disorder. 92nd Annual Convention of the American Psychological Association. *Psychotherapy in Private Practice*, **3**, 4: 43–7.

Bisson, J.I. (1993). Automatism and post-traumatic stress disorder. *British Journal of Psychiatry*. **163**: 830–32.

Bisson, J. and Deahl, M. (1994). Psychological debriefing and prevention of post-traumatic stress. More research is needed. [Editorial] *British Journal of Psychiatry*, **165**, 6: 717–20.

Blake, D.D., Albano, A.M. and Keane, T.M. (1992). Twenty years of trauma: Psychological Abstracts through 1989. *Journal of Traumatic Stress*, **5**, 3: 477–84.

Borus J.F. (1974). Incidence of maladjustment in Vietnam returnees. *Archives of General Psychiatry*, **30**: 554–7.

Bram, I. (1927). Psychic trauma and pathogenesis of exophthalmic goitre. *Endocrinology*, **11**: 106–16

Braverman, M. (1977). Validity of psychotraumatic reactions. *Journal of Forensic Sciences*, **22**, 3: 654–62.

Brende, J.O. (1981). Combined individual and group therapy for Vietnam veterans. *International Journal of Group Psychotherapy*, **31**, 3: 367–78.

Brett, E. A. (1993). Classification of PTSD in DSM-IV: Anxiety Disorder, Dissociative Disorder, or Stress Disorder. In *PTSD: DSM-IV and Beyond*, Ed. J.R. Davidson and E.B. Foa. Washington: American Psychiatric Press.

Brom, D. and Kleber, R.J. (1989). Prevention of post-traumatic stress disorders. *Journal of Traumatic Stress*, **2**, 3: 335–51.

Brom, D., Kleber, R.J. and Defares, P.B. (1989). Brief psychotherapy for posttraumatic stress disorders. *Journal of Consulting and Clinical Psychology*, **57**, 5: 607–12.

Brooks, N. and McKinlay, W.W. (1992). Mental health consequences of the Lockerbie disaster. *Journal of Traumatic Stress*, **5**, 4: 527–43.

Burstein, A. (1986a). Can monetary compensation influence the course of a disorder? *American Journal of Psychiatry*, **143**, 1: 112.

Burstein, A. (1986b). Treatment length in post-traumatic stress disorder. *Psychosomatics*, **27**, 9: 632–7.

Choy, T. and de Bosset, F. (1992). Post-traumatic stress disorder: An overview. *Canadian Journal of Psychiatry*, **37**, 8: 578–83.

Cline, W.R. and Rath, F.H. (1982). The concept of an army as a psychiatric casualty. *Journal of the Royal Army Medical Corps*, **128**, 2: 79–88.

Daly, R.J. (1983). Samuel Pepys and post-traumatic stress disorder. *British Journal of Psychiatry*, **143**: 64–8.

Davidson, J.R. and Foa, E.B. (1991). Diagnostic issues in posttraumatic stress disorder: Considerations for the DSM-IV. Special issue: Diagnoses, dimensions, and DSM-IV: The science of classification. *Journal of Abnormal Psychology*, **100**, 3: 346–55.

Davidson, J.R., Roth, S. and Newman, E. (1991). Fluoxetine in post-traumatic stress disorder. *Journal of Traumatic Stress*, **4**, 3: 419–23.

Duffy, J.D. and Malloy, P.F. (1994). Efficacy of buspirone in the treatment of post-traumatic stress disorder: An open trial. *Annals of Clinical Psychiatry*, **6**, 1: 33–7.

Erlinder, C.P. (1984). Paying the price for Vietnam: post traumatic stress disorder and criminal behavior. *Boston College Law Review*, **25**, 2: 305–47.

Fleming, R.H. (1985). Post Vietnam syndrome: Neurosis or sociosis? *Psychiatry*, **48**, 2: 122–3.

Foa, E.B. and Rothbaum, B.O. (1989). Behavioural psychotherapy for post-traumatic stress disorder. Special issue: Behavioural psychotherapy into the 1990s. *International Review of Psychiatry*, **1**, 3: 219–26.

Frank, J.B., Kosten, T.R., Giller, E.L. and Dan, E. (1988). A randomized clinical trial of phenelzine and imipramine for posttraumatic stress disorder. *American Journal of Psychiatry*, **145**, 10: 1289–91.

Friedman, M.J. (1981). Post-Vietnam syndrome: recognition and management. *Psychosomatics*, **22**, 11: 931–43.

Gersons, B.P. and Carlier, I.V. (1992). Post-traumatic stress disorder: The history of a recent concept. *British Journal of Psychiatry*, **161**: 742–8.

Greenwald, E. and Leitenberg, H. (1990). Posttraumatic stress disorder in a nonclinical and nonstudent sample of adult women sexually abused as children. *Journal of Interpersonal Violence*, **5**, 2: 217–28.

Hillsborough Officers Lose Trauma Claim Hillsborough Football Disaster (1995). *The Times*, 11 April.

Hillsborough Police Claims 'Repugnant' (1995). *The Daily Telegraph*, 29 March: 4.

Horowitz, M.J. (1973). Phase oriented treatment of stress response syndromes. *American Journal of Psychotherapy*, **27**, 4: 506–15.

Horowitz, M.J., Weiss, D.S. and Marmar, C. (1987). Diagnosis of posttraumatic stress disorder. *Journal of Nervous and Mental Disease*, **175**, 5: 267–8.

Jones F. D. (1967). Experiences of a Division Psychiatrist in Vietnam. *Military Medicine*, **132**, 12: 1003–8.

Keiser L. (1968). *The Traumatic Neurosis*. Philadelphia: J. B. Lippincott & Co.

Kelly, W.E. (1985). *PTSD and the War Veteran Patient.* Brunner Mazel Psychosocial Stress Series No. 5. New York: Brunner Mazel.

Kemp, A., Green, B.L., Hovanitz, C. and Rawlings, E.I. (1995). Incidence and correlates of PTSD in battered women shelter and community samples. *Journal of Interpersonal Violence,* **10**: 1.

Kolb, L.C. (1989). Chronic post-traumatic stress disorder: implications of recent epidemiological and neuropsychological studies. *Psychological Medicine,* **19**, 4: 821–4.

Kutz, I., Shabtai, H., Solomon, Z., Neumann, M. and David, D. (1994). Post-traumatic stress disorder in myocardial infarction patients: prevalence study. *Israeli Journal of Psychiatry and Related Sciences,* **31**, 1: 48–56.

Law Commission (1995). *Liability for Psychiatric Illness. Law Commisson Consultation Paper No. 137.* London: HMSO.

Lundin, T. (1994). The treatment of acute trauma: Post-traumatic stress disorder prevention. *Psychiatric Clinics of North America,* **17**, 2: 385–91.

Madakasira, S. and O'Brien, K.F. (1987). Acute posttraumatic stress disorder in victims of a natural disaster. *Journal of Nervous and Mental Disease,* **175**, 5: 286–90.

Malt, U. (1988). The long term psychiatric consequences of accidental injury; a longitudinal study of 107 adults. *British Journal of Psychiatry,* **153**: 810–18.

Marciniak, R.D. (1986). Implications to forensic psychiatry of post-traumatic stress disorder: A review. *Military Medicine,* **151**, 8: 434–7.

Mareth, T.R. and Brooker, A.E. (1985). Combat stress reaction: A concept in evolution. *Military Medicine,* **150**, 4: 186–90.

McFarlane, A.C. and Papay, P. (1992). Multiple diagnoses in posttraumatic stress disorder in the victims of a natural disaster. *Journal of Nervous and Mental Disease,* **180**, 8: 498–504.

McGorry, P.D., Chanen, A., McCarthy, E., Van, R.R., McKenzie, D. and Singh, B. (1991). Posttraumatic stress disorder following recent onset psychosis: an unrecognized postpsychotic syndrome. *Journal of Nervous and Mental Disease,* **179**, 5: 253–9.

Mendelson, G. (1982). Not 'cured by a verdict'. Effect of legal settlement on compensation claimants. *Medical Journal of Australia,* **2**, 3: 132–4.

Mendelson, G. (1987). The concept of posttraumatic stress disorder: A review. *International Journal of Law and Psychiatry,* **10**, 1: 45–62.

Menefee, S.P. (1985). The 'Vietnam syndrome' defense: a G.I. bill of criminal rights?. *Army Lawyer,* 1–28.

Mossman, D. (1994). At the VA, it pays to be sick. (Department of Veterans Affairs). *The Public Interest,* 114: 35–48.

Mott F.W. (1917). Mental hygiene and shell shock. *British Medical Journal,* **2**: 39–42.

Muse, M. (1986). Stress-related, posttraumatic chronic pain syndrome: Behavioral treatment approach. *Pain,* **25**, 3: 389–94.

Muss, D.C. (1991). A new technique for treating post-traumatic stress disorder. *British Journal of Clinical Psychology,* **30**, 1: 91–2.

O'Donohue, W. and Elliott, A. (1992). The current status of post-traumatic stress disorder as a diagnostic category: Problems and proposals. *Journal of Traumatic Stress,* **5**, 3: 421–39.

Packer, I.K. (1983). Post-traumatic stress disorder and the insanity defense: A critical analysis. *Journal of Psychiatry and Law,* **11**, 2: 125–36.

Parry-Jones, B. and Parry-Jones, W.L. (1994). Post-traumatic stress disorder: Supportive evidence from an eighteenth century natural disaster. *Psychological Medicine*, **24**, 1: 15–27.

Pitman, R.K., Van der Kolk, B.A., Orr, S.P. and Greenberg, M. (1990). Naloxone-reversible analgesic response to combat-related stimuli in posttraumatic stress disorder: A pilot study. *Archives of General Psychiatry*, **47**, 6: 541–4.

Rado, S. (1942). Pathodynamics and treatment of traumatic war neurosis (traumatophobia). *Psychosomatic Medicine*, **4**: 362–8.

Report of the War Office Committee of Enquiry on Shell Shock (1922). London: HMSO.

Rivers, W.H.R. (1920). *Instinct and the Unconscious*. Cambridge: Cambridge University Press.

Salmon, T.W. (1917). *The Care and Treatment of Mental Diseases and War Neuroses 'Shell Shock' in the British Army*. New York: War Work Committee of the National Committee for Mental Hygiene .

Scott, M.J. and Stradling, S.G. (1994). Post-traumatic stress disorder without the trauma. *British Journal of Clinical Psychology*, **33**, 1: 71–4.

Shannon, M.P., Lonigan, C.J., Finch, A.J. and Taylor, C.M. (1994). Children exposed to disaster: I. Epidemiology of post-traumatic symptoms and symptom profiles. *Journal of the American Academy of Child and Adolescent Psychiatry*, **33**, 1: 80–93.

Shapiro, F. (1989). Eye movement desensitization: A new treatment for post-traumatic stress disorder. *Journal of Behavior Therapy and Experimental Psychiatry*, **20**, 3: 211–17.

Shaw, D.M., Churchill, C.M., Noyes, R. and Loeffelholz, P. (1987). Criminal behavior and post-traumatic stress disorder in Vietnam veterans. *Comprehensive Psychiatry*, **28**, 5: 403–11.

Sierles, F.S., Chen, J.J., McFarland, R.E. and Taylor, M.A. (1983). Posttraumatic stress disorder and concurrent psychiatric illness: a preliminary report. *American Journal of Psychiatry*, **140**, 9: 1177–9.

Sierles, F.S., Chen, J., Messing, M., Besyner, J. and Taylor, M.B. (1986). Concurrent psychiatric illness in non-Hispanic outpatients diagnosed as having posttraumatic stress disorder. *Journal of Nervous and Mental Disease*, **174**, 3: 171–3.

Silver, S.M. and Iacono, C.V. (1984). Factor analytic support for Diagnostic and Statistical Manual of Mental Disorders III PTSD for Vietnam veterans. *Journal of Clinical Psychology*, **40**, 1: 5–14.

Solomon, Z. (1989). Untreated combat-related PTSD: Why some Israeli veterans do not seek help. *Israel Journal of Psychiatry and Related Sciences*, **26**, 3: 111–23.

Solomon, Z., Benbensihty, R., Waysman, M. and Bleich, A. (1994). Compensation and psychic trauma: a study of Israeli combat veterans. *American Journal of Orthopsychiatry*, **64**, 1: 91–102.

Solomon, Z., Kotler, M., Shalev, A. and Lin, R. (1989). Delayed onset of PTSD among Israeli veterans of the 1982 Lebanon War (post traumatic stress disorder). *Psychiatry of Interpersonal and Biological Processes*, **52**, 4: 428–37.

Spiegel, D., Hunt, T. and Dondershine, H.E. (1988). Dissociation and hypnotizability in posttraumatic stress disorder. *American Journal of Psychiatry*, **145**, 3: 301–5.

Spiro, A., Schnurr, P. and Aldwin, C. (1994). Combat-related posttraumatic stress disorder symptoms in older men. *Psychology of Aging*, **9**, 1: 17–26.

Stuart, R. (1982). Veteran's case puts focus on Vietnam syndrome. *The New York Times*, 26 February: 11.

Stutman, R.K. and Bliss, E.L. (1985). Posttraumatic stress disorder, hypnotizability, and imagery. *American Journal of Psychiatry*, **142**, 6: 741–3.

Tarrier, N. (1995). Psychological morbidity in adult burns patients: Prevalence and treatment. *Journal of Mental Health*, **4**, 1: 51–62.

The Cap Badge Says Death or Glory, Not 'Or Compensation' (1994). *The Daily Telegraph*, 28 February: 18.

Trimble, M.R. (1981). *Post-traumatic Neurosis: From Railway Spine to the Whiplash*. Chichester: John Wiley & Sons.

Tyndel, M. and Tyndel, F.J. (1984). Post-traumatic stress disorder: A nomogenic disease. *Emotional First Aid: A Journal of Crisis Intervention*, **1**, 3: 5–10.

Veale, D. (1991). Special treatment for post traumatic stress. *MIMS Magazine*, 15 November: 32.

Walker, J.I. (1981). The psychological problems of Vietnam veterans. *Journal of the American Medical Association*, **246**, 7: 781–2.

Weisaeth L. and Eitinger, L. (1991). Research on PTSD and other post-traumatic reactions: European literature Part 1. *PTSD Research Quarterly*, **2**: 2.

Wolfe, J. and Keane, T.M. (1990). The diagnostic validity of PTSD. In *PTSD, Aetiology, Phenomenology and Treatment*. Ed J. Wolfe and A.D. Mosnaim. Washington: American Psychiatric Press.

Yule, W. and Udwin, O. (1991). Screening child survivors for post-traumatic stress disorders: Experiences from the "Jupiter" sinking. *British Journal of Clinical Psychology*, **30**, 2: 131–8.

Zeiss, R.A. and Dickman, H.R. (1989). PTSD 40 years later: Incidence and person–situation correlates in former POWs. *Journal of Clinical Psychology*, **45**, 1: 80–7.

CHAPTER 2

NORMAL REACTIONS TO TRAUMA

Before we can examine normal reactions to trauma, it is necessary to come to some understanding of what is and is not normal. This may seem pedantic or simplistic, but it is not as simple as it seems.

The Oxford English Dictionary contains a large number of definitions of the word normal. Some are specific to physics or chemistry and are not relevant. Others include:

- the usual state or condition
- constituting, conforming to, not deviating or differing from, the common type or standard; regular, usual
- a normal variety of anything; that which, or a person who, is healthy and is not impaired in any way.

It is a little depressing to see that even *The Oxford English Dictionary* uses the word normal in the definition of the word normal. It seems that there are two relevant definitions of normal. One refers to the frequency of occurrence of the matter under study, that it is or is not the usual or common state. The other refers to an absence of disease. The two are not synonymous. For example, acne is probably statistically normal in adolescence but is not a healthy-normal. More dramatically, the statistically normal response to ingestion of an inoculum of *Vibrio cholerae* is probably to develop cholera.

It is fairly easy to define a concept of statistical normality. For example, the modal response might be considered to be the statistical norm. The same is less clear for a concept of health-normal. Following a traumatic event, what constitutes disease or abnormality in health terms, and what is a normal response or health-normal? This is precisely the area to be addressed in this chapter.

Is PTSD an illness or a normal response?

This question is not as simple as it first seems. The answer is influenced strongly by the identity of both the questioner and the respondent. If a client with PTSD symptoms asks a social worker if they are ill, they will probably be told that what they are suffering from is a normal reaction to an abnormal situation. A psychiatrist may say the same, but if the client is clutching a private health insurance form or is a litigant in a personal injury case, then the psychiatrist may need to modify this opinion as only the presence of a defined illness may allow provision of care or recompense for personal injury. When trying to gain public acceptance, supporters of the concept may emphasise the normative nature of the PTSD response, although in negotiation with those responsible for commissioning purchase of health services they may focus on the condition as a significant illness. This is of major importance in negotiation both with health maintenance organisations or insurers, and with nationalised health providers such as the National Health Service in Britain. In the latter, there is a clearly stated intention to focus mental health services on those with 'severe and enduring mental illness'. In essence, the 'worried well' or 'normal responders' need not apply.

The author has been asked the specific question of whether PTSD is normal response or illness many times, particularly by lawyers. Indeed it has been a major topic at a number of seminars for personal injury lawyers. This group demonstrates nicely the importance of the argument. If PTSD is an illness or disease, then it may, in certain circumstances, be eligible for compensation at law. If it is a health-normal response, then it is not so eligible whatever the circumstances or its statistical normality or abnormality. The normal vicissitudes of life, including distress and normal response to events, are generally to be borne without recompense.

Mental disorder

In DSM-IV, a mental disorder is considered to be 'a clinically significant behavioural or psychological syndrome or pattern that occurs in an individual and that is associated with present distress (a painful symptom) or disability (impairment in one or more important areas of functioning) or with a significantly increased risk of suffering death, pain, disability, or an important loss of freedom.' (Williams, 1994). However, the definition continues, to say 'In addition, this syndrome or pattern must not be merely an expectable and culturally sanctioned response to a particular event'.

Thus a mental disorder is a recognisable pattern of behaviour change which is associated with, or which increases the risk of distress or disability.

However, DSM-IV also contains a 'cautionary statement'. In addition to pointing out that the official classificatory system in the USA, like elsewhere, is ICD, it also points out that the classification does not necessarily contain all conditions for which people may receive treatment. It reminds us that the inclusion of a diagnostic category does not necessarily imply 'that the condition meets legal or other non-medical criteria for what constitutes a mental disease, mental disorder, or mental disability'.

DSM-IV also contains a category of 'Other conditions that may be a focus of clinical attention'. These represent situations in which it is appropriate for a patient to seek help or assistance even though there is no mental disorder present. A list of such situations is given in the manual, including problems related to bereavement, occupational problems, and phase of life difficulties. These are not defined as mental disorders even though they may lead to patients seeking specialist help.

PTSD as an illness

There appears to exist clear evidence that PTSD is an illness or disorder, and thus that it is not 'normal'.

- At its simplest, the fact that PTSD is included in DSM-IV as a mental disorder indicates that it is one.
- There is considerable support for the contention that there is a recognisable pattern of symptoms, even if none is pathognomonic.
  There is a body of evidence that the symptoms of PTSD do occur together, and also that they are consistent across populations. This latter is a necessary requirement for establishment of a diagnosis (Davidson and Foa, 1991; Davidson, 1993). There is plenty of evidence that, in victims of crime, in veterans, and in disaster victims, there is a common pattern of symptoms that occurs despite the differing types of trauma. The symptoms of PTSD have been shown to have good internal cohesion and high interrelation (Silver and Iacono, 1984; Green, 1993; Keane, 1993; Kilpatrick and Resnick, 1993).
- PTSD is clearly a source of distress and disability. The new diagnostic criteria of DSM-IV demand that there be identifiable disability in occupational, social, or other important area of functioning, in order to make the diagnosis.

PTSD as a normal reaction

There is also evidence to suggest that PTSD is not a disorder, but a normal reaction. Some workers have strongly argued this position, such as Blank (1985) who sees PTSD as really being a fixation or freezing of a normal stress reaction. Others (Rozynko and Dondershine, 1991) see PTSD as being as much a process as a disorder, and as such being compatible with leading a normal life. This last is an interesting concept. While DSM-IV demands some degree of disability for the diagnosis to be made, this does not mean that the diagnosis is synonymous with total incapacity. The effect of PTSD may be very variable.

That PTSD is different from other conditions defined in DSM-IV is quite clear. PTSD does not follow the atheoretical approach vaunted for the classificatory system and its aetiology is part of the definition. Although disability is a requirement for mental disorders in general, PTSD is unusual in having a separate requirement in the definition that there is significant disability. Why is it that in PTSD alone there is a need to have a separate diagnostic criterion of disability in addition to the symptom profile? It certainly seems to suggest, at least by implication, that it is possible to have the symptom profile of PTSD, even after qualifying trauma, in the absence of significant disability, and therefore in the absence of significant illness or disorder. In contrast to the gradual redefinition of the stressor criterion through the revisions of DSM, this addition to the diagnostic criteria in DSM-IV has been the subject of comparatively little discussion in the specialist press. It seems entirely reasonable that individuals should have some form of disability or problem if they have a disorder but nobody implies that it is possible to suffer from the symptom complex that is major affective disorder without having significant disability and therefore disorder.

Yehuda and McFarlane (1995) have recently produced a review of the problems with the current status of PTSD. They point out that the status of PTSD has changed and discuss in depth whether PTSD can be considered to be normal or pathological.

Much of the original impetus for the definition of PTSD was based on the idea that the PTSD response to traumatic events was essentially a normative one (Green, Wilson and Lindy, 1985; Horowitz, 1986). This was to move away from the idea expressed in earlier editions of DSM that chronic responses to trauma were generally an expression of pre-existing vulnerability whereas those who did not have such vulnerability might suffer from what might later be called uncomplicated or simple PTSD and would be expected to recover and resume normal functioning. DSM-III broke away from this idea and postulated that PTSD was a chronic condition which could be expected to develop in otherwise normal people in the absence of any vulnerability. The implication was that PTSD was part of a natural process of adaptation to severe stressors, and did not require previous vulnerability. It was the stressor that counted.

The definition of PTSD was at least as much a socio-political move as a medical one. There were political, social, and moral issues about the treatment and recognition of those who were considered to have been abused in a wide variety of ways – although clearly the groups of first concern were Vietnam veterans and rape victims, with the survivors of the Holocaust also remaining in view to trouble the collective conscience. There was felt to be a need to separate out responses to severe and 'abnormal' trauma from illness following stress in general. The definition of PTSD was clearly intended to help validate the experience of victims and consider their responses to be a means of coping with trauma. At one level this was intended as an alternative to seeing their responses as a psychiatric illness precipitated by stress, instead recognising an understandable and accepted response to an impossible position.

The evidence does not really support this point of view. PTSD does not actually seem to be one extreme of an adaptive response to stress, but to be qualitatively as well as quantitatively different. Study of the biological response to trauma has not supported the idea that there is a continuous spectrum of changes following stress, with PTSD at one extreme. Study of biochemical and hormonal responses in PTSD shows changes which would not be predicted from previous stress research (Mason, et al., 1994; Yehuda, et al., 1995a). There are differences in direction as well as magnitude of biochemical and neuroendocrinological responses in PTSD patients when compared with those in subjects who were exposed to the same stressor but did not develop PTSD, and in those who develop other illnesses after trauma (Mason, 1986; Pitman et al., 1987; Kosten, et al., 1987; Shalev, Orr and Pitman, 1993; Yehuda et al., 1993, 1995b). These results taken together suggest that PTSD is not simply part of the normal response to adverse stress, but something qualitatively different. This is an area which will be discussed in more detail in Chapter 4 when considering the aetiology of post-traumatic illness.

Epidemiological studies have shown that PTSD is not the normative response to any particular degree of severity of trauma, or to any specific type of trauma. Certainly all of the major epidemiological studies (Breslau et al., 1991) have found that although serious trauma is all too common, PTSD as a response is much less often seen.

In contrast to the idea that it was the trauma in itself which was paramount, a range of investigators (Davidson *et al.*, 1985; Helzer, Robins and McEvoy, 1987; Barrett and Mizes, 1988; Solomon, Mikulincer and Avitzur, 1988; McFarlane, 1989; Solomon, Waysman and Mikulincer, 1990; Schnurr, Friedman and Rosenberg, 1993; Bremner *et al.*, 1993) have demonstrated the part played by other factors not related to the trauma, such as personality, genetics, family history, social support, history of abuse or trauma, previous history, and subsequent events. This also strongly suggests that PTSD is other than a normal or normative response.

There have nevertheless been a number of authors who have continued to propose the idea that PTSD really is a normal or normative response. These include Weiss (1993) who argues that PTSD is one extreme on a continuum of normal responses to traumatic stress.

Austin-Cardona (1994) wrote an interesting article in a journal which is not generally considered to be in the mainstream of the mental health literature, the *Journal of Biological Photography*. The source of the article is significant as it was intended to be read by medical photographers themselves with reference to their own potential exposure to trauma. The author describes PTS (sic) as synonymous with his preferred term of critical incident stress. He defines it as a 'normal emotional and physiological response to trauma', and describes methods by which people experiencing such phenomena can gain assistance. The importance of this article seems to be that it supports a view that, at least with this particular target audience, there is more likely to be acceptance of the concept and existence of PTSD if it is described as a normal response rather than as an illness.

A number of clinical treatment or help programmes have emphasised the need to see and to portray PTSD as 'a normal reaction to a very abnormal event' (Bowen *et al.*, 1992). The staff of a Veterans Administration outreach programme described themselves as 'not so much treaters of pathology but rather as facilitators and catalysts of a normal stress recovery process' (Gelsomino and Mackey, 1988). In this situation it is clear that it is considered by the health care providers, and presumably the recipients, that there is considerable advantage in avoiding the concept of mental illness. It seems that both in terms of gaining patient acceptance and in public attitude there is benefit associated with the stance that PTSD is not so much an illness as a normal reaction. Anecdotal observation would suggest that this has been successful to some extent, with PTSD being one of the few, if not the only, psychiatric diagnosis that it is 'respectable' to receive.

So is PTSD a normal response or an illness?

Despite the obvious political, social and cultural advantages of presenting it as a normal response to an abnormal situation, and despite the wholly understandable, and probably fairly accurate, expectation of a relative ease in getting people to accept assistance with 'readjustment' (Kelly, 1985) rather than illness, the evidence remains that PTSD is not really a normal reaction, but that it is a mental disorder.

- It is not statistically normal in that it is relatively uncommon even in those exposed to major trauma.
- It has a relatively well-circumscribed clinical picture which is relatively well maintained across populations.
- It certainly can cause both distress and disability.
- The biological research suggests that patients with PTSD have changes which would not be predicted by the normal response to stress.
- Study of vulnerability factors suggests that PTSD is more like an illness in that additional factors play a major part in causation.
- The course of the condition is not generally that which would be expected in a normal response.
- There is a large excess of comorbidity in patients with PTSD.

While it may be appropriate and helpful in the process of engaging with patients and in actual therapy to normalise the PTSD response, the conclusion seems to be inescapable that there is a mental disorder called post-traumatic stress disorder which sometimes follows traumatic stress and which is different from the normal response.

Are acute stress reactions normal responses?

The archetype of acute stress disorders is surely battle shock or combat stress reaction (CSR). It is curious to see how this concept has swung from being considered to be criminal behaviour to illness to normal reaction, and back to illness, over time.

In the First World War, for example, much that would now be called CSR was seen as cowardice and a significant number of probable sufferers were executed (Report of the War Office Committee of Enquiry on Shell Shock, 1922). At least in part as a result of what was recognised as a callous and inhuman response to real problems, CSR came to be largely accepted as a normal and anticipated reaction. In the Second World War there was a mixed attitude of acceptance of illness and normalisation of CSR. This latter was for the same reasons that years later PTSD was 'normalised'. It was felt that addressing the issue, accepting that it could happen to anyone, and that sufferers could become normal again, would result in a degree of acceptance as well as an expectation of recovery.

During the Second World War, previous lessons about CSR had needed to be relearned. In the years of the cold war, when there was detailed planning for a major tank-led war across Western Europe. It was recognised that such conditions might well result in psychological casualties and CSR, but also that such casualties could be expected to recover rapidly with intervention. It was recognised that the potential numbers involved could be huge and that not only would this cause a major strain on the medical services, but such individuals, if they recovered, could be a significant source of reinforcements. There was therefore some planning for the future presentation of such problems. Certain principles of management were developed, namely proximity, immediacy, expectancy, and simplicity. Of most importance in the question of normality or normalisation of responses is expectancy. This principle stated that there was an expectation that the CSR sufferer would continue to act as a soldier and would return quickly to normal duties rather than adopting a sick role.

Solomon is one of many workers who, over the years, have advocated this approach which has been accepted policy in most military medical services (Solomon and Benbenishty, 1986).

With the definition of PTSD, many people began to see CSR as being, almost automatically, a subset or variant of the same condition (Bleich, 1986; Garb *et al.*, 1987). Indeed, it began to be the case that the two were considered to be synonymous (Turnbull, 1993). This is despite the fact that CSR was considered to be a brief reaction from which the expectation was recovery, and PTSD, by definition, had to last at least one month. It was also despite the significant point that the presentations of CSR were more protean than those of PTSD and did not conform to it; not to mention the fact that the large numbers of Vietnam veterans with PTSD had not presented with, and apparently not suffered from, CSR. With similar causation but different duration and presentations, it seems less than totally justified to consider them to be synonymous.

Prior to the definition of PTSD, and even for some time after, CSR was seen as a brief, essentially normative, reaction, from which recovery could be expected with simple management. The main move against this view came from the extensive work done by Solomon and others after the Yom Kippur and Lebanon wars. The received wisdom at the time was that most victims of CSR could be treated and returned to normal duties, and this was exactly what they found. However, the Israelis also carried out research projects following up large numbers of recovered CSR patients as well as those who did not recover. CSR patients had higher rates of later psychiatric problems in general (Solomon, 1989a; Benbenishty, 1991) than controls who had been in combat but had not been treated for CSR . In addition, they had dramatically higher rates of PTSD (Solomon, 1989b) in the long term than did those who had not suffered a CSR, and this even included those with CSR who had apparently recovered and had effectively returned to duties as soldiers.

These findings did not support the view that CSR was a normal or adaptive response to an abnormal situation. CSR was not inevitably followed by PTSD or other psychiatric illness in the longer term, but it greatly increased this risk, even following the expected apparent rapid resolution of the CSR. This lent considerable weight to the idea that CSR and acute stress reactions were not normal reactions, but were, like PTSD, mental disorders.

With the publication of DSM-IV, CSR and other acute stress reactions were firmly placed back into the arena of mental disorder as PTSD had been since DSM-III. The diagnostic category 308.3 acute stress disorder was defined and a similar one (F43.0 acute stress disorder) was defined in ICD-10. There were now both acute and chronic stress disorders in both classificatory systems.

Initially it seemed to the author that acute stress disorder was an artificial and unhelpful diagnostic category, medicalising what was essentially a brief and self-limiting situation which did not usually need medical intervention. It was a response in which it seemed clear that, at least outside the combat situation, most people recovered and did not go on to suffer long-term illness. It seemed that one of the major reasons for the development of the diagnosis was so that those victims who suffered brief distress following trauma but did not fulfil diagnostic criteria for PTSD because their symptoms settled, could claim relief at law or from society.

In fact, although the symptom pattern of acute stress disorder is indeed what might be predicted as part of an adaptation to an abnormal event, the observation that it has a high predictive value for both PTSD and other psychological illness and distress indicates that it is a maladaptive or illness state rather than a normal one.

Some authors have recognised that acute stress disorders may be followed by PTSD or other illness, but nevertheless continue to describe them as being 'a psychological adaptation to a stressful event' (Koopman et al., 1995). The same authors have pointed out (Classen, Koopman and Spiegel, 1993; Spiegel, Koopman and Classen, 1994) that the severe dissociative symptoms of acute stress disorder predict PTSD. It is accepted that the dissociative and avoidance symptoms which predominate in acute stress disorder may well be protective in that they help enable the victim to function, albeit at a reduced level. However, it is also clear that recent work by the same authors suggests that although most of those who suffer acute stress disorder actually do recover quickly and do not develop PTSD, most of those who develop PTSD after acute trauma have suffered an acute stress disorder to some degree. This makes it hard to accept that acute stress disorder is an adaptive process rather than a pathological reaction.

Thus the evidence is that brief symptomatic reactions such as CSR and acute stress disorder, while they may be comparatively common following trauma, do not represent a health-normal response, but a brief illness which may or may not be followed by chronic disability.

So what is a normal reaction?

This seems a much more difficult question to answer than whether or not PTSD and acute stress disorders are normal. Not surprisingly, there has been very little research into the symptomatology and reactions to trauma of those who do not have illness or disability. There is a considerable body of work concerning factors which may or may not be protective against acute and chronic PTI, but it naturally concentrates on the pre-existing and current differences between those who do and do not develop disability, and upon the nature of the disability suffered by those who do become ill, rather than the changes of behaviour after trauma in those who do not. It seems understandable that investigators and those who fund investigations will be more likely to study those who have problems than those who do not.

It seems to be generally accepted, although I am not sure on what grounds, that we are all of us affected by exposure to trauma to some extent. It has been convincingly demonstrated that the majority do not develop illness after trauma, and that the patterns of illness in those who do so suffer can be identified. However, the nature of the claimed normal changes in those who do not develop illness is unclear.

There is evidence that in those who survive trauma but do not develop illness there is a transient high level of distress associated with the incident, as demonstrated in Israeli civilians following the missile attacks during the Gulf War (Bleich *et al.*, 1991).

A description of the normal response to disaster

The nature of the distress suffered by those who are not seen as ill but as adapting to a traumatic event has been described in some detail by Forster (1992) in a book designed to help mental health professionals plan for, and deal with, disasters. He points out that normal reactions can include symptoms of anxiety, insomnia, hyperarousal, and mild depressive symptoms. He reminds us that McGee has pointed out (McGee, 1984) that flashbacks, nightmares and hyperarousal may be a normal consequence of the process of laying down traumatic memories and need not be considered pathological, at least in the immediate aftermath.

Forster describes the normal course of adjustment:

1. response phase
    a) outcry
    b) repair and early recovery
2. adaptation phase
    a) intrusive
    b) alternating intrusion and denial
    c) denial and avoidance predominate
3. recovery.

Response phase

The initial phase of outcry and alarm usually lasts only minutes in most situations in which the trauma is sudden and discrete, because of the need for reaction to order the situation and seek or offer help.

The vast majority of people are able to mobilise themselves to act appropriately in the repair and early recovery stage (Duffy, 1988). A normal response shown by perhaps a quarter of victims is to show little response, to be extremely calm and rational, and to appear to function even more effectively than before the event. However, the majority do what needs to be done while nevertheless experiencing some degree of intermittent anxiety, fear, denial, anger, withdrawal, or even psychomotor retardation. These things need not be indicative of illness or abnormality. Those who cannot find a focus for action because they are helpless or because there is nothing that can be done are more likely to show psychomotor slowing or withdrawal (Rahe, 1988) than their peers.

Overall, the response phase may last hours or days depending upon the trauma and the subject. However, moving on to the next phase may be delayed if there is a need to concentrate on survival or repair above all else (McFarlane and Raphael, 1984; McFarlane, 1988). The second, adaptation, phase usually takes longer and this is where the conflict caused by DSM-III's definition of PTSD after one month's symptomatology may be eased by the inclusion in DSM-IV of the need for demonstrable disability. It seems clear that some changes can last longer than four weeks without serious dysfunction and without poor prognosis or predisposition to later illness in the absence of further events. It is suggested that symptoms or behavioural changes can continue with benign prognosis for about three months after major disasters or trauma (Atkeson *et al.*, 1982; Fairley, Langeluddecke and Tennant, 1986; Saigh, 1988; Holen, 1991).

Adaptation phase

The adaptation phase is typified by alternating states of denial and intrusion, as described by Horowitz (1986). Initially, intrusive phenomena tend to dominate, intruding into normal activities to some extent but not preventing function. There may be insomnia and nightmares, hypervigilance and startle, and painful thoughts and memories.

It seems likely that the denial and avoidance symptoms which predominate later are a response to, or a means of coping with, these intrusive symptoms. There may be decrease in emotional contact, avoidance of others, and a reluctance to talk about what has happened. Again, in the normal reaction, function is generally preserved. However, at this stage there may be increasing irritability, intolerance and complaint.

Several authors have noted that in this later part of the normal adaptation phase there is an increase in vague or ill-defined physical symptoms, with headaches, fatigue, muscle aches and gastrointestinal upsets (Gleser, Green and Winget, 1981; Dahl, 1989; Feinstein, 1989). Following the Mount St Helens eruption there was a documented increase in medical consultation for a range of complaints and conditions in the weeks and early months after the disaster (Adams and Adams, 1984).

The border between normal reaction and illness

It can clearly be seen from the description above that the differentiation of the normal response from PTI is not that easy. This is complicated by the fact that the description of the normal response is not operationally defined. While there is a general consistency in the course, experience of talking to survivors will quickly demonstrate that in addition to a wide range of severity of actual mental disorder following trauma, there is also a vast range in the degree and duration of normal response which does not incapacitate and does not lead to disorder in the long-term.

The course of the normal response is predictable only in the broadest terms. It is affected in populations and individuals by the nature of the trauma, its duration, its meaning; and by the individual's personality, experience, support, and personal role in society and the family. It may differ in duration, intensity, and specific symptom constellation.

Although DSM-III put a lower time limit of one month on symptoms, it is clear that normal reactions can last longer than this. In any event, DSM-IV has allowed a definition of disorder in acute stress disorder which requires only a minimum of 48 hours of symptomatology.

Similarly, many of the symptoms described in the definitions of disorder and in the accounts of normal responses by Forster and Horowitz are common to both.

The key to differentiation must rest in the DSM-IV criterion for both PTSD and acute stress disorder of significant disability in an important area of function in addition to symptomatology. For other PTI which does not explicitly contain a disability criterion, the diagnostic criteria do not completely overlap with the normal response to trauma and it should be possible to differentiate the latter from disorder. For example, the criteria for major affective disorders require marked depressive symptomatology most of the day, every day, for at least two weeks. This is unlike the usual fluctuating course of the normal response to trauma.

Summary

- Despite political and social pressures to the contrary, the empirical evidence is that PTSD cannot be considered, in mental health terms, to be a normal response to trauma, but a significant disorder.
- However, it seems, at least by implication, that it is possible to have the symptoms of PTSD without any demonstrable disability. In this case DSM-IV criteria state that the disorder is not present. People may have symptoms without disability and without disorder.
- Similarly, other mental disorders presenting as PTI should properly be considered as disorders and not somehow diminished as being normal.
- Acute stress disorder is a mental disorder rather than a normal reaction as it causes dysfunction and is strongly predictive of PTSD.
- The normal stress response can be differentiated by an effective lack of significant dysfunction or disability.
- There is a general picture of the normal response, which can presumably be developed with research, which consists of the phases of response and adaptation.

- This normal response is, however, only a general picture and both course and nature can be significantly affected by individual, community and trauma factors.
- The evidence is that normal symptomatology may continue, though decreasing, for several months after the event, without being followed by chronic symptomatology or significant dysfunction.
- Despite the above, there remain significant arguments for normalising even formal post-traumatic illness. While the evidence is that this represents disorder rather than normal response, focus upon the 'normal response to an abnormal situation' is likely to confer significant benefits in actual practice:
  - it may help gain allocation of funds from governments
  - it may increase acceptance by the general public, and particularly by important others such as family and employers
  - it may facilitate early intervention by increasing acceptance in the traumatised population or individual
  - it may help mobilise individual strengths and coping strategies.
- There may, however, also be negative effects of the normalisation and general acceptance of post-traumatic responses:
  - familiarity may lead to trivialisation of the problem
  - there may be a backlash against what is seen as a 'getting on the bandwagon' or a weakness in those whose jobs involve exposure to severe stress (The Cap Badge Says Death or Glory, Not 'Or Compensation', 1994; Hillsborough Police Claims 'Repugnant', 1995) such as police officers after Hillsborough and soldiers following combat
  - if responses are seen as normal rather than illness, then under the present law in England their consequences will, without doubt, be excluded from relief at law.

References

Adams, P. and Adams, G. (1984). Mount St Helens ashfall: evidence for a disaster stress reaction. *American Psychologist*, **3**: 252–60.

Atkeson, B.M., Calhoun, K.S., Resnick, P.A. and Ellis, E.M. (1982). Victims of rape; repeated assessment of depressive symptoms. *Journal of Consulting and Clinical Psychology*, **50**: 96–102.

Austin-Cardona, R. (1994). Critical incident stress and the medical photographer: its causes and effects. *Journal of Biological Photography*, **62**, 4: 119–21.

Barrett, T.W. and Mizes, J.S. (1988). Combat level and social support in the development of posttraumatic stress disorder in Vietnam veterans. *Behavior Modification*, **12**, 1: 100–115.

Benbenishty, R. (1991). Combat stress reaction and changes in military medical profile. *Military Medicine*, **156**, 2: 68–70.

Blank, A.S. (1985). Psychological treatment of war veterans: A challenge for mental health professionals. *Medical Hypnoanalysis*, **6**, 3: 91–6.

Bleich, A., Kron, S., Margalit, C., Inbar, G., Kaplan, Z., Cooper, S. and Solomon, Z. (1991). Israeli psychological casualties of the Persian Gulf war: characteristics, therapy, and selected issues. *Israeli Journal of Medical Science*, **27**, 11–12: 673–6.

Bleich, G. (1986). Combat stress disorder and the military physician: An approach to a category of PTSD. *Journal of the Royal Army Medical Corps*, **132**: 54–7.

Bowen, D.J., Carscadden, L., Beighle, K. and Fleming, I. (1992). Post-traumatic stress disorder among Salvadoran women: Empirical evidence and description of treatment. Special Issue: Refugee women and their mental health: Shattered societies, shattered lives: II. *Women and Therapy*, **13**, 3: 267–80.

Bremner, J.D., Southwick, S.M., Johnson, D.R., Yehuda, R. and Charney, D.S. (1993). Childhood physical abuse and combat-related posttraumatic stress disorder in Vietnam veterans. *American Journal of Psychiatry*, **150**, 2: 235–9.

Breslau, N., Davis, G.C., Andreski, P. and Peterson, E. (1991). Traumatic events and posttraumatic stress disorder in an urban population of young adults. *Archives of General Psychiatry*, **48**, 3: 216–22.

Classen, C., Koopman, C. and Spiegel, D. (1993). Trauma and dissociation. *Bulletin of the Menninger Clinic*, **57**, 2: 178–94.

Dahl, S. (1989). Acute response to rape: A PTSD variant. Special issue: Traumatic stress: Empirical studies from Norway. *Acta Psychiatrica Scandinavica*, **80**, 355: 56–62.

Davidson, J. (1993). Issues in the diagnosis of PTSD. In *APP Review of Psychiatry*, Vol. 12. Ed. J. Oldham, M. Riba and A. Tasman, Chapter 6. Washington: American Psychiatric Press.

Davidson, J.R. and Foa, E.B. (1991). Diagnostic issues in posttraumatic stress disorder: Considerations for the DSM-IV. Special issue: Diagnoses, dimensions, and DSM-IV: The science of classification. *Journal of Abnormal Psychology*, **100**, 3: 346–55.

Davidson, J., Swartz, M., Storck, M., Krishnan, R.R. and Hammett, E. (1985). A diagnostic and family study of posttraumatic stress disorder. *American Journal of Psychiatry*, **142**, 1: 90–93.

Duffy, J.C. (1988). The Porter Lecture: Common psychological themes in societies' reaction to terrorism and disasters. Association of Military Surgeons of the United States Annual Convention, 1987, Las Vegas, Nevada. *Military Medicine*, **153**, 8: 387–90.

Fairley, M., Langeluddecke, P. and Tennant, C. (1986). Psychological and physical morbidity in the aftermath of a cyclone. *Psychological Medicine*, **16**: 671–6.

Feinstein, A. (1989). Posttraumatic stress disorder: A descriptive study supporting DSM-III—R criteria. *American Journal of Psychiatry*, **146**, 5: 665–6.

Forster, P. (1992). Nature and treatment of acute stress reactions. *In Responding to Disaster: A Guide for Mental Health Professionals*. Ed. L. Austin, pp. 25–52. Washington: American Psychiatric Press.

Garb, R., Kutz, I., Bleich, A. and Solomon, Z. (1987). Varieties of combat stress reaction: An immunological metaphor. *British Journal of Psychiatry*, **151**: 248–51.

Gelsomino, J. and Mackey, D. (1988). Clinical interventions in emergencies: war related events. In *Mental Health Response to Mass Emergencies:Theory and Practice*. Ed. M. Lystad, pp. 211–38. New York: Brunner/Mazel.

Gleser, G., Green, B. and Winget, C. (1981). *Prolonged Psychosocial Effects of Disaster: A Study of Buffalo Creek*. New York: Academic Press.

Green, B.L. (1993). Disasters and PTSD. In *PTSD: DSM-IV and Beyond*, pp. 75–97. Ed. J. Davidson and E. Foa. Washington: American Psychiatric Press.

Green, B.L., Wilson, J.P. and Lindy, J.D. (1985). Conceptualizing Post Traumatic Stress Disorder: a Psychosocial Framework. In *Trauma and Its Wake: the Study and Treatment of PTSD*, pp. 53–70. Ed. C. R. Figley, *Brunner/Mazel Psychosocial Stress Series, No. 4*. New York: Brunner/Mazel.

Helzer, J.E., Robins, L.N. and McEvoy, L. (1987). Post-traumatic stress disorder in the general population: Findings of the Epidemiologic Catchment Area survey. *New England Journal of Medicine*, **317**, 26: 1630–4.

Hillsborough Police Claims 'Repugnant' (1995). *The Daily Telegraph*, 29 March: 4.

Holen, A. (1991). A longitudinal study of the occurrence and persistence of post-traumatic health problems in disaster survivors. *Stress Medicine*, **7**: 11–17.

Horowitz, M.J. (1986). Stress-response syndromes: A review of posttraumatic and adjustment disorders. *Hospital and Community Psychiatry*, **37**, 3: 241–9.

Keane, T.M. (1993). Symptomatyology of Vietnam veterans with PTSD. In *PTSD: DSM-IV and Beyond*, pp. 99–111. Ed. J. Davidson and E. Foa. Washington: American Psychiatric Press.

Kelly, W.E. (1985). *PTSD and the War Veteran Patient*. Brunner Mazel Psychosocial Stress Series No. 5. New York: Brunner Mazel.

Kilpatrick, D.G. and Resnick, H.S. (1993). PTSD associated with exposure to criminal victimisation in clinical and community populations. In *PTSD; DSM-IV and Beyond*, pp. 113–46. Ed. J.R. Davidson and E.B. Foa. Washington: American Psychiatric Press.

Koopman, C., Classen, C., Cardena, E. and Spiegel, D. (1995). When disaster strikes, acute stress disorder may follow. *Journal of Traumatic Stress*, **8**, 1: 29–46.

Kosten, T.R., Mason, J.W., Giller, E.L., Ostroff, R.B. and Harkness, L. (1987). Sustained urinary norepinephrine and epinephrine elevation in post-traumatic stress disorder. *Psychoneuroendocrinology*, **12**, 1: 13–20.

Mason, J.W. (1986). Urinary free-cortisol levels in posttraumatic stress disorder patients. *Journal of Nervous and Mental Disease*, **174**, 3: 145–9.

Mason, J., Southwick, S., Yehuda, R., Wang, S., Riney, S., Bremner, D., Johnson, D., Lubin, H., Blake, D. and Zhou, G. (1994). Elevation of serum free tri-iodothyronine, total triiodothyronine, thyroxine-binding globulin, and total thyroxine levels in combat-related posttraumatic stress disorder. *Archives of General Psychiatry*, **51**, 8: 629–41.

McFarlane, A.C. (1988). The longitudinal course of posttraumatic morbidity: The range of outcomes and their predictors. *Journal of Nervous and Mental Disease*, **176**, 1: 30–39.

McFarlane, A.C. (1989). The aetiology of post-traumatic morbidity: Predisposing, precipitating and perpetuating factors. *British Journal of Psychiatry*, **154**: 221–8.

McFarlane, A.C. and Raphael, B. (1984). Ash Wednesday: The effects of a fire. *Australian and New Zealand Journal of Psychiatry*, **18**, 4: 341–51.

McGee, R. (1984). Flashbacks and memory phenomena: a comment on 'Flashback phenomena – Clinical and Diagnostic Dilemmas'. *Journal of Nervous and Mental Disease*, **172**: 273–8.

Pitman, R.K., Orr, S.P., Forgue, D.F., de Jong, J. and Claiborn, J.M. (1987). Psychophysiologic assessment of posttraumatic stress disorder imagery in Vietnam combat veterans. Second Annual Meeting of the Society for Traumatic Stress Studies (1986, Denver, Colorado) and the 140th Annual Meeting of the American Psychiatric Association (1987, Chicago, Illinois). *Archives of General Psychiatry*, **44**, 11: 970–75.

Rahe, R.H. (1988). Acute versus chronic psychological reactions to combat. *Military Medicine*, **153**, 7: 365–72.

Report of the War Office Committee of Enquiry on Shell Shock (1922). London: HMSO.

Rozynko, V. and Dondershine, H.E. (1991). Trauma focus group therapy for Vietnam veterans with PTSD . Special issue: Psychotherapy with victims. *Psychotherapy*, **28**, 1: 157–61.

Saigh, P.A. (1988). Anxiety, depression, and assertion across alternating intervals of stress. *Journal of Abnormal Psychology*, **97**, 3: 338–41.

Schnurr, P., Friedman, M. and Rosenberg, S. (1993). Premilitary MMPI scores as predictors of combat-related PTSD symptoms. *American Journal of Psychiatry*, **150**, 3: 479–83.

Shalev, A.Y., Orr, S.P. and Pitman, R.K. (1993). Psychophysiologic assessment of traumatic imagery in Israeli civilian patients with posttraumatic stress disorder. *American Journal of Psychiatry*, **150**, 4: 620–24.

Silver, S.M. and Iacono, C.V. (1984). Factor analytic support for Diagnostic and Statistical Manual of Mental Disorders III PTSD for Vietnam veterans. *Journal of Clinical Psychology*, **40**, 1: 5–14.

Solomon, Z. (1989a). Psychological sequelae of war: a 3 year prospective study of Israeli combat stress reaction casualties. *Journal of Nervous and Mental Disorders*, **177**, 6: 342–6.

Solomon, Z. (1989b). A 3-year prospective study of post-traumatic stress disorder in Israeli combat veterans. *Journal of Traumatic Stress*, **2**, 1: 59–73.

Solomon, Z. and Benbenishty, R. (1986). The role of proximity, immediacy, and expectancy in frontline treatment of combat stress reaction among Israelis in the Lebanon War. *American Journal of Psychiatry*, **143**, 5: 613–17.

Solomon, Z., Mikulincer, M. and Avitzur, E. (1988). Coping, locus of control, social support, and combat-related posttraumatic stress disorder: A prospective study. *Journal of Personality and Social Psychology*, **55**, 2: 279–85.

Solomon, Z., Waysman, M. and Mikulincer, M. (1990). Family functioning, perceived societal support, and combat-related psychopathology: The moderating role of loneliness. *Journal of Social and Clinical Psychology*, **9**, 4: 456–72.

Spiegel, D., Koopman, C. and Classen, C. (1994). Acute stress disorder and dissociation. *Australian Journal of Clinical and Experimental Hypnosis*, **22**, 1: 11–23.

The Cap Badge Says Death or Glory, Not 'Or Compensation' (1994). *The Daily Telegraph*, 28 February: 18.

Turnbull, G. (1993). How we helped the freed hostages. *General Practitioner*, 19 March: 62.

Weiss, D.S. (1993). Psychological processes in traumatic stress. *Journal of Social Behavior and Personality*, **8**: 5.

Williams J.B. (1994). Psychiatric classification. In *APP Textbook of Psychiatry*, 2nd edn, pp. 201–24. Ed. R. Hales, S. Yudofsky and J. Talbott. Washington: American Psychiatric Press.

Yehuda, R., Giller, E., Levengood, R., Southwick, S. and Siever, L. (1995a). Hypothalamic–pituitary–adrenal functioning in PTSD: expanding the concept of the stress response spectrum. In *Neurobiological and Clinical Consequences of Stress*. pp. 351–66. Ed. M. Friedman, D. Charney and A. Deutch. Philadelphia: Lippincott-Raven.

Yehuda, R., Kahana, B., Binder Brynes, K., Southwick, S.M., Mason, J.W. and Giller, E.L. (1995b). Low urinary cortisol excretion in Holocaust survivors with posttraumatic stress disorder. *American Journal of Psychiatry*, **152**, 7: 982–6.

Yehuda, R. and McFarlane, A.C. (1995). Conflict between current knowledge about posttraumatic stress disorder and its original conceptual basis. *American Journal of Psychiatry*, **152**, 12: 1705–13.

Yehuda, R., Southwick, S.M., Krystal, J.H., Bremner, D., Charney, D.S. and Mason, A.W. (1993). Enhanced suppression of cortisol following dexamethasone administration in posttraumatic stress disorder. *American Journal of Psychiatry*, **150**, 1: 83–6.

CHAPTER 3

EPIDEMIOLOGY OF POST-TRAUMATIC STRESS DISORDER AND POST-TRAUMATIC ILLNESS

As with so much else, the vast majority of the research into the epidemiology of post-traumatic illness has looked at post-traumatic stress disorder specifically. However, whereas the combat studies tend to concentrate solely on this, there are a number of civilian trauma-related and disaster-related studies which have looked at the incidence and prevalence of other conditions following trauma exposure.

There are generally three types of epidemiological study which have been carried out in post-traumatic research:

- those looking at patients presenting for treatment
- those looking at identified high-risk groups or at those otherwise selected
- genuine community studies of prevalence.

The last of these seems to be the most important and is the least common. It is unsurprising that community studies of a 'new' condition would be preceded by studies of complainants and of high-risk groups. However, there can be no doubt that the only way to estimate the real relevance and importance of the condition is to measure its prevalence in the general population. Such studies do now exist.

Kulka (Kulka *et al.*, 1991) has commented upon the rapid expansion of epidemiological research from relatively small studies in clinical settings, via the congressionally mandated post-Vietnam studies, into population-based or 'community' studies. He points out that studies outwith treatment settings present both opportunities and potential hazards. He focuses upon the importance of the diagnostic methods and treatment design used. The differences in prevalence rates in different studies, particularly of Vietnam veterans, are described and explanations considered. He presents a general strategy for assessing PTSD in the community, emphasising the use of multiple assessment methods and multiple information sources.

Most of the military studies give their results as current prevalence rates of PTSD or lifetime rates of PTSD, or both.

Studies of patients

Some of the influential early papers on the problems of Vietnam veterans were not empirical studies but reports of series of cases (Van Putten and Emory, 1973). Apart from the obvious likelihood of over-representation of conditions in subjects who are help-seeking or are identified as patients, there may be other pressures which influence prevalence rates. For example, if it becomes known that there is a clinician with a special interest in a particular syndrome or condition, then that knowledge is likely to lead to sufferers and possible sufferers gravitating to such a unit. There may be an effectively irresistible unconscious tendency to have a low threshold for detection of the particular disorder and to have a relatively high diagnostic rate.

Problems with patient studies

There may be a need for the identified patient to have specific symptoms in order to gain treatment or to gain treatment which is free at point of provision. One unusual example (Salloway, Southwick and Sadowsky, 1990) concerns a patient in an opiate withdrawal state who managed to gain methadone and also shelter by complaining of symptoms of PTSD. This is of particular interest because of the similarity between some of the symptoms of PTSD and opiate withdrawal as mediated by abnormalities of noradrenergic function.

There may be financial incentives to presentation as a patient, such as pensions or compensation. There may also be some degree of reduction of responsibility for alleged criminal behaviour or for personal and family obligations (Lacoursiere, 1993).

There is the possibility of investigator bias or presumption. For example, a number of the original investigators associated with work on Vietnam veterans were themselves Vietnam veterans. They would therefore certainly identify strongly with the subjects and perhaps have a lower index of suspicion for PTSD. Indeed, Lees-Haley (1986) has argued that in a legal context there are major pressures to apply the diagnosis of PTSD to serve the needs of the patient, to whom the clinician will inevitably feel some loyalty or obligation to assist. He suggests that not only does this lead to overdiagnosis, but also that it produces what he calls 'pseudo-PTSD' in which symptoms are gradually fabricated over time in patients because of medical and psychological intervention. In a study of 22 subjects previously assessed in a medicolegal setting following the sinking of the Aleutian Enterprise (Rosen, 1995), it was found that 86% were given a diagnosis of PTSD which was maintained for at least six months. It is pointed out that this is an extremely high prevalence compared with virtually all other studies. It is suggested that this is probably erroneous, and that 'attorney advice' and the 'sharing' of symptoms may have led to this extremely high frequency of diagnosis.

There are some limited data about the significance of what has been called priming set. La Guardia (LaGuardia *et al.*, 1983) showed that veterans could be influenced in their response to questions about the effect of Vietnam experience by prior priming with either negative or positive perceptions of the effect of the experience on the psyche. When a group of non-complaining veterans was prepared for a questionnaire about the effects of Vietnam with an introduction suggesting that the belatedly recognised negative effects of PTSD were being investigated, they tended to endorse a large number of possible ill-effects. On the other hand, when they were primed with an introduction about how recent media reporting had exaggerated the negative effects of Vietnam service and totally failed to acknowledge the benefits to the personality of this growth and maturational experience, they endorsed far fewer symptoms and far more positive responses.

There are a few, but only a few, studies reporting cases of factitious PTSD in which subjects present complaining that they have PTSD but have not been exposed to the trauma which they report. Sparr described five cases, of whom three claimed to have been prisoners of war in Vietnam (Sparr and Pankratz, 1983). In fact none had been a prisoner of war, four had not been in Vietnam, and two had never been in the military. In another study of seven cases (Lynn and Belza, 1984) claiming Vietnam-related PTSD, none had been in combat but all had acquired enough knowledge of the symptomatology of PTSD to present in such a way as to be accepted as patients.

Despite the above, there are still genuine studies which report the incidence and prevalence of PTSD in patients who have been exposed to traumatic stress. Intentional fabrication of PTSD appears to be relatively rare.

Studies of patients seeking treatment

Studies of Vietnam veterans, not surprisingly, reported a high prevalence of PTSD in veterans who were presenting for psychiatric help, mostly at Veterans

Administration units. In addition, there were other studies which looked at veterans who had presented for assessment with a view to allocation of financial support or compensation, and it is not surprising that such studies show much higher rates of PTSD than are seen in general population studies, even those of Vietnam veterans.

A study of Australian Vietnam veterans engaged in psychiatric treatment (n=108) found a 45% current prevalence of PTSD (Kidson, Douglas and Holwill, 1993). Of 62 American World War II veterans in long-term care facilities (Herrmann and Eryavec, 1994), 23% had a lifetime prevalence of PTSD. Other studies of elderly veterans have found high rates of PTSD amongst psychogeriatric patients admitted with other diagnoses.

There have also been studies of other groups of patients presenting seeking help. A study based on a new community mental health service established in Northern Ireland (Allen, Cassidy and Monaghan, 1994) showed that about 8% of new referrals presented with complaints directly resulting from 'the troubles' as the state of unrest in Ulster has been called. Such cases were not all PTSD and a diagnosis of PTSD did not predict whether or not patients were still in treatment two years later.

Some studies have looked at PTSD in patients with atypical or unexplained physical complaints rather than overt psychiatric presentations. One example is a study of 34 patients with chronic idiopathic orofacial pain (Aghabeigi, Feinmann and Harris, 1992), in which 15% were found to have PTSD which was thought to underlie their pain.

A study of psychiatric patients with a recent history of schizophrenia suggested that a surprising number of the 36 subjects who had recently suffered a psychotic illness seemed to have PTSD in which their psychotic illness was considered to be the traumatic event. The rate was 46% at four months, and 35% at 11 months (McGorry et al., 1991). In an anxiety disorders research project, 10% of 711 subjects interviewed had PTSD (Fierman et al., 1993) at the time.

Substance-abuse patients have generally been found to have rates of PTSD of up to 25% (Brown, Recupero and Stout, 1995), while the specific group of inpatient Vietnam veteran substance-abuse patients have rates of 58% (Triffleman et al., 1995).

The connection between a history of physical or sexual abuse and PTI in identified patients seeking crisis intervention, support, or formal mental health service provision has been investigated in both children and adult women. In a study of 98 children who were psychiatric inpatients, the rates of PTSD were found to be 43% in those subjected to sexual abuse, 20% in those subjected to physical abuse, and 28% in those subjected to both (Adam, Everett and O'Neal,

1992). In another study the rate of PTSD in sexually abused children was essentially the same at 42.3%, and that for non-abused children was only 8.7% (McLeer *et al.*, 1994).

Probably the highest reported rates of PTSD anywhere are seen in some of the studies of battered, sexually abused, or raped women. In a study of female psychiatric inpatients (Craine *et al.*, 1988), 51% of women gave a history of sexual abuse, and of these 66% fulfilled diagnostic criteria for PTSD. In two studies of women actively seeking help or treatment following sexual abuse or battering, rates of PTSD in excess of 40% were found, but there were also raised rates of depression, other anxiety disorders, deliberate self-harm, and substance abuse (Briere and Runtz, 1987; Gleason, 1993). Another, multiple source, but also essentially self-selected, study found an 81% rate of PTSD in physically abused women.

High-risk group studies

Vietnam veterans

There has been a whole series of studies on Vietnam veterans in the community, although individual studies have varied in size, in design and in robustness. It is of considerable importance when considering such studies to examine the methodology, not only in diagnostic methods, but also in sampling and selection procedures.

Some of the pre-PTSD studies were relatively crude and insensitive. For example, Borus (1974), in a study of 577 Vietnam veterans and 172 other soldiers, used unit disciplinary records and mental health services referral as the indicators of 'maladjustment'. He found a 23% rate of maladjustment, with no significant differences between groups.

Card (1987) studied a group of approximately 500 Vietnam veterans, 500 non-Vietnam veterans, and 500 non-veterans who were all 36 years old and had completed high school in 1963. Vietnam veterans reported significantly more problems related to nightmares, loss of control over behaviour, emotional numbing, withdrawal from the external environment, hyperalertness, anxiety, and depression. Card estimated that the lifetime prevalence of PTSD in Vietnam veterans was 19%, while that in non-veterans and those who had not been in South East Asia was about 12%. However, the diagnostic method used did not conform exactly to either DSM-III or DSM-IIIR criteria for PTSD and it is difficult to draw firm conclusions about true prevalence.

Snow's team, in 1988 (Snow *et al.*, 1988), looked at a total of 2858 randomly selected American Legion members who had served in South East Asia. Subjects were investigated by questionnaire, with consideration of military service and personal health factors as well as a variety of mental health outcomes. Current prevalence rates for PTSD ranged all the way from 1.8% to 15.0%, depending upon how strictly 'exposure' to combat, and therefore criterion A eligibility, was defined. There were a number of problems with this study. First, there is no support for the suggestion that Legion members are representative of all veterans. It may well be that veterans join, or are actively involved in, the Legion for reasons related to service. Secondly, the response rate in this postal study was low. Thirdly, only a single self-report questionnaire which had not been validated against clinical diagnoses was used to make diagnoses and thus estimate prevalence.

Green and her team (Green *et al.*, 1990a) studied 'a general sample' of 200 Vietnam veterans and found a rather higher current prevalence of 17%, but also the interesting finding of a 28% current prevalence in civilian survivors of a flood disaster. It is unusual for natural disaster PTSD rates to be estimated to be higher than those in Vietnam veterans.

Goldberg and others (Goldberg *et al.*, 1990) looked at 2092 male–male, monozygotic, pairs of twins who served in the US armed forces, using postal and telephone interviews carried out in 1987. In the paper quoted, they looked specifically at pairs (n=715) who were discordant for military service in South East Asia. They found a prevalence of PTSD of 5% in co-twins who did not serve in South East Asia, and of 16.8% in twins who did serve there. The difference in rates was increased for those twins who had experienced high levels of combat in Vietnam, but in general, simply having been a Vietnam veteran increased prevalence rates of PTSD for these monozygotic male twins.

In Helzer's epidemiological catchment area study (see below), 64 of the 965 men studied had been in Vietnam. Of this small sample, only 6.3% fulfilled diagnostic criteria for lifetime PTSD using the diagnostic interview schedule (DIS), although if only those exposed to combat were looked at, the rate rose to 9.3%, and rose again to 20% in the very small group of those wounded.

The Vietnam Experience Study

The Vietnam Experience Study (VES) (Centers for Disease Control Vietnam Experience Study, 1988) was a major study run by the Centers for Disease Control on the instructions of Congress. The aim was to study the overall health effects of military service in Vietnam, and it looked at a large sample (n= 15 288, with a response rate of 86% of those eligible) of men who had joined the army between 1965 and 1972. Subjects were located using the services of a private contractor, with 87% of Vietnam and 84% of non-Vietnam veterans being traced. The initial survey was carried out by telephone but a smaller sub-sample was randomly invited for examination. In this phase, 75% (n=2490) of Vietnam veterans and 63% (n=1972) of non-veterans actually participated. All of the medical and psychological examinations were carried out at a single facility. Mental health examinations were carried out by 'specially trained psychology technicians under the supervision of licensed clinical psychologists'. They used the DIS and the Minnesota Multiphasic Personality Inventory (MMPI).

The study found a lifetime prevalence for combat-related PTSD of 15% and a current prevalence of 2% in Vietnam veterans. No current relevant symptoms were reported by 79% of Vietnam veterans. Their definition of 'current' illness was that diagnostic criteria were met within the last month. They only looked at combat-related PTSD and did not examine the prevalence of PTSD in the group of non-Vietnam veterans.

In addition, the study looked at other conditions diagnosed by the DIS. In general, Vietnam veterans were more likely than Vietnam era veterans to be currently suffering from a range of mental health problems which could be considered to be PTI. Depression (4.5% versus 2.3%), generalised anxiety (4.9% versus 3.2%) and alcohol-related problems (13.7% versus 9.2%) were all more commonly seen in Vietnam veterans. Those who had served in Vietnam were also more likely to have multiple diagnoses and to have more abnormal MMPI scales.

In contradiction to some other studies, the VES found similar economic and social function in both groups, with no excess of marital breakdown in the Vietnam group, 90% general satisfaction with family life in both groups, and 90% of all subjects being in some form of current employment.

The National Vietnam Veterans Readjustment Study
The National Vietnam Veterans Readjustment Study (NVVRS) (Kulka *et al.*, 1990; Weiss *et al.*, 1992; Schlenger *et al.*, 1992) is described as having been the most comprehensive population study of PTSD in Vietnam veterans ever conducted. It too was congressionally mandated and specifically aimed at studying psychosocial adjustment rather than all health issues. It involved face-to-face interview of a representative sample of over 3000 people: 1632 Vietnam veterans, 716 veterans who had not been to Vietnam, and 668 non-veterans. Spitzer's Structured Clinical Interview for DSM-IIIR, a comprehensive diagnostic tool of good reliability, was used in conjunction with validated self-administered questionnaires including the MMPI PTSD scale of Keane (Keane, Malloy and Fairbank, 1984), the Mississippi Scale for combat-related

Table 3.1. *NVVRS Current PTSD rates*

	Current PTSD	
Group	Male (%)	Female (%)
Vietnam veterans	15.2	8.5
High combat exposure	38.5	17.5
Other exposure	8.5	2.5
Civilian controls	1.3	0.3
Non-Vietnam veterans	2.5	1.1

PTSD (Keane, Caddell and Taylor, 1988), and the Impact of Events Scale of Horowitz (Horowitz, 1979). Lifetime and current prevalences were estimated, although current was taken to mean meeting diagnostic criteria at some time during the previous six months. Unlike the VES, they did look at the prevalence of PTSD in their control groups.

The lifetime prevalence of PTSD was found to be 30.9% among male theatre veterans and 26% among females. Current rates were found to be 15.2% and 8.5% respectively. These were significantly higher than for the non-theatre veterans or the civilian controls, as shown in Table 3.1.

According to this study it could be calculated by extrapolation that 480 000 of the 3 200 000 who served in Vietnam had PTSD in 1988. When NVVRS looked at what they called 'partial PTSD', or significant symptomatology falling short of a formal diagnosis, they estimated that as many as 830 000 Vietnam veterans were continuing to experience clinically significant distress and disability from symptoms of PTSD 15 years after the war ended.

Apart from staggering under the magnitude of this postulated problem and what it means to health provision if there are really an additional 830 000 patients who theoretically needed mental health services, there are also other messages to be read. This finding has some bearing on the prognosis of PTSD in that it suggests that at this stage, some 15 years after the event, 49% of those who had ever had significant symptomatology were still significantly distressed.

VES versus NVVRS

In general most reviewers accept the NVVRS figures over those of the VES (Kulka *et al.*, 1991; Schlenger *et al.*, 1992; Davidson and Fairbank, 1993; Fairbank *et al.*, 1995), although it must be recognised that the reviews tend to come from a small number of sources and sometimes from those involved to some extent in the NVVRS. One argument against the VES is that it used 'a smaller subset of the population', although there were 2490 Vietnam veterans examined in the VES. Selection methods do not explain the discrepancy.

Fairbank *et al.*, have stated when reviewing the studies that it is recognised that 'in spite of large variations in methodology between the major epidemiological studies of PTSD among Vietnam veterans, the findings are surprisingly consistent. The estimates of the majority of studies lie within the 95% confidence interval of the NVVRS estimates'. However, elsewhere they attribute the much lower rates in the VES to the use of 'trained lay interviewers' and to the use of the DIS which they say would only diagnose one in four of the current cases in the NVVRS, 'indicating a degree of sensitivity insufficient to detect true cases in a community population'. It is notable that when Helzer's community study did use the same tool (the DIS), they did indeed find levels similar to that of the VES.

The argument is that the VES, using DIS, was simply not sensitive enough to detect the majority of cases of PTSD. This is certainly true if the NVVRS is accepted as the gold standard. However, there is as yet no way of confirming the 'gold standard'. The VES also produced the then surprising results of a lack of social, occupational, and marital disability in Vietnam veterans when compared with non-Vietnam veterans. This perhaps raises a question of the clinical relevance of some of the PTSD diagnosed in the NVVRS and elsewhere. The NVVRS talks of hundreds of thousands of people needing treatment but does not directly demonstrate disability or help-seeking. The question which to a large extent remains less than fully answered is what is the significance of positive responses to queries about PTSD symptomatology in non-complainers.

Race and PTSD in Vietnam veterans

The NVVRS looked at the prevalence of current PTSD amongst male veterans according to race or ethnicity and found certain differences. Prevalence rates were highest for Hispanic veterans at 27.9%, were 20.6% among black veterans, and were 13.7% among Caucasians and others.

However, Green *et al.* went further and studied the relationship between race and trauma exposure (Green *et al.*, 1990b) rather than just race and PTSD. They looked at a fairly small sample of 181 Vietnam war veterans, of whom 80% were white and 20% were black. Black subjects reported higher levels of war-related traumatic stressors and of symptoms. In fact there was a common regression line which defined the relationship between exposure and outcome in both groups. Higher symptom levels in black subjects were accounted for by higher levels of stressors during their war experience, with more intense combat experiences. There was no requirement to postulate a racial sensitivity to PTSD. Rather, this study suggested that black soldiers saw or perceived more stressful combat exposure than white soldiers.

Studies of veterans of other wars

Many of the studies of veterans of other wars have looked only at one particular group – those who had been prisoners of war. These studies will be considered separately.

One of the largest studies (Spiro, Schnurr and Aldwin, 1994) of combat veterans in general looked at World War II and Korean veterans up to 45 years after combat. It was a postal study using a number of measures, and rates of PTSD varied between 0% and 12.4% depending upon the instruments used and also upon the reported degree of exposure to combat.

A small study of 32 Second World War naval veterans (Hamilton *et al.*, 1987) found a PTSD rate of 15%.

A number of studies have been carried out upon Dutch World War II resistance fighters many years on (Hovens *et al.*, 1992, 1994). The numbers investigated have varied between 147 and 822 in the different studies, and different diagnostic methods have been used. In a study of 147 veterans which, like the NVVRS, used the Structured Clinical Interview for DSM-III (SCID) as a diagnostic tool, the PTSD rate was 56%. However, in another which used a locally produced validated instrument in the larger sample group, the lifetime rates were 27% for men and 20% for women.

A Finnish study of soldiers (Molgaard *et al.*, 1991) who had and had not been in combat in World War II found no significant difference in rates of mental illness generally between the two groups. There was a non-specific trend for those who had seen combat to have more mental illness. However, the effect was small. Only by comparing those who had been actively involved in nine or more battles with those without such experience, and by grouping them into categories of 'any mental illness' versus 'no mental illness' could a significant difference be identified.

Studies of British Falklands veterans have been small scale. Orner (Orner, Lynch and Seed, 1994) sought out volunteers using a networking model for a postal study without controls. He found a 60% rate of PTSD in 53 respondents, although there is no evidence that this was a representative sample. The author (O'Brien and Hughes, 1991) compared 64 Falklands veterans still serving five years after the war with closely matched controls. On a questionnaire, 22% responded positively to questions about symptoms indicative of PTSD as defined by DSM-III. However, neither self-report nor investigation of records demonstrated any evidence of an excess over the controls of social or occupational disability, or of increased use of health services, so that the significance of the symptoms must be in some doubt.

Studies of prisoners of war

There have been a number of studies of former prisoners of war from various conflicts other than Vietnam. Friedman and others (Friedman, Schnurr and McDonagh-Coyle, 1994) have produced a review of studies of PoWs.

Of particular interest are studies of World War II PoWs who were assessed 40 years later. The quality of the studies is very variable, as is the sample size. Some studies involved retrospective reviews of case notes, some postal questionnaires, and some face-to-face interviews. One problem with much of the research into such particular groups is sample bias. To obtain representative samples 40 years later is by no means easy. It is tempting to use groups such as the Burma Star Association or the American Legion. However, those who are members of such organisations 40 years on are likely to be a highly selected group. Even if subjects are approached directly and randomly, there may be confounding factors influencing the decision to agree to take part in the study.

The study, too, may have its own effects. An ex-Far East prisoner of war was seen as a patient for the first time 46 years after his release. He gave a history of some disturbance in the first year after his release but had then coped well for 45 years until he was approached unexpectedly by a historian who was researching a book about the Japanese attack upon the British Military Hospital in Changi, Singapore where the patient worked until he was captured and abused. He spent many hours going over details of the incident which he, for whatever reason, had not considered for many years. Within weeks he was suffering severe distress as a result of PTSD symptomatology, and a year later he sought help for the first time in over 45 years.

A small Australian study found lifetime and current rates of 82% and 27% in eleven ex-PoWs (Watson, 1993).

American studies of 62 World War II PoWs found that 81% had a lifetime mental illness diagnosis on the SADS-L, and 91% had abnormal MMPIs, while 50% now gave histories suggestive that they had suffered PTSD in the first year after release, and 29% still reported such symptoms after 40 years (Speed *et al.*, 1989; Engdahl *et al.*, 1991).

In a larger study of 188 US PoWs from World War II 67% had a lifetime diagnosis of PTSD, of whom 8% had not recovered at all and 24% had significant residual symptoms (Kluznik *et al.*, 1986). In a sample of 442, there was a

56% lifetime rate of PTSD which was said to have a waxing and waning course (Zeiss and Dickman, 1989). Le Crocq and others looked at 817 Wermacht conscripts held prisoner by the Russians (Crocq *et al.*, 1991). They found that 71% had symptoms consistent with PTSD, and that the rate increased in association with increased duration of captivity.

Sutker and her team have produced a whole series of studies of ex PoWs. They found that in a group of 20 Korean War PoWs subjected to particularly severe abuse the rate of PTSD was between 90% and 100%, with 75% also having mood disorders, and 45% anxiety disorders (Sutker *et al.*, 1990). They looked at 36 World War II PoWs and 29 high combat exposure veterans (Sutker, Allain and Winstead, 1993), and found that both groups had higher than expected rates of depression and anxiety. Lifetime and current rates of PTSD were 78% and 70% for PoWs and 29% and 18% for the controls. This suggests that the chronic and particularly severe stresses of captivity and privation suffered by prisoners of war can lead to higher rates of PTSD and to chronicity. Such opinion is supported by a number of studies which have shown that severe weight loss in captivity, presumably a good measure of privation, is the strongest predictor of chronic psychological morbidity (Eberly and Engdahl, 1991).

In their study of 30 captured aircrew, Sutker and Allain, (1995) found 33% lifetime and current rates for PTSD. They suggested that the greater training, education and status of aircrew were protective in comparison with other servicemen.

One important study is a longitudinal one of Israeli PoWs from the 1973 Yom Kippur War. Three groups were followed up, consisting of 164 PoWs, 112 veterans treated for CSR, and 184 combat-exposed controls (Solomon *et al.*, 1994). Lifetime and current rates of PTSD were 23% and 13% for PoWs, 37% and 13% for CSR cases, and 14% and 3% for controls. This is interesting in that it shows lower rates for PoWs than were found in World War II and Korea. It is tempting to speculate that this was associated with briefer periods of captivity in much briefer conflicts and therefore a relative absence of chronic, inescapable, privation. The results seemed to suggest, however, that PoW-induced PTSD was less likely to resolve than that which followed CSR or uncomplicated exposure to combat.

Studies of victims of natural disasters

It is difficult effectively to define natural disasters. While earthquakes and tornadoes are essentially uncontrollable 'acts of God', humans may well influence fires and floods. The intention here is to differentiate between events which are essentially accidental, even if influenced by humans, and events which are intentional consequences of human activities. For example, the sinking of a ship in war would not be included in this section, but the accidental sinking of the Herald of Free Enterprise car ferry at Zeebrugge would be included.

Shore and colleagues studied survivors of the Mount St Helens volcanic eruption, comparing them with nearby residents not affected by the event. They studied over a thousand people and, like the VES, used the DIS as their main diagnostic tool. They found relative increases in rates of depression and generalised anxiety disorder in the sample exposed to the eruption. The over-representation of PTSD was much less impressive than that for these two disorders, with a lifetime rate for PTSD of 3.6% in the sample exposed to the eruption, and 2.6% in those not exposed (Shore, Tatum and Vollmer, 1986; Shore, Vollmer and Tatum, 1989).

Survivors of the Buffalo Creek dam collapse have been studied in detail over the years (Erikson, 1976; Green et al., 1991, 1994). In particular, a group of 99 children were followed up 17 years later. They were found to have initial rates of PTSD of 32%, falling to 7% at follow-up. Girls were more commonly affected than boys.

Earthquake victims have been studied in a number of areas. There was evidence of increased PTI following an Armenian earthquake (Goenjian et al., 1994) and in an interesting study, Armenian earthquake victims were compared with Azerbaijani victims of political violence, with both groups showing similar raised rates of PTSD. This seems to suggest that the nature of the stressor is not important, although any assumption that 'doses' of trauma exposure are equivalent is not based on known evidence.

Earthquakes in California and Chile have been used to compare and contrast the effects of such phenomena and the rate of PTI (Durkin, 1993) in the two sites. Three groups were studied, 288 households in California, 116 households in a housing project in Chile, and control households in California. In both affected areas the rate of major depression after the earthquake was increased to 2.7 times that found in controls. However, although the rate for PTSD in Chile following the earthquake was seven times that found in controls, the rate found in Californian survivors was little increased. This certainly seems to suggest that the effect of trauma in causing or precipitating PTI is not a simple homogeneous one, but may vary in intensity of effect for different disorders and in different groups of victims. In this study, even if the effects of the two earthquakes were of quite different intensity, what is of interest is that they had similar effects upon depression but very different effects upon PTSD.

Studies of rescuers or emergency services personnel

There have been a number of studies of emergency services personnel, with differing results.

The Australian fires

Probably the best-known studies of emergency workers are those carried out by McFarlane following the Ash Wednesday bush fires in New South Wales in 1983. He has produced at least 15 papers, principally looking at a group of 469 fire-fighters who were studied at 4, 11, and 29 months. A subgroup of 147 considered to be at high risk were also studied at 42 months after the fires (Spurrell and McFarlane, 1993) when 48% appeared to have PTSD, 30% an affective disorder, and 46% an anxiety disorder. The studies are particularly well known because of McFarlane's finding that the degree of exposure to the fires played only a small part in predicting subsequent PTI, and because in some respects chronic illness was more common than acute disturbance.

Other studies of emergency workers

Self report instruments were used to study the relationship between recognised work stresses and psychological distress in 145 fire-fighters (Boxer and Wild, 1993). It was found that about 40% reported significant psychological distress and that a significant number used alcohol to cope with such symptoms so that there was a possible alcohol abuse rate of 29%. However, neither of these outcomes was significantly associated with the occurrence of any one of the ten most commonly reported significant work stresses.

Seventy-nine rescue workers were assessed following an explosion (Durham, McCammon and Allison, 1985), and significant symptomatology was found in 10%.

An interesting study used pre-existing assessment data to measure change in police officers who participated in body-handling duties following the Piper Alpha oil rig fire (Alexander and Wells, 1991). A control group of officers who were not so deployed was also used. The study failed to demonstrate any increased incidence of PTSD or of psychiatric morbidity or distress in the officers involved in the body-handling duties. This is perhaps surprising given the horrific nature of the incident and the injuries, and when one considers the progress of legal claims for psychiatric injury in groups of police officers following other major disasters such as the mass deaths by crushing at Hillsborough.

Following the explosion of a gun turret on the USS Iowa, 54 volunteer body-handlers were studied at 1, 4 and 13 months, and were compared with volunteers not involved in body handling (Ursano *et al.*, 1995). In the body-handler group there were rates of PTSD of 11%, 10% and 2% at the three assessment points. There was no excess of depression at any assessment. This study, like that of the Piper Alpha, supports the idea that PTI is relatively uncommon in rescue workers who are exposed to death and destruction as part of their duties.

Studies of victims of terrorist activity

Terrorist attacks and violent crime are common features of today's society. There have been a number of specific studies, although thankfully none has been able to look at very large numbers of victims from a single incident.

Survivors of a number of terrorist attacks in France were studied, with extent of physical injury being used to classify them into no, moderate and severe injury groups, which seems at least a reasonable indicator of severity of the incident or at least of proximity to the bombs. This was a postal study aimed at 324 victims (Abenhaim, Dab and Salmi, 1992) which used a specifically designed questionnaire and had a response rate of 78.4%. Rates of PTSD for the three groups were 10.5%, 8.3%, and 30.7% respectively. The rate of depression was 13.3% across all three groups. There was no difference according to sex or age. As with the American earthquakes, the results showed that the effects of the traumatic event upon depression and upon PTSD were different. In this study the rate of depression was relatively high in all three groups but did not vary with exposure, while the rate of PTSD was increased across the board but was further increased markedly by increased exposure.

Shalev has reported on a number of small groups of survivors of terrorist bombings in Israel (Shalev 1992). Twelve out of 14 survivors of a bus bombing were assessed at ten months and four were found to have PTSD.

In a study of acute presentations in Israel, all accident and emergency department attendances directly related or attributed to the missile attacks on Israel during the Gulf War were looked at (Rotenberg, Noy and Gabbay, 1994). Of the 103 such attendances, 70 were for acute psychiatric reactions. That more people should have presented at hospital with acute stress reactions to the missile attacks than with physical injuries is actually rather surprising and is not something that has been shown elsewhere.

A study of 129 survivors of a bomb blast focused on the 35 survivors who were buried in the rubble for more than one hour (Fraser, Leslie and Phelps, 1943). It was found that 66% had significant acute psychiatric symptoms, and that 40% were off work for more than three weeks. While it was accepted that many of those studied had some brief psychological difficulties, it was suggested that those with essentially normal personalities all recovered within a few weeks. This would, of course, be in keeping with the received wisdom in the forties that stress reactions were brief and chronic problems were due to pre-existing vulnerability.

A Dutch study looked at 138 victims and their families from a series of eight hostage incidents up to nine years previously (Van der Ploeg and Kleijn, 1989). It was found that about one third still had some sort of problems, and that 12% of the hostages and 11% of their family members were considered to be in need of professional intervention at the time of the assessment. This study therefore shows that only a third of those reporting problems were considered to have disability and need intervention. It adds weight to the idea that report of symptoms does not necessarily equate with disability and a need for treatment.

Victims of violence

Kilpatrick and Resnick, who have researched PTSD after rape in particular, produced a detailed review of the evidence of PTSD in crime victims in general, and rape victims in particular (Kilpatrick and Resnick, 1993). They provide a detailed analysis of about 20 papers based on 11 different sample groups. They point out that although a number of the studies carried out on crime in general have formed part of random population surveys, nearly all of the specific rape studies have looked only at people referred for help or assessment. Thus members of this group will, by definition, have been identified by a professional or by the individual, as having a problem. There can be no doubt at all that PTSD after rape is common, and it is therefore not surprising that rates of PTSD for rape victims in these studies were very high, with some studies showing lifetime prevalence of over 80% and others showing current prevalence rates of 70%. For the wider group of all violent crime victims, rates varied considerably, with lifetime rates between 19% and 75%, and current rates between 5% and 39%

Rates of PTSD in children

McNally (1993) produced a review of the occurrence of PTSD in children in 1993. He reports that although there were a considerable number of papers about children and PTSD, only 13 could be described which used structured interviews and DSM criteria. There have been more such studies since.

One of the striking things about the studies of children is perhaps the wide range of rates of PTSD following various types of incident. The various studies, which have had different methodologies and different sample sizes, have had rates for PTSD between zero and 100% for different traumata. There have also sometimes been major differences from different studies of apparently similar traumatic situations.

The DSM-IV diagnostic criteria for PTSD contain a couple of notes to the effect that symptoms may present in different ways in children. There has even been suggestion that the concept or specific diagnosis may be of limited use in children (Armsworth and Holaday, 1993), although this is not a majority view. There are a number of reports of different forms of suggested symptoms in children, either in addition to or instead of adult PTSD symptoms. An opportunistic study of Bangladeshi children following a major flood (Durkin et al., 1993) was possible because an epidemiological study of 2- to 9-year-old children had recently been carried out. When 162 were re-examined five months after the flood, the rate of aggressive behaviour had risen from zero to 10%, and 34% of those previously dry had developed enuresis. It was suggested that these were signs of PTSD.

Certain specific tools have been developed for the diagnosis of PTSD and related conditions in children. The PTSD Reaction Index is a self-report measure which has been used following the Armenian earthquake (Goenjian et al., 1995) and elsewhere. The Diagnostic Interview for Children and Adolescents is a structured interview which is not solely designed for PTSD, and which has versions to be used both with child and parent. It has been used in studies of PTSD (Famularo, Kinscherff and Fenton, 1992).

Some stressors seem to be extremely potent at causing PTSD in children. In particular, witnessing violent assault on parents seems to be relevant. Two small studies have examined ten children who witnessed a sexual assault on their mothers (Pynoos and Nader, 1989) and 16 who witnessed the murder of one or other parent (Malmquist 1986). Each found a PTSD prevalence of 100%.

In some situations the border between witnessing and being involved is less than clear. A study of 159 children involved or witnessing a sniper attack in a school playground (Pynoos et al., 1987) found that proximity predicted PTSD and that 77% of those actually in the playground had PTSD.

When children are the defined victims, as, for example, in child sexual abuse, it might be expected that PTSD would be a frequent outcome. The evidence is, however, mixed. There is much evidence of disturbance but the rates of PTSD per se have been very variable. In a group of 17 consecutive adolescent sexual abuse victims being admitted for psychiatric care (Sansonnet-Hayden et al., 1987), all, not surprisingly, had psychiatric diagnoses, but none had PTSD.

Livingston (1987) used the Diagnostic Interview for Children and Adolescents to assess 13 sexually abused children and found high rates of a variety of psychiatric illnesses, but no PTSD. A much larger study (Sirles, Smith and Kusama, 1989) looked at 207 child abuse victims seen in outpatients. The overall rate of illness was lower at 38% and the most common diagnosis was of an affective disorder. There was no PTSD. In marked contrast, Kiser *et al.* (1988) found PTSD in 9 out of 10 children aged two to six who were assessed at a day centre and believed to be victims of sexual abuse. In a wider age group McLeer *et al.* (1988) found that 48% of 31 victims had PTSD.

For a range of other traumatic incidents there have been small-scale studies of varying detail. Martini *et al.* (1990) said that three out of five children injured in a boating accident had PTSD. Stoddard found a lifetime rate of 30% and a current rate of 6.9% after severe burns (Stoddard, Norman and Murohy, 1989). Natural disasters have tended to show relatively low rates of PTSD, with the very large studies of children after Hurricane Hugo (Shannon *et al.*, 1994) finding a PTSD prevalence of 5%.

The evidence is, therefore, that children certainly can and do develop PTSD. There is record of even small children showing signs of PTSD. It seems clear that witnessing extreme violence, particularly to a parent, is likely to cause PTSD and studies of children involved in war have shown intermediate levels. As in adults, there is a variable rate of PTSD following varying degrees of exposure to danger and violence, with lower rates after natural disasters. While the evidence in the case of sexual abuse and PTSD is contradictory, all of the studies showed high rates of PTI in general and this may add fuel to the suggestion that in some circumstances the DSM-IV type concept of PTSD may not be the most useful model of PTI in children.

Specific British studies

No large-scale epidemiological studies of PTSD or PTI have as yet been published from the UK. Most relevant papers have either referred to specific groups or to specific traumata, or have been reviews or overviews.

There are a small number of papers written about British soldiers involved in the Falklands War. Two of these have been referred to above.

Northern Ireland

Not surprisingly, there have been a number of papers written about PTI associated with the problems of Northern Ireland and the troubles there over the past 25 years or so. There are three studies of rates of illness which consider

PTSD. However, the results need careful interpretation. In most of the studies the samples studied were all assessed for medicolegal purposes rather than being a random sample or even a sample seeking treatment.

One exception was Fraser's retrospective look at the rate of psychiatric presentations and admissions following civil violence. Areas of Belfast with different rates of violence were compared with each other following an increase in civil unrest. In fact there was little evidence of an increase in psychiatric referral or attendance (Fraser, 1971). This study does not tell us whether there was an increase in symptomatology or morbidity, but there was no significant increase in the numbers of those being recognised as needing help or deciding to seek it.

Loughrey et al. (1988) carried out a retrospective case-note study of 499 consecutive people assessed for the Criminal Injuries Compensation Board (CICB) following terrorist violence. The CICB is a governmental board which compensates victims of violent crime for their injuries without reference to whether the perpetrator was identified or convicted. It was estimated that 23.2% of the claimants would have fulfilled diagnostic criteria for PTSD.

A second paper looked at the same sample plus those seeking compensation for violence which was not of terrorist origin. The sample size was 643 cases in total. Again 23% were considered retrospectively to have had PTSD so that terrorist violence was not more likely to be followed by PTSD in those who sought CICB compensation. The PTSD cases were older, more likely to be female, and more likely to be widowed.

The study of survivors of the Eniskillen bombing on Remembrance Sunday, November 1987 (Curran et al. 1990), looked at 26 adults seeking compensation. The original incident killed 11 and 60 were physically injured when a bomb was exploded near the cenotaph at a Remembrance Day service. However, of the sample studied, only five had serious physical injuries. Fifty per cent of the group studied were diagnosed as having PTSD at six months. Interestingly, the PTSD group had significantly lower physical injury scores than those without PTSD. This should perhaps be considered in light of the knowledge that in the absence of such physical injury the only way in which people who had been victims of this outrage could possibly gain the compensation for their injuries which they were seeking was if they had psychiatric injury. Presumably, if they did not have either physical or psychiatric injury they would not have been seeking compensation and the fact that they were seeking such compensation meant that they did have one or the other.

Thus the Northern Ireland studies, in the main, give information only about the rate of PTSD in compensation claimants.

The Herald of Free Enterprise

This disaster, in which a car ferry rolled over outside the harbour in Zeebrugge killing 193 people, has been the focus of ongoing study by the Institute of Psychiatry. Again, in some studies subjects were referred for medicolegal assessment for compensation rather than for treatment or as a community sample.

A study published in the *British Journal of Psychiatry* in 1991 detailed results of full or partial assessments of 20 claimants (Joseph *et al.*, 1991). and a further study on a similar group was also published (Joseph, Yule and Williams, 1994).

Two papers published in 1993 and 1994 studied a group of 73 (18%) of the surviving population (Joseph *et al.*, 1993, 1994), using postal questionnaires. They found high levels of disturbance on the IES and GHQ, but did not give actual rates for PTSD, presumably as formal assessment for PTSD was not carried out.

The Lockerbie plane crash

In December 1988 a terrorist bomb exploded on a jumbo jet over Lockerbie in Scotland. All those on the plane and 11 of those in the town over which it crashed were killed. The studies have generally involved medicolegal assessments.

Brooks and McKinlay examined 66 adults seeking compensation at about 12 months after the event (Brooks and McKinlay, 1992). PTSD of significant degree was found in 44%. The 27% who had never had any PTSD were found to have no significant mental illness.

Two studies have looked at 31 elderly survivors of Lockerbie (Livingston *et al.*, 1992; Livingston, Livingston and Fell, 1994), who were recruited in an unusual way. Elderly survivors attending their general practitioner were screened with the GHQ-28. Those who scored positive were asked if they wished to be assessed for financial compensation and this was the sample. Not surprisingly, 84% were considered to have PTSD. Coexisting major depression was present in 51%. At three years the prevalence of depression had fallen to 5.3%, and that of PTSD had fallen to 16%.

Other disasters

Two papers about the King's Cross underground station fire in 1987 described the psychiatric response and individual cases but did not give rates of PTI (Rosser, Dewar and Thompson, 1991; Sturgeon, Rosser and Shoenberg, 1991).

Twenty-five survivors of the Marchioness disaster, in which a pleasure cruiser sank in the river Thames, were studied (Thompson, Chung and Rosser, 1994). Again the subjects were seen for medicolegal assessment.

Papers following the Hillsborough disaster in which 95 football supporters were killed in a crush at the start of a match have not studied actual survivors, but have looked at those who lived near the scene (Wright, Binney and Kunkler, 1994).

A paper about the Piper Alpha oil rig disaster did not give rates of PTI.

In summary

The British studies are very heavily weighted towards investigation of those actively seeking compensation and identified as claimants. By definition someone must think that these people have, or are likely to have, physical or psychiatric injury, or both. It would be most surprising if such studies did not show very high rates of PTI and PTSD in survivors. They should not be considered to be representative of the population of survivors. There are no significant epidemiological studies which have been carried out in the UK, and estimates of the prevalence of PTSD and PTI in the UK must be based on studies elsewhere, principally the USA.

Community studies

A number of genuine community studies have been carried out in the USA.

Helzer *et al.* reported part of the Epidemiological Catchment Area Study (Helzer, Robins and McEvoy, 1987). This was a study of the prevalence and incidence of psychiatric services plus the uptake of services in five different areas, with up to 5000 households and 500 residents of institutions in each site. The diagnostic instrument used was the DIS as used in the VES study. In 1983, 2493 of the 3004 people initially interviewed in St Louis were assessed for the third time. The interviews were face to face. The lifetime rate for prevalence of PTSD was 1%. A lifetime diagnosis of PTSD was associated with an increased risk of some other psychiatric diagnosis. In particular, risk was much raised for obsessive compulsive disorder and affective disorders. There was no increased risk of schizophrenia or anorexia nervosa.

Davidson *et al.* reported a similar study to that of Helzer, carried out in North Carolina. Again the DIS was used. The sample size was 2985 and the lifetime rate for PTSD was 1.3%. The rate of current PTSD, defined as within the past six months, was 0.44% (Davidson *et al.*, 1991). The results for other diagnoses in patients with PTSD were, however, different from those in St Louis. Particularly PTSD patients were found to be 20 times as likely to have had a diagnosis of schizophrenia, whereas certain affective disorders and substance abuse were not over-represented. This was markedly in contrast with Helzer's work.

In 1992, Breslau *et al.* published a study, using the DIS, of 1007 young adults who were members of a health maintenance scheme in Detroit (Breslau and Davis, 1992). They found that almost 40% of these young people had been exposed to a traumatic event. The lifetime rates for PTSD were 9% in the whole populations studied, and 24% for those with a history of exposure to trauma. More than half those who had had PTSD suffered chronic illness, and chronicity was associated with increased anxiety and affective disorders.

Resnick *et al.* looked at women only. The sample was a USA national one, with 4008 subjects. The DIS was used. Perhaps surprisingly, they found that almost 70% had suffered a traumatic event. In this group the lifetime and current PTSD rates were 17.9% and 6.7%. When the minority who had not suffered trauma were included, rates fell to 12.3% and 4.6% (Resnick *et al.*, 1993).

Summary

There is a relative paucity of true epidemiological studies of PTSD. Those that have been done have been prevalence rather than incidence studies and there are no general incidence studies on whole populations.

There is a single national US study of PTSD in women. This found point and lifetime prevalences of 12.3% and 4.6% respectively. However, the rate of traumatic experience in the sample was nearly 70% and this seems surprising. While it is not at variance with the DSM-IV definition of the stressor criterion, it seems a far cry from the earlier description of catastrophic events in DSM-III as being events 'outside the range of normal human experience'.

The major catchment area studies have each looked at people from individual small areas of the United States and, although the numbers studied have been in the low thousands, these are still very small samples from which to extrapolate to the whole population of the United States or other countries. Having said that, the results for PTSD, if not those for comorbidity, were remarkably similar. The best estimate of the lifetime prevalence of PTSD in the community today is 1%, and that for current PTSD is about 0.5%. These are probably the figures upon which work should be based. However, it should be noted that these figures are of the same order as those for life prevalence of schizophrenia. PTSD does not seem to present as a treatment problem with the same frequency. This reinforces the idea that the positive response to probe questions about symptoms does not necessarily equate with significant disorder and disability.

There are no really useful British epidemiological studies. Much of the research has been based on identified claimants and litigants and it is not at all safe to make assumptions about populations from these studies.

Most of the research has been based on soldiers exposed to combat, and specifically to Vietnam veterans. There is a series of studies epitomised by the NVVRS which indicates lifetime rates of 30% and current rates of 15%. On the other hand, the VES study and others found lower rates, for example lifetime 15% and current 2%. It has been suggested that the VES was too strict or too specific. In the absence of a gold standard for diagnosis of PTSD, however, it is certainly possible that the NVVRS was too sensitive. Not until there is some external measure of PTSD will this controversy be finally settled. Until then, it depends what one wishes to use the prevalence rates for. If they are to plan provision of services then the NVVRS figures, which may well be accurate, will almost certainly overestimate the demand for service provision.

Rates of PTSD following civilian traumata vary widely. Although there was a significant amount of pathology reported after a volcano, the rate of PTSD was little raised. However, an earthquake was followed by a sevenfold rise in one city while in another city a similar event did not produce any significant excess of PTSD. Virtually all sorts of traumatic event have been demonstrated to be followed by PTSD or PTI. For most civilian events the rate is lower than that for combat. This may well be associated with the usually shorter duration of civilian events. The biggest exception is the violent crime of rape which has been reported to be followed by very high rates of PTSD.

Studies are consistent in showing an excess of other psychiatric morbidity following trauma, either as comorbidity or as separate PTI, in those who do not have PTSD. Perhaps surprisingly, while all studies have found trauma to be a risk factor for other psychiatric illnesses, they tend to have found it a risk for different psychiatric illnesses. For example, while one study found no excess of schizophrenia, another found a twentyfold increase. The most robust findings have been an excess of affective and anxiety disorders.

It is important to note that results in selected studies can certainly be selected by expectations, either the expectations of the subjects or the investigators. Papers reporting prevalence rates should be carefully examined to consider the sample selection methods and the tools used for diagnosis.

There is still a need for a large-scale epidemiological study in the USA and for others in Europe and elsewhere. There is also a need for a major prospective incidence study, and for further examination of comorbidity and PTI other than PTSD.

References

Abenhaim, L., Dab, W. and Salmi, L.R. (1992). Study of civilian victims of terrorist attacks (France 1982, 1987). *Journal of Clinical Epidemiology*, **45**, 2: 103–9.

Adam, B.S., Everett, B.L. and O'Neal, E. (1992). PTSD in physically and sexually abused psychiatrically hospitalized children. *Child Psychiatry and Human Development*, **23**, 1: 3–8.

Aghabeigi, B., Feinmann, C. and Harris, M. (1992). Prevalence of postraumatic stress disorder in patients with chronic idiopathic facial pain. *British Journal of Oral Maxillofacial Surgery*, **30**, 6: 360–4.

Alexander, D. and Wells, A. (1991). Reactions of police officers to body-handling after a major disaster. A before-and-after comparison. *British Journal of Psychiatry*, **159**: 547–55.

Allen, J., Cassidy, C. and Monaghan, C. (1994). A community mental health team in Northern Ireland: New referrals as a result of civil disorder. *Irish Journal of Psychological Medicine*, **11**, 2: 67–9.

Armsworth, M.W. and Holaday, M. (1993). The effects of psychological trauma on children and adolescents. *Journal of Counseling and Development*, **72**, 1: 49–56.

Borus, J.F. (1974). Incidence of maladjustment in Vietnam returnees. *Archives of General Psychiatry*, **30**: 554–7.

Boxer, P., and Wild, D. (1993). Psychological distress and alcohol use among fire fighters. *Scandinavian Journal of Work and Environmental Health*, **19**, 2: 121–5.

Breslau, N., and Davis, G.C. (1992). Posttraumatic stress disorder in an urban population of young adults: Risk factors for chronicity. *American Journal of Psychiatry*, **149**, 5: 671–75.

Briere, J., and Runtz, M. (1987). Post sexual abuse trauma: Data and implications for clinical practice. *Journal of Interpersonal Violence*, **2**, 4: 367–9.

Brooks, N. and McKinlay, W.W. (1992). Mental health consequences of the Lockerbie Disaster. *Journal of Traumatic Stress*, **5**, 4: 527–43.

Brown, P.J., Recupero, P.R. and Stout, R. (1995). PTSD substance abuse comorbidity and treatment utilization. *Addictive Behaviors*, **20**, 2: 251–4.

Card, J.J. (1987). Epidemiology of PTSD in a national cohort of Vietnam veterans. *Journal of Clinical Psychology*, **43**, 1: 6–17.

Centers for Disease Control Vietnam Experience Study (1988). Health status of Vietnam veterans; I. psychosocial characteristics. *Journal of the American Medical Association*, **259**, 18: 2701–8.

Craine, L.S., Henson, C.E., Colliver, J.A. and MacLean, D.G. (1988). Prevalence of a history of sexual abuse among female psychiatric patients in a state hospital system. *Hospital and Community Psychiatry*, **39**, 3: 300–04.

Crocq, M.A., Hein, K.D., Duval, F. and Macher, J.P. (1991). Severity of the prisoner of war experience and post-traumatic stress disorder. *European Psychiatry*, **6**, 1: 39–45.

Curran, P.S., Bell, P., Murray, A. Loughrey, G., Roddy, R. and Rocke, L.G. (1990). Psychological consequences of the Enniskillen bombing. *British Journal of Psychiatry*, **156**, 479–82.

Davidson, J.R. and Fairbank, J.A. (1993). The epidemiology of PTSD. *In PTSD-DSM-IV and Beyond*, pp. 147–72. Ed. J.R. Davidson and E.B. Foa. Washington: American Psychiatric Press.

Davidson, J.R., Hughes, D., Blazer, D.G. and George, L.K. (1991). Post-traumatic stress disorder in the community: An epidemiological study. *Psychological Medicine*, **21**, 3: 713–21.

Durham, T.W., McCammon, S.L. and Allison, E.J.J. (1985). The psychological impact of disaster on rescue personnel. *Annals of Emergency Medicine*, **14**, 7: 664–8.

Durkin, M.E. (1993). Major depression and post traumatic stress disorder following the Coalinga and Chile earthquakes: a cross cultural comparison. *Journal of Social Behavior and Personality*, **8**: 5.

Durkin, M, Khan, N., Davidson, L., Zaman, S. and Stein, Z. (1993). The effects of a natural disaster on child behavior: evidence for posttraumatic stress. *American Journal of Public Health*, **83**, 11: 1549–53.

Eberly, R.E. and Engdahl, B.E. (1991). Prevalence of somatic and psychiatric disorders among former prisoners of war. *Hospital and Community Psychiatry*, **42**, 8: 807–13.

Engdahl, B.E., Speed, N., Eberly, R.E. and Schwartz, J. (1991). Comorbidity of psychiatric disorders and personality profiles of American World War II prisoners of war. *Journal of Nervous and Mental Disease*, **179**, 4: 181–7.

Erikson, K.T. (1976). *Everything in its Path – Destruction of a Community in the Buffalo Creek Flood*. New York: Simon & Schuster.

Fairbank, J.A., Schlenger, W.E., Saigh, P.A. and Davidson J.R. (1995). An epidemiologic profile of post traumatic stress disorder. In *Neurobiological and Clinical Consequences of Stress*, pp. 415–27. Ed. M.J. Friedman, D.S. Charney and A.Y. Deutch. Philadelphia: Lippincott–Raven.

Famularo, R., Kinscherff, R. and Fenton, T. (1992). Psychiatric diagnoses of maltreated children: Preliminary findings. *Journal of the American Academy of Child and Adolescent Psychiatry*, **31**, 5: 863–7.

Fierman, E.J., Hunt, M.F., Pratt, L.A. Warshaw, M.G., Yonkers, K.A., Peterson, L.G., Epstein, K.T. and Norton, H.S. (1993). Trauma and posttraumatic stress disorder in subjects with anxiety disorders. 144th Annual Meeting of the American Psychiatric Association, 1991, New Orleans, Louisiana. *American Journal of Psychiatry*, **150**, 12: 1872–974.

Fraser, R.M. (1971). The cost of commotion: an analysis of the psychiatric sequelae of the 1969 Belfast riots. *British Journal of Psychiatry*, **118**, 544: 257–64.

Fraser, R., Leslie, I.M. and Phelps, D. (1943). Psychiatric effects of personal experiences during bombing. *Proceedings of the Royal Society of Medicine*, **36**: 119–23.

Friedman, M.J., Schnurr, P.P. and McDonagh-Coyle, A. (1994). Post-traumatic stress disorder in the military veteran. *Psychiatric Clinics of North America*, **17**, 2: 265–77.

Gleason, W.J. (1993). Mental disorders in battered women: An empirical study. *Violence and Victims*, **8**, 1: 53–68.

Goenjian, A.K., Najarian, L.M., Pynoos, R.S., Steinberg, A.M., Tavosian, G., Manoukian, G.T.A. and Fairbanks, L.A. (1994). Posttraumatic stress disorder in elderly and younger adults after the 1988 earthquake in Armenia. *American Journal of Psychiatry*, **151**, 6: 895–902.

Goenjian, A.K., Pynoos, R.S., Steinberg, A.M., Najarian, L.M., Asarnow, J.R., Karayan, I., Ghurabi, M. and Fairbanks, L.A. (1995). Psychiatric comorbidity in children after the 1988 earthquake in Armenia. *Journal of the American Academy of Child and Adolescent Psychiatry,* **34,** 9: 1174–84.

Goldberg, J., True, W.R., Eisen, S.A. and Henderson, W.G. (1990). A twin study of the effects of the Vietnam War on posttraumatic stress disorder. *Journal of the American Medical Association,* **263,** 9: 1227–32.

Green, B.L., Grace, M.C., Lindy, J.D., Gleser, G.C. and Leonard, A. (1990a). Risk factors for PTSD and other diagnoses in a general sample of Vietnam veterans. *American Journal of Psychiatry,* **147,** 6: 729–33.

Green, B.L., Grace, M.C., Lindy, J.D. and Leonard, A.C. (1990b). Race differences in response to combat stress. *Journal of Traumatic Stress,* **3,** 3: 379–93.

Green, B.L., Grace, M.C., Vary, M.G., Kramer, T.L., Gleser, G.C. and Leonard, A.C. (1994). Children of disaster in the second decade: A 17–year follow-up of Buffalo Creek survivors. *Journal of the American Academy of Child and Adolescent Psychiatry,* **33,** 1: 71–9.

Green, B.L., Korol, M., Grace, M.C., Vary, M.G., Leonard, A.C., Gleser, G.C. and Smitson, C.S. (1991). Children and disaster: Age, gender, and parental effects on PTSD symptoms. *Journal of the American Academy of Child and Adolescent Psychiatry,* **30,** 6: 945–51.

Hamilton, J.D., Canteen, W., Beigel, A. and Yost, D. (1987). Posttraumatic stress disorder in World War II naval veterans. *Hospital and Community Psychiatry,* **38,** 2: 197–9.

Helzer, J.E., Robins, L.N. and McEvoy, L. (1987). Post-traumatic stress disorder in the general population: Findings of the Epidemiologic Catchment Area survey. *New England Journal of Medicine,* **317,** 26: 1630–34.

Herrmann, N. and Eryavec, G. (1994). Posttraumatic stress disorder in institutionalized World War II veterans. *American Journal of Geriatric Psychiatry,* **2,** 4: 324–31.

Horowitz, M.J. (1979). Brief therapy of the stress response syndrome. *Psychiatric Clinics of North America,* **2,** 2: 365–77.

Hovens, J.E., Falger, P.R.J., Op, d.V.W., De Groen J.H. and Van Duijn, H. (1994). Posttraumatic stress disorder in male and female Dutch Resistance veterans of World War II in relation to trait anxiety and depression. *Psychological Reports,* **74,** 1: 275–85.

Hovens, J.E., Falger, P.R. Op, d.V.W., Schouten, E.G. and Van Duijn, H. (1992). Occurrence of current post traumatic stress disorder among Dutch World War II resistance veterans according to the SCID. *Journal of Anxiety Disorders,* **6,** 2: 147–57.

Joseph, S., Brewin, C., Yule, W. and Williams, R. (1991). Causal attributions and psychiatric symptoms in survivors of the Herald of Free Enterprise disaster. *British Journal of Psychiatry,* **159:** 542–46.

Joseph, S., Yule, W. and Williams, R. (1994). The Herald of Free Enterprise disaster: The relationship of intrusion and avoidance to subsequent depression and anxiety. *Behaviour Research and Therapy,* **32,** 1: 115–17.

Joseph, S., Yule, W., Williams, R. and Hodgkinson, P. (1993). The Herald of Free Enterprise disaster: Measuring post-traumatic symptoms 30 months on. *British Journal of Clinical Psychology,* **32,** 3: 327–31.

Joseph, S., Yule, W., Williams, R. and Hodgkinson, P. (1994). Correlates of post-traumatic stress at 30 months: The Herald of Free Enterprise disaster. *Behaviour Research and Therapy,* **32,** 5: 521–4.

Keane, T.M., Caddell, J.M. and Taylor, K.L. (1988). Mississippi Scale for combat-related posttraumatic stress disorder: Three studies in reliability and validity. *Journal of Consulting and Clinical Psychology*, **56**, 1: 85–90.

Keane, T.M., Malloy, P.F., and Fairbank, J.A. (1984). Empirical development of an MMPI subscale for the assessment of combat-related posttraumatic stress disorder. *Journal of Consulting and Clinical Psychology*, **52**, 5: 888–91.

Kidson, M., Douglas, J. and Holwill, B. (1993). Post-traumatic stress disorder in Australian World War II veterans attending a psychiatric outpatient clinic. *Medical Journal of Australia*, **158**, 8: 563–6.

Kilpatrick, D.G. and Resnick, H.S. (1993). PTSD associated with exposure to criminal victimisation in clinical and community populations. In *PTSD; DSM-IV and Beyond*, pp. 113–46. Ed. J.R. Davidson and E.B. Foa. Washington: American Psychiatric Press, 113–46.

Kiser, L.J., Ackerman, B.J. Brown, E. and Edwards, N.B., McColgan, E., Pugh, R. and Pruit, D.B. (1988). Post-traumatic stress disorder in young children: A reaction to purported sexual abuse. *Journal of the American Academy of Child and Adolescent Psychiatry*, **27**, 5: 645–49.

Kluznik, J.C., Speed, N. Van, V.C. and Magraw, R. (1986). Forty-year follow-up of United States prisoners of war. Annual Meeting of the World Psychiatric Association, 1985, Athens, Greece. *American Journal of Psychiatry*, **143**, 11: 1443–6.

Kulka, R.A., Schlenger, W.E., Fairbank, J.A., Hough, R.L., Jordan, B.K., Marmar, C. and Weiss, D.S. (1990). Brunner Mazel Psychosocial Stress Series No. 18. *Trauma and the Vietnam War Generation: Report of Findings from the National Vietnam Veterans Readjustment Study*. New York: Brunner Mazel.

Kulka, R.A., Schlenger, W.E., Fairbank, J.A. and Jordan, B.K. (1991). Assessment of posttraumatic stress disorder in the community: Prospects and pitfalls from recent studies of Vietnam veterans. Special Section: Issues and methods in assessment of posttraumatic stress disorder. *Psychological Assessment*, **3**, 4: 547–60.

Lacoursiere, R.B. (1993). Diverse motives for fictitious post-traumatic stress disorder. *Journal of Traumatic Stress*, **6**, 1: 141–9.

LaGuardia, R.L., Smith, G., Francois, R. and Bachman, L.. (1983). Incidence of delayed stress disorder among Vietnam era veterans: the effect of priming on response set. *American Journal of Orthopsychiatry*, **53**, 1: 18–26.

Lees-Haley, P.R. (1986). Pseudo-posttraumatic stress disorder. *Trial Diplomacy Journal*, **9**, 4: 17–20.

Livingston R. (1987). Sexually and physically abused children. *Journal of the American Academy of Child and Adolescent Psychiatry*, **26**: 413–15.

Livingston, H.M., Livingston, M.G., Brooks, D.N. and McKinlay, W.W. (1992). Elderly survivors of the Lockerbie air disaster. *International Journal of Geriatric Psychiatry*, **7**, 10: 725–9.

Livingston, H.M., Livingston, M.G. and Fell, S. (1994). The Lockerbie disaster: A 3-year follow up of elderly victims. *International Journal of Geriatric Psychiatry*, **9**, 12: 989–94.

Loughrey, G.C., Bell, P., Kee, M., Roddy, R.J. and Curran, P.S. (1988). Post-traumatic stress disorder and civil violence in Northern Ireland. *British Journal of Psychiatry*, **153**: 554–60.

Lynn, E.J., and Belza, M. (1984). Factitious posttraumatic stress disorder: The veteran who never got to Vietnam. *Hospital and Community Psychiatry.* **35**, 7: 697–701.

Malmquist, C.P. (1986). Children who witness parental murder: Posttraumatic aspects. *Journal of the American Academy of Child Psychiatry,* **25**, 3: 320–25.

Martini, D.R., Ryan, C., Nakayama, D. and Ramenofsky, M. (1990). Psychiatric sequelae after traumatic injury: The Pittsburgh Regatta accident. *Journal of the American Academy of Child and Adolescent Psychiatry,* **29**, 1: 70–5.

McGorry, P.D., Chanen, A., McCarthy, E., Van Riel R., McKenzie, B. and Singh, B.S. (1991). Posttraumatic stress disorder following recent-onset psychosis: An unrecognized postpsychotic syndrome. *Journal of Nervous and Mental Disease,* **179**, 5: 253–8.

McLeer, S.V., Callaghan, M., Henry, D. and Wallen, J. (1994). Psychiatric disorders in sexually abused children. *Journal of the American Academy of Child and Adolescent Psychiatry,* **33**, 3: 313–19.

McLeer, S.V., Deblinger, E., Atkins, M.S., Foa, E.B. and Ralphe, D.L. (1988). Posttraumatic stress disorder in sexually abused children. Annual Meeting of the Academy of Child and Adolescent Psychiatry, 1987, Washington, DC. *Journal of the American Academy of Child and Adolescent Psychiatry,* **27**, 5: 650–54.

McNally, RJ. (1993). Stressors that produce post traumatic stress disorder in children. *In Posttraumatic Stress Disorder: DSM-IV and Beyond,* pp. 57–74. Ed. J.R. Davidson and E.B. Foa. Washington: American Psychiatric Press.

Molgaard, C, Poikolainen, K., Elder, J., Nissinen, A., Pekkanen, J., Golbeck, A.L., deMoor C., Lahtela, K. and Puska, P. (1991). Depression late after combat: a follow-up of Finnish World War Two veterans from the seven countries East-West cohort. *Military Medicine,* **156**, 5: 219–22.

O'Brien, L.S. and Hughes, S.J. (1991). Symptoms of post-traumatic stress disorder in Falklands veterans five years after the conflict. *British Journal of Psychiatry,* **159**: 135–41.

Orner, R.J., Lynch, T. and Seed, P. (1994). Long term stress reactions in British Falklands veterans. *British Journal of Clinical Psychology,* **33**, 2: 258.

Pynoos, R.S., Frederick, C., Nader, K., Arroyo, W. Eth, S., Nunez, F. and Fairbanks, L. (1987). Life threat and posttraumatic stress in school-age children. Annual Meeting of the American Psychiatric Association, 1985, Dallas, Texas. *Archives of General Psychiatry,* **44**, 12: 1057.

Pynoos, R.S., and Nader, K. (1989). Children who witness the sexual assaults of their mothers. *Annual Progress in Child Psychiatry and Child Development,* 165–178.

Resnick, H.S., Kilpatrick, D.G., Dansky, B.S., Saunders, B.E. and Best C.L. (1993). Prevalence of civilian trauma and posttraumatic stress disorder in a representative national sample of women. *Journal of Consulting and Clinical Psychology.* **61**, 6: 984–91.

Rosen, G.M. (1995). The Aleutian Enterprise sinking and posttraumatic stress disorder: Misdiagnosis in clinical and forensic settings. *Professional Psychology: Research and Practice.* **26**, 1: 82–7.

Rosser, R., Dewar, S. and Thompson, J. (1991). Psychological aftermath of the King's Cross fire. *Journal of the Royal Society of Medicine,* **84**, 1: 4–8.

Rotenberg, Z., Noy, S. and Gabbay, U. (1994). Israeli ED experience during the Gulf War. *American Journal of Emergency Medicine,* **12**, 1: 118–19.

Salloway, S., Southwick, S.M. and Sadowsky, M. (1990). Opiate withdrawal presenting as posttraumatic stress disorder. *Hospital and Community Psychiatry*, **41**, 6: 666–7.

Sansonnet-Hayden, H., Haley, G., Marriage, K. and Fine, S. (1987). Sexual abuse and psychopathology in hospitalized adolescents . *Journal of the American Academy of Child and Adolescent Psychiatry*, **26**, 753–757.

Schlenger, W.E., Kulka, R.A., Fairbank, J.A. and Hough, R.L. (1992). The prevalence of post-traumatic stress disorder in the Vietnam generation: A multimethod, multi-source assessment of psychiatric disorder. *Journal of Traumatic Stress*, **5**, 3: 333–63.

Shalev, A.Y. (1992). Posttraumatic stress disorder among injured survivors of a terrorist attack: Predictive value of early intrusion and avoidance symptoms. *Journal of Nervous and Mental Disease*, **180**, 8: 505–9.

Shannon, M.P., Lonigan, C.J., Finch, A.J. and Taylor, C.M. (1994). Children exposed to disaster: I. Epidemiology of post-traumatic symptoms and symptom profiles. *Journal of the American Academy of Child and Adolescent Psychiatry*, **33**, 1: 80–93.

Shore, J.H., Tatum, E.L. and Vollmer, W.M. (1986). Psychiatric reactions to disaster: The Mount St. Helens experience. *American Journal of Psychiatry*, **143**, 5: 590–5.

Shore, J.H., Vollmer, W.M. and Tatum, E.L. (1989). Community patterns of post-traumatic stress disorders. *Journal of Nervous and Mental Disease*, **177**, 11: 681–5.

Sirles, E., Smith, J. and Kusama, H. (1989). Psychiatric status of intrafamilial child sexual abuse victims. *Journal of the American Academy of Child and Adolescent Psychiatry*, **28**, 225–9.

Snow, B.R., Stellman, J.M., Stellman, S.D. and Sommer, J.F.J. (1988). Post traumatic stress disorder among American Legionnaires in relation to combat experience in Vietnam: associated and contributing factors. *Environmental Research*, **47**, 2: 175–92.

Solomon, Z., Neria, Y., Ohry, A., Waysman, M. and Ginzburg, K.I. (1994). PTSD among Israeli former prisoners of war and soldiers with combat stress reaction: A longitudinal study. *American Journal of Psychiatry*, **151**, 4: 554–9.

Sparr, L. and Pankratz, L.D. (1983). Factitious posttraumatic stress disorder. *American Journal of Psychiatry*, **140**, 8: 1016–19.

Speed, N., Engdahl, B., Schwartz, J. and Eberly, R. (1989). Posttraumatic stress disorder as a consequence of the POW experience. *Journal of Nervous and Mental Disease*, **177**, 3: 147–53.

Spiro, A., Schnurr, P. and Aldwin, C. (1994). Combat-related posttraumatic stress disorder symptoms in older men. *Psychology of Aging*, **9**, 1: 17–26.

Spurrell, M.T. and McFarlane, A.C. (1993). Post-traumatic stress disorder and coping after a natural disaster. *Social Psychiatry and Psychiatric Epidemiology*, **28**, 4: 194–200.

Stoddard, F.J., Norman, D.K. and Murohy, J.M. (1989). A diagnostic outcome study of children and adolescents with severe burns. *Journal of Trauma*, **29**, 4: 471–7.

Sturgeon, D., Rosser, R. and Shoenberg, P. (1991). The King's Cross fire. Part 2: The psychological injuries. *Burns*, **17**, 1: 10–13.

Sutker, P. B. and Allain, A.N. (1995). Psychological assessment of aviators captured in World War II. *Psychological Assessment*, **7**, 1: 66–8.

Sutker, P.B., Allain, A.N.J. and Winstead, D.K. (1993). Psychopathology and psychiatric diagnoses of World War II Pacific theater prisoner of war survivors and combat veterans. *American Journal of Psychiatry*, **150**, 2: 240–246.

Sutker, P.B., Winstead, D.K., Galina, Z.H. and Allain, A.N. (1990). Assessment of long-term psychosocial sequelae among POW survivors of the Korean Conflict. *Journal of Personality Assessment*, **54**, 1–2: 170–80.

Thompson, J., Chung, M. and Rosser, R. (1994). The Marchioness disaster: preliminary report on psychological effects. *British Journal of Clinical Psychology*, **33**, 1: 75–77.

Triffleman, E.G., Marmar, C.R., Delucchi, K.L. and Ronfeldt, H. (1995). Childhood trauma and posttraumatic stress disorder in substance abuse inpatients. *Journal of Nervous and Mental Disease*, **183**, 3: 172–6.

Ursano, R.J., Fullerton, C.S., Kao, T.-C. and Bhartiya, V. (1995). Longitudinal assessment of posttraumatic stress disorder and depression after exposure to traumatic death. *Journal of Nervous and Mental Disease*, **183**, 1: 36–42.

Van, der Ploeg H.M., and Kleijn, W.C. (1989). Being held hostage in The Netherlands: A study of long-term aftereffects. *Journal of Traumatic Stress*, **1**, 2: 153–69.

Van Putten, T. and Emory, W.H. (1973). Traumatic neuroses in Vietnam returnees. A forgotten diagnosis? *Archives of General Psychiatry*, **29**, 5: 695–8.

Watson, I.B. (1993). Post-traumatic stress disorder in Australian prisoners of the Japanese: A clinical study. *Australian and New Zealand Journal of Psychiatry*, **27**, 1: 20–29.

Weiss, D.S., Marmar, C.R., Schlenger, W.E. and Fairbank, J.A. (1992). The prevalence of lifetime and partial post-traumatic stress disorder in Vietnam theater veterans. *Journal of Traumatic Stress*, **5**, 3: 365–76.

Wright, J.C., Binney, V. and Kunkler, J. (1994). Psychological distress in the local Hillsborough or 'Host' community following the Hillsborough Football Stadium disaster. *Journal of Community and Applied Social Psychology*, **4**, 2: 77–89.

Zeiss, R.A., and Dickman, H.R. (1989). PTSD 40 years later: Incidence and person–situation correlates in former POWs. *Journal of Clinical Psychology*, **45**, 1: 80–87.

CHAPTER 4

AETIOLOGY AND
PREDISPOSING FACTORS

At first glance there seems little point in studying the aetiology of PTI. The very definition includes the cause. As Brett and Ostroff (1985) have pointed out, the hypothesis that a unique pattern of symptoms is caused by the experience of extremely stressful events is central to the inclusion of PTSD in the DSM. The threat and feelings of helplessness and vulnerability are thought to be uniquely destabilising of the victim's previous function. PTSD is defined as being the consequence of a traumatic event. In DSM-IV (American Psychiatric Association, 1994), PTSD is one of the few disorders for which the atheoretical approach is abandoned and the definition includes presumed aetiology. It is stated that 'the essential feature of PTSD is the development of characteristic symptoms following exposure to an extreme traumatic stressor'. In the differential diagnosis section it is recorded that the stressor must be of an extreme (i.e. life-threatening) nature. This is in keeping with the definition in ICD-10 (World Health Organisation, 1992).

It seems clear that the aetiology of PTI is connected with trauma, even though Scott (Scott and Stradling, 1994) has suggested that PTSD can occur in the absence of extreme trauma, and there has been serious debate about the necessity or otherwise of the stressor criterion (March, 1993). Breslau and Davis (1987a) have pointed out that there is 'insufficient data to show that the set of symptoms characteristic of PTSD is strongly and uniquely associated with extraordinary stressors'. PTSD has been associated with a wide range of events which would not be considered extraordinary or particularly severe stressors. These include idiopathic illness (McGorry et al., 1991), apparently uncomplicated medical procedures, and 'normal' loss events. Scott, like others, has said that there are patients who have all of the symptoms of PTSD but in whom no single 'extreme' stressor can be identified although their symptoms seem to be related to a series of less severe stressors or one chronic stressful situation. March, on the other hand has reviewed the studies on the stressor criterion to examine the possibility of a dose response, to consider the role of personal perception, and to look at ways of refining the stressor criterion for PTSD.

If trauma causes PTSD and PTI, then the aetiology – 'the causes and origins of the disease' – is defined. This does not, however, explain the cause of PTI fully. The simple equation trauma → PTI does not hold good. By no means everyone exposed to trauma develops PTI. Even those exposed to the same trauma do not all develop PTI. There are a number of questions which need to be answered.

- Why is it that not everybody who is exposed to trauma develops PTI? Is there a dose effect of trauma, with increasing levels of trauma causing increasing rates of PTI?
- Is there a threshold level of trauma below which PTI does not occur?
- Do other illnesses play a part?
- Does personality play a part?
- Does previous history or family history play a part?
- Is there an inherited or genetic component?
- What is the role of experience after the trauma?

There are other questions to be answered about the teleology or final causation of PTI. We will focus on the underlying substrate of PTSD as the biological changes of other PTIs are described in works on the individual conditions such as affective disorder or specific phobia, and have been investigated for many years. This chapter will explore the question of whether or not there are specific physical changes or signs associated with the development of PTSD.

- Are there neuronal changes?
- Are there hypothalamic–pituitary–adrenal (HPA) axis changes?
- Are there other pathological or biochemical changes?
- Are there physiological changes?
- Is there a Grand Unified Theory which will explain the observed changes?

There will be an attempt to answer these questions, coming to some sort of view of the aetiology of PTI and PTSD, and of the teleology of PTSD in particular. There is a somewhat arbitrary but nevertheless necessary categorisation of the biological questions. It is not really possible to discuss neuronal changes without encroaching upon endocrinology, neuroendocrinology and physiology.

However, initially to discuss all aspects of the biological findings in a single section would be confusing. The aim is therefore to look at various aspects before trying to produce some sort of synthesis.

When considering the causation of PTSD it may be helpful to look briefly at a very different medical condition as a model for the problem. If we take tuberculosis as an example, then this seems very different indeed from PTI. It is caused by the tubercle bacillus. If the bacillus is there, then we have tuberculosis, if not then we do not.

The situation is not that simple, however, even with this apparently straightforward medical illness about which far more is known than is known about PTI. Simple contact with the micro-organism does not guarantee that tuberculosis will be contracted. Other factors play a part. The subject may have some degree of natural or acquired immunity. There is a dose–response relationship so that a certain innoculum of the bacillus is required to contract the disease and a single bacillus is insufficient. Intercurrent and previous illnesses play a part, as do other factors in life such as nutrition, medical support and social situation. The course and presentation are affected by factors in the patient and his environment.

Having taken this cautionary look at what seems a much more simple disease of known aetiology, we will look at the case of PTSD in particular and PTI in general .

Why is it that not everybody who is exposed to trauma develops PTI, and is there a dose effect of trauma?

Reported incidences of PTSD following trauma vary considerably but, apart from a very few papers, do not approach anywhere near 100%. The very highest rates, and also the widest variation, have been found in some of the studies of female survivors of sexual abuse, rape and physical abuse. Rates have varied from 4% (Greenwald and Leitenberg, 1990) through 58% (Astin *et al.*, 1995) and 70% (Bownes, O'Gorman and Sayers, 1991), to 81% (Kemp *et al.*, 1995), depending upon methodology and population studied. Following physical injury in individual or small-scale accidents, PTSD rates have varied from less than 1% following accidental injury (Malt 1988) to 45% in burn victims (Tarrier 1995).

In studies of combat veterans Vietnam has, not surprisingly, tended to dominate. There have been a number of large-scale studies. Current PTSD rates vary between 2.2% in the congressionally mandated Vietnam Experience Study (Centers for Disease Control Vietnam Experience Study 1988) and 17% (Green *et al.*, 1990a, 1990b). Lifetime rates vary from 6.3% (Helzer, Robins and

McEvoy, 1987) to 30.9%. The wide variation in rates has probably been attributable to different diagnostic methods and thresholds for diagnosis. The most widely accepted study is the NVVRS study, which claims a male current rate of 15.2% and lifetime rate of 30.9% (Kulka *et al.*, 1990).

Studies of other veterans have been less systematic. There have been a number of studies of elderly veterans in various circumstances. Rates in general groups of elderly veterans varied from 12% (Spiro, Schnurr and Aldwin, 1994), while rates were as high as 56–67% in ex-prisoners of war (Zeiss and Dickman, 1989) many years after incarceration (Muse 1986).

There have been a host of studies of PTI, or more specifically PTSD, in other situations. For example, those exposed to natural disasters had reported rates varying from 5% in children who survived a hurricane (Shannon *et al.*, 1994) to 60% in survivors of a tornado (Madakasira and O'Brien, 1987).

These widely varying rates are of considerable interest. Even though it is clear that methodology can result in wide variation in rates of detection of PTI and PTSD in subjects apparently exposed to similar stressors, nevertheless it is seen that in general most survivors do not develop PTI. Clearly, trauma does not have the same effect on all people. This may be due to factors inherent in the traumatic event, to factors in the person or the environment, or to a mixture of both. Specific aspects of the stressor itself will be addressed in Chapter 5.

Quite apart from the variations due to detection methods, or perhaps to the orientation and bias of investigators, there is clearly a variation in PTI which is not explained by the trauma itself. There have been a number of attempts to discover how much of the variance of PTI, or more commonly PTSD, can be ascribed to variations in the stressor. Most of this work has been done where combat is the stressor. There are a number of reasons for this. Combat is all too common. The Vietnam War was the major impetus to the development of the concept of PTSD. Combat involves large numbers of people. A great deal is known about those involved in combat. Depending upon their employment and location, different military personnel will be exposed to varying degrees of combat, allowing for natural control groups. It is interesting that one of the few groups studied in detail other than soldiers, fire fighters in Australia, has produced results at variance with much of that from combat work.

The role of severity of trauma exposure in PTI

A number of studies have found that degree of combat exposure is related to incidence and/or severity of PTSD. Foy *et al.* (1984) found PTSD to be associated in help-seekers with combat exposure and, to a lesser extent, other mili-

Table 4.1. *Matched pair odds-ratio for discordant pairs*

Group	Odds-ratio	95% confidence limits
Non-theatre	1.0	
Theatre	4.5	2.9–7.0
Theatre, no combat	1.7	1.5–2.1
Theatre, low combat	3.0	2.2–4.2
Theatre, moderate combat	5.3	3.2–8.6
Theatre, high combat	9.2	4.8–17.6

tary factors, but not pre-military factors. A non-clinical study also found that PTSD was associated with combat exposure (Foy and Card, 1987). A study of orthopaedic Vietnam veteran patients also found that duration of PTSD symptoms was associated with duration and intensity of exposure to combat (Buydens-Branchey, Noumair and Branchey, 1990).

The Vietnam Era Twin Registry (see below), has been used to provide effective controls in exploring the effects of trauma exposure.

In 1990, Goldberg *et al.* published details of a study using the sample of 2092 male-male monozygotic twin pairs. They were interested in the 715 pairs which were discordant for service in South East Asia, i.e. one served in theatre and one did not. One of the main spurs to this research was the need to find valid controls for Vietnam veterans. Clearly, a monozygotic twin who was in the military but did not go to Vietnam is a good control.

Initially they compared the discordant twins with concordant twin pairs who either did or did not serve in South East Asia. The former group had a presumptive PTSD prevalence of 12.9%, while the latter had a rate of 5%. In the discordant groups the rates were 5% for non-theatre veterans and 16.8% for theatre veterans.

They studied the odds-ratio for having PTSD in theatre veteran twins compared with non-theatre twins, using a matched-pair odds-ratio. With the non-theatre veterans being considered to have an odds-ratio of one, the theatre veterans had an odds-ratio of 4.5. This varied with combat exposure, as shown in Table 4.1.

None of the studies has actually found that the whole of the variance of PTSD or PTI symptomatology is explained by degree of exposure to trauma. Foy *et al.* suggested that 40% of the variance was explained by combat exposure (Foy *et al.*, 1987), while a replication study on a non-clinical sample (Foy and Card, 1987) found that only 28% of the variance was explained by combat exposure and by military adjustment. Breslau and Davis (1987b), studying 69 Vietnam veterans inpatients with PTSD, found that 35% of the variance was explained by combat exposure factors, with 29% being explained by participation in atrocities alone.

Hennessy's study of Australian Vietnam veterans (Hennessy and Oei, 1991) found that intensity of combat exposure did not predict PTSD. However, this study was carried out 23 years after the tour of duty. It may well be that the differential effect of exposure is eroded by time, or negated by intervening traumatic events. Some small studies, such as that of Iranian soldiers (Ghods, 1992), have failed to show an important role for combat exposure in predicting PTI.

A study of burn victims (Perry *et al.*, 1992), perhaps surprisingly, found that PTSD was not positively correlated with severity of injury. In fact, they found that at two months PTSD was predicted by smaller burn surface area.

McFarlane's work with Australian fire-fighters has tended to indicate that much less of the variance in PTI symptomatology and in PTSD is explained by trauma variables than that found in studies of Vietnam veterans. It must be remembered that his study was of 469 fire-fighters following a single brief, 15-hour, traumatic event in which there was little personal loss for them. However, he found that in studies at 4, 11 and 29 months, disaster-related variables accounted for a maximum of 8% of the symptom variance as measured by the GHQ (McFarlane 1989). While the GHQ is not synonymous with PTSD, in this study GHQ scores had a 90% specificity for detecting PTSD.

In contrast, the Mount St Helen's studies showed a dose response when dose was measured by property loss or bereavement (Murphy 1984; Shore, Tatum and Vollmer, 1986). In addition, the Buffalo Creek research showed some relationship between life threat and chronic PTI in children (Green *et al.*, 1991).

Fontana and Rosenheck's study of a causal model

There have been a number of reviews of the role of trauma in causation of PTI, some combined with empirical study. Very helpful indeed is a study of 381 Vietnam veterans, 77.5% of whom had PTSD (Fontana and Rosenheck, 1993). This study used a process of structural equation modelling as an improvement over the multiple regression analysis used in previous studies. The authors also provide a very useful review of the situation, pointing out that a number of previous studies had taken an adversarial stance between trauma exposure and pre-existing vulnerability as potentially almost mutually exclusive causes of PTSD. They note that Atkinson (Atkinson *et al.*, 1982), Borus (Borus, 1974) and McFarlane (McFarlane, 1989) side with vulnerability factors, while Foy (*op. cit.*),

Table 4.2. *Factors studied by Fontana and Rosenheck*

	Range	Label
Premilitary variables		
Childhood physical or sexual abuse	0–3	ABUSE
Psychiatric treatment before age 18	0–1	PSYCH
Parental psychiatric hospitalisation	0–1	PAR-PSY
Father exposed to combat	0–1	FATH-COM
Family instability	0–11	FAM-INST
Previous drug abuse	0–1	DRUG
Ethnic minority status	0–1	ETHNIC
Probable childhood conduct disorder	0–11	CONDUCT
Military entry variables		
Willing or volunteer soldier	0–1	WILLING
Age on entry	years	AGE
War zone variables		
Combat exposure from Revised Combat Scale		
and Combat Exposure Scale	score	COMBAT
Witnessing abusive violence	0–1	WITNESS
Taking part in abusive violence	0–1	PARTICIP
Disciplinary problems in theatre	0–1	DISCIP
Dissociation		
Mean of five structured questions	0–1	DISSOC
PTI variables		
Sum of SCID PTSD Symptom Score and		
Mississippi Scale score	score	PTSD
Brief Symptom Inventory and		
Addiction Severity Index	score	PTI

Figley (Figley and Leventman, 1980), and Wilson (Wilson, 1978) championed the cause of the severity and extent of trauma. Such a split is not surprising if one takes into account the politics of the 'post-Vietnam syndrome' and the fact that a number of the most outspoken investigators were, themselves, Vietnam veterans.

The study under discussion reported that the work of Foy and Card and of others had failed to show any significant role for predisposing vulnerabilities, while that of Nace *et al.* (1978) and Vinokur (1987) had shown a positive relationship between pre-existing vulnerabilities and subsequent PTSD following combat exposure in Vietnam. It also pointed out that most of this work used a composite index of pre-existing vulnerability which made it difficult to see if some factors but not others were relevant.

Their study allowed for sharing of variance, and for examination of the connections between variables. Although it was, inevitably, retrospective, they formed the reasonable view that as the factors studied were clearly sequential and easily separated in time, it was appropriate to consider the effect of earlier variables upon later variables. They looked at pre-existing vulnerabilities and history, history of entry to the service, military adjustment as evidenced by disciplinary problems, war zone experience, dissociative experiences, and subsequent PTI, both PTSD and other psychiatric illness (Table 4.2).

There were three hypotheses:

- that trauma contributed more to PTI than did premilitary variables
- that war zone exposure contributed more to PTSD than to other PTI
- that each set of variables studied affected each subsequent set.

From the results they constructed a model of aetiology of PTSD and another for other psychiatric illness (PTI). These models accounted for 59% of the variance for PTSD, and for 60% of that for PTI.

Common features of the models

Factors affecting entry to the military:
FATH-COM and FAM-INST were both associated with lower age on entry, while DRUG was associated with higher age.
DRUG and ETHNIC were associated with reluctance to join up.
Factors affecting military experience:
CONDUCT and low AGE were associated with disciplinary problems.
PSYCH and ABUSE were associated with low combat exposure, whereas low AGE was associated with high combat exposure.
FATH-COM and WILLING were associated with participation in abusive violence.
WILLING was associated with less witnessing of abusive violence.

Effects of factors on PTSD

The following factors had a positive association with PTSD, in decreasing order of importance:

PARTICIP
WITNESS

DISSOC
COMBAT
FATH-COM.

Parental psychiatric illness played no part in the model, and discipline problems had no effect upon PTSD.

Effects of factors on PTI

The following factors had a positive association with PTI in decreasing order of importance:

PARTICIP
WITNESS
DISSOC
FAM-INST
FATH-COM
DISCIP.

Combat exposure had no direct effect on PTI. A history of drug use before service was, surprisingly, negatively associated with PTI.

The study, therefore, supports the three hypotheses:

- although pre-military variables did have an effect, trauma variables contributed more to PTSD
- war zone factors, particularly combat exposure, had more effect in predicting PTSD than PTI
- the study did show mediating effects of each set of variables on subsequent variables.

Overall, therefore, the evidence is that by no means everybody develops PTI after trauma. There is evidence about a range of factors which influence the likelihood of PTI. It seems likely that the effect of the various factors may not be the same after combat as it is after civilian disasters which are usually more short-lived. There seems to be good evidence that in combat there is a dose–response effect of exposure to trauma, but the evidence is much less solid for other traumatic events.

Is there a threshold level of trauma below which PTI does not occur?

According to the definitions of PTSD at least, there should certainly be a minimum level of trauma required to induce PTI. The definitions in both

DSM-IV and ICD-10 refer to major or catastrophic stressors. Earlier definitions of PTSD specifically excluded the role of less severe stressors. However, there is no good empirical evidence that this is the case if the symptomatology of PTSD is considered without the precondition that symptoms must be related to extreme stressors. Burstein found that in a study of 73 outpatients (Burstein, 1985a), eight fulfilled diagnostic criteria for PTSD except for the stressor criterion, criterion A. The sort of problems which were associated with their symptomatology included marital difficulties, the behaviour of children, the collapse of plans to adopt children, and 'normal' bereavement. In an epidemiological catchment area study, events such as miscarriage and an extramarital affair by a spouse were associated with PTSD symptomatology, albeit at lower frequency than rape or other criminal violence (Helzer, Robins, and McEvoy 1987). Solomon and Canino (1990) have suggested that everyday stressors such as money problems and illness or injury in the household have a greater association with PTI symptomatology than do natural disasters.

Two studies of aircraft crashes have produced interesting results which again perhaps suggest that PTSD does not follow a minimum stressor level, or threshold trauma. In a Canadian military aircraft crash (Lukasik, 1991) nobody was killed. Subsequent study showed that spouses of those involved, who were not there, had higher rates of PTI symptoms, particularly intrusive symptoms, than did those who were involved. A study following an incident where a military jet crashed into a hotel with ten fatalities (Smith *et al.*, 1990) found that although psychological problems were more common in those employees actually in the hotel at the time of the disaster, nevertheless PTI symptomatology did occur in some of those who were not on the site and were not supposed to be there.

Although DSM-IV and ICD-10 require particular forms or severity of stressors to be present before a diagnosis of PTSD can be made, there is no empirical evidence that this is anything but an arbitrary decision. The evidence suggests that even 'normal' stressors can be associated with the symptomatology seen in PTSD.

Do other illnesses play a part?

This is a question which, like so much else in PTI research, is a focus of great controversy. It perhaps illustrates the polarity between the 'stress evaporation' theory of Worthington (1978) and the 'residual stress' theory of Figley (1978). These theories, which were both published shortly before the DSM-III definition of PTSD, consolidated the previously existing contrasting views of the pathogenesis of PTI. Worthington's theory suggests that PTI should be a short-lived response to trauma and only becomes chronic if there is some pre-existing 'maladjustment' or vulnerability factor. Figley, however, focuses on the effect of the traumatic experience itself, and suggested that PTI could exist for many years even in those of normal personality and adjustment. In fact, of course, the argument is far from being that simple. There are many studies which show that trauma exposure is a factor in severity and chronicity of PTI, while others demonstrate the role of pre-existing or previous problems.

One of the problems of studying the effect of pre-existing psychiatric illness is that much of the research has, of course, been carried out in relation to combat exposure of soldiers. This is hardly surprising when war is so common; most of the impetus to PTI research came from concern about veterans, and soldiers provide a population about whom much data is available. However, combat exposure is not necessarily equivalent to civilian trauma, which is usually of much shorter duration. In addition, soldiers are far from being a representative sample of the general population. They are highly selected. It will be remembered that after the First World War experience the Americans made great efforts to select out those considered to be likely to suffer mental health problems in combat. As a result, they had a rejection rate of draftees on psychological grounds which was four times that seen before. That they failed seriously to reduce combat stress reaction rates is less important for this discussion than the observation that those with a current and previous history of psychiatric problems were excluded and to varying degrees this has been the case in all armies since then. Thus the average soldier is a young physically healthy male, which means that he is not in a group with the highest prevalence of psychiatric illness. In addition, current psychiatric illness or a history of serious psychiatric illness will exclude him from service. One sometimes sees soldiers who have enlisted by concealing a serious psychiatric history. However, the self-selection factors involved in such a decision must mean that they are even less representative of the 'normal' population.

Given the above, it is not that surprising that few of the military studies have directly studied previous or pre-existing mental illness rather than a history of behavioural problems or maladjustment. Of those which have made such enquiry, few have shown a major effect. Those that have shown an effect have, not surprisingly, related *previous* rather than *pre-existing* mental illness to PTI. The study of Fontana and Rosenheck (*op. cit.*) showed that childhood mental ill health affected both PTSD and other PTI indirectly and to a small degree by affecting combat exposure. Other studies following World War II have demonstrated some effect of previous illness. On the other hand, Holloway and

Ursano (1984) have indicated that pre-existing psychiatric illness is neither a necessary nor sufficient precursor of PTSD. In another military study there was no difference between rates of previous psychiatric illness between those with and without PTSD (McFarlane, 1988)

The study quoted above in which a military jet hit a hotel was used to study the importance of pre-existing rather than previous psychiatric illness. The aim was to interview the 62 surviving employees of the hotel using the Diagnostic Interview Schedule. Fifteen per cent were not found, and 13% refused to take part. Eventually 74% of the eligible personnel took part. Seventeen had been on site at the time, while 29 had not. The study looked at a range of PTI rather than just PTSD. It also looked at pre-incident diagnoses. Perhaps the most surprising finding was that 43% of the hotel employees had at least one Axis-I diagnosis at the time of the incident. Relevant diagnoses were PTSD, alcohol abuse, depression, and generalised anxiety disorder. Fifty-four per cent had at least one diagnosis four to six weeks after the disaster. Not surprisingly, given the very high pre-existing illness rate, such illness was the best predictor of post-disaster illness, with a sensitivity of 72% and specificity of 90%.

A number of other studies of the effects of civilian trauma have also found that previous or pre-existing psychiatric illness is the best predictor of PTI (Bromet *et al.*, 1980, 1982; Lopez-Ibor, Carras and Rodriguez-Gamazo, 1985; Smith *et al.*, 1986).

Does personality play a part?

There are two questions about the connection between personality and PTI (Reich, 1990). The first is whether or not PTI or PTSD is associated with personality change or personality difficulty, and the second is whether or not personality factors predispose to the occurrence of PTI.

Personality change in PTI

The former seems quite uncontentious, with there being little or no disagreement about the contention that PTI does result in changes of behaviour and of personality. Cavenar and Nash (1976) presented a series of case histories.

Sherwood, Funari and Piekarski, (1990) examined 189 Vietnam veterans admitted to a specialist inpatient treatment programme. These subjects had suffered problems for up to 20 years or more and it was hypothesised that this chronic disability would be associated with personality change. Seventy-two per cent were diagnosed as suffering from PTSD. The patients were assessed using

94

the Millon Clinical Multiphasic Personality Inventory, and Minnesota Multiphasic Personality Inventory, and 148 useable profiles were received. Scores suggestive of passive–aggressive, avoidant and schizoid personality disorders were significantly associated with PTSD.

Personality changes associated with the PTI that followed the Buffalo Creek disaster were described (Titchener and Kapp, 1976; Lindy and Titchener, 1983).

A number of papers have explored the relationship between PTSD and antisocial personality disorder in particular, both from a clinical (Sierles *et al.*, 1983; Behar, 1984; Rosenheck and Nathan, 1985) and from a legal (Erlinger, 1983) point of view.

It seems generally accepted, therefore, that personality change is associated with chronic PTSD. Indeed, ICD-10 contains a specific diagnostic entity of the personality change which can follow PTSD and can become permanent.

Personality factors as predictors of PTI

Hendin *et al.* (1983) produced a review of personality as a predisposing factor in 1983. They noted the fact that up until World War II it was accepted that chronic PTI had more to do with personality vulnerabilities than with the trauma, whereas later work, including that of Kardiner (1941), found little connection between premorbid personality and PTI. That pre-existing factors had little or no relevance was the point of view extant when Hendin's paper was written. However, in contrast with Kardiner, they pointed out that after treating about 100 patients they had come to be of the opinion (which was not supported by empirical data) that personal view of life and the perception of events were of major importance.

There are studies indicating the importance of personality factors and other pre-existing factors, including that of Weisaeth following an industrial disaster (Weisaeth, 1989). Sudak and others (1984) produced a paper about 'antecedent personality factors' but it was a series of case reports and described signs of abnormal behaviour prior to the trauma rather than specific personality features.

McFarlane produced a number of papers examining a large cohort of firefighters involved in a brief but severe natural disaster. Overall his work, unlike that on the more chronic stress in Vietnam, did not find that stressor severity explained much of the variance of PTI (McFarlane, 1989). He used the Eysenck Personality Inventory (EPI) and found that premorbid factors accounted for more of the variance than trauma exposure. The most important factor was neuroticism, as measured on the EPI. In a study of a subgroup (McFarlane

1988) he found that a PTSD group scored significantly higher on the EPI neuroticism scale and lower on the extroversion scale than a non-PTSD group. Davidson's study of 30 chronic PTSD patients from World War II, Korea and Vietnam also used the EPI (Davidson, Kudler and Smith, 1987). PTSD veterans were significantly more introverted and neurotic than non-psychiatric controls or matched non-psychiatric veterans. They also had higher neuroticism scores than patients with depression assessed after treatment. PTSD patient scores did not change significantly with treatment.

Henderson, following the Three Mile Island nuclear incident also emphasised the importance of neuroticism (Henderson, Byrne and Duncan-Jones, 1981).

A study of burn victims (Tucker, 1987) also used the EPQ (a later modified version of the EPI). It too found that neuroticism predicted psychosocial outcome.

In Czechoslovakia (Pavlovsky, 1972) it was found that PTI in 200 burns patients was associated with premorbid 'asthenic' personality.

In a study of traumatised and non-traumatised college students (Bunce, Larsen and Peterson, 1995) it was found that traumatised individuals were more introverted, scored higher on neuroticism, and were less emotionally stable, even in this non-clinical sample.

In much earlier work, Brill and Beebe (1955) looked at 955 Second World War cases of psychoneurosis and stated that 20% had 'pathological personalities'.

A single case history (Johnson, 1995) highlighted the role of premorbid narcissistic personality in exacerbating PTSD.

Schnurr *et al.* (Schnurr, Friedman and Rosenberg, 1993) produced an essentially unique paper in that they presented the PTSD symptomatology and pre-service MMPI scores of 50% of a cohort of 1483 college students first tested on entry to college in 1963 and 1964. The study was carried out between 1985 and 1987. It was determined that 52% of the sample had remained civilians, 3% had been conscientious objectors, 28% had done military service but had not been in combat, and 17% were combat veterans. A subsample were interviewed. Thirty-eight veterans had not seen combat, 56 combat veterans had no PTSD, 13 had some PTSD symptoms, 14 had subthreshold PTSD, and 10 had full PTSD. In general, they all had average pre-combat MMPI scores within the normal range. However, despite this, certain subscales did differentiate between those with no PTSD and all those with any PTSD symptomatology. Relevant subscales were, in decreasing order of significance, psychopathic deviancy, hypochondriasis, and masculinity–femininity. The fact that the MMPI had been measured many years before the trauma means that this can be seen as significant evidence of some effect of premorbid personality factors. Shulman (1994) questioned the methodology and stated that it was far from surprising that personality was seen as influencing PTSD, but Schnurr, Friedman and Rosenberg, (1994) responded by pointing out that in 1994 there was still considerable controversy about the importance or otherwise of premorbid personality or other pre-existing factors.

On balance, the evidence is, therefore, that certain personality traits, specifically neuroticism and perhaps some of the MMPI subscales such as psychopathic deviancy, are associated with the development of PTSD following trauma. Card (1983) did not show any significant effect of personality but it is noted that he looked at behaviours rather than pathological personality variables. Wilson and Krauss's study (Wilson, 1985), which examined some of the DSM-III Axis II personality disorders, found that, contrary to their hypothesis, there was a connection between premorbid personality and PTSD symptoms. However, although the evidence is that premorbid personality does play some part, there is no evidence for the point of view held up to World War II, that only those with personality defects or other pathology could develop other than brief PTI. Personality is only one factor amongst many.

What is the effect of previous history and family history?

A number of individual pre-trauma factors have been investigated with regard to their effect upon PTI following combat exposure. Where a composite index of pre-military factors has been used, the results have been conflicting, as recorded above. However, a large number of studies, of varying size and value, have studied individual factors and, in general, have found that pre-existing factors do have some bearing on the development of PTSD and PTI, even if the effect is smaller than that of trauma exposure. In general, studies of survivors of civilian disasters have shown a larger effect of these pre-existing factors.

1. Academic difficulties in veterans have been associated with PTI in six studies (Health status of Vietnam veterans; I. psychosocial characteristics. (Worthington, 1977; Helzer *et al.*, 1979; Helzer, 1981; Centers for Disease Control Vietnam Experience Study 1988; True, Goldberg and Eisen, 1988; Kulka, *et al.*, 1990) but were found not to have an effect in one (Card, 1983).

2. Family instability or other problems have been found to have an effect in six studies including those of Chemtob *et al.* (1990), Egendorf *et al.* (1981), and Emery *et al.* (1991)

3. A childhood history of being the victim of physical or sexual abuse was found to be relevant in all of three studies, including those of Carmen (1984) and of Swett (1990).

4. Having a father who was exposed to combat was associated with PTI in four studies (Rosenheck and Nathan, 1985 Rosenheck, 1986; Harkness, 1990; Kulka, *op. cit.*).

5. Davidson *et al.* (Davidson, Smith and Kudler, 1989) produced one of four papers showing that a significant history of mental illness in a parent was a risk factor for PTI.

6. All relevant studies have shown that a personal history of mental illness as a child or adolescent increased the risk of PTI (Swank, 1949; Brill and Beebe, 1955; Wilson, 1985).

7. Behaviours indicative of conduct disorder as a child were associated with PTI in four studies.

8. Two studies indicated that a history of illicit drug use before military service was associated with PTI, while that of Fontana and Rosenheck (*op. cit.*) found pre-service drug users less likely to develop non-PTSD PTI .

9. The situation for ethnic minority status is less clear, with six studies finding a positive effect (e.g. Penk, *et al.*, 1989; Green, *et al.*, 1990) and two finding no relationship.

10. Five studies agreed that joining the military at a younger age was associated with post-Vietnam PTI (Hastings, 1991)

11. The two studies to consider willingness to serve have both shown that those who volunteered or were pleased to be drafted were more likely to develop PTI.

Is there an inherited or genetic component to PTI ?

As with so much else in PTI, most of the research into genetic factors has been associated with Vietnam veterans and PTSD.

One exception is the study by Skre *et al.* (1993). This was a study of the involvement of environmental and genetic factors in anxiety disorders. The design involved diagnostic assessment and interviewing of twenty 30–48-year-old monozygotic (MZ) and twenty-nine 21–53-year-old dizygotic (DZ) co-twins of anxiety disorder probands. A comparison group of co-twins of twelve 19–50-year-old MZ and twenty 31–52-year-old DZ twin probands with other non-psychotic mental disorders was also studied. The results showed that simple and social phobias were equally represented in co-twins of anxiety disorder and comparison probands. However, panic disorder, generalized anxiety disorder and PTSD were more prevalent in co-twins of probands with a history of the same disorder. Furthermore, PTSD was more prevalent in MZ than in DZ co-twins. This supports the hypothesis that there is a genetic component to the aetiology of panic disorder, generalised anxiety disorder and PTSD .

The Vietnam veterans research is mostly based on studies of the Vietnam Era Twin Registry (VETR; Eisen, 1993) whose aim was to assess the genetic, common environmental, and unique environmental contributions to the impact of Vietnam service on the medical, psychological, and psychosocial aspects of health of veterans. The VETR contains approximately 7400 male–male monozygotic and dizygotic twin pairs who were born between 1939 and 1953 where both siblings served in the armed forces of the United States during the Vietnam War. Data were obtained by interview of registry members, and by questionnaire or telephone assessment. Although funding for the VETR study officially ended in 1989, the Hines Cooperative Studies Coordinating Center continued the statistical analyses.

True et al. published a study in 1993 (True et al., 1993) which assessed genetic and environmental contributions to the liability for developing PTSD in 4042 monozygotic and dizygotic twin pairs both of whom were in military service during the Vietnam War, and found a genetic influence on PTSD. They used questionnaire responses to quantify the relative contributions of heredity, shared familial environment, and unique environment to the development of PTSD. When they looked at the individual symptom clusters in PTSD, inherited factors contributed to susceptibility for nearly all symptoms. Combat exposure was a strong predictor only of the 're-experiencing' symptom cluster and of the single symptom 'avoiding activities' in the 'avoidance and numbing' cluster. Shared family experiences did not contribute to susceptibility to PTSD symptoms. True et al. suggested that the finding of a genetic influence on PTSD symptoms might be expected to generalise to non-Vietnam trauma, although they had no evidence of this. Their findings were not universally accepted in that Lurie and Geyer (1994) claimed that their study was flawed because it assumed that non-combat environmental influences were not more highly correlated in monozygotic twins than in dizygotic twins. The authors' response (True, Rice and Heath, 1994) was that shared environments were unlikely to affect such a severe disorder as PTSD.

The studies which have shown that PTI is associated directly and indirectly with having a father who was exposed to combat do not, of course, provide weight to the genetic argument, but this association is at least as likely to represent an effect or effects of environmental experience.

The evidence suggests that there may well be a genetic or inherited susceptibility to some anxiety disorders including PTSD. However, the size of the
effect is really not known yet and there is need for further study.

What is the effect of post-trauma environment and experience?

There seems to be general agreement that events following exposure to trauma
have a bearing upon whether or not a victim develops PTI. Such agreement
adds force to the argument that trauma is a necessary, but not a sufficient, cause
of PTI.

The two areas of post-trauma experience that have been most studied have
been those of homecoming and of social support. The former clearly applies
in the main to soldiers who go away to war and then return. It is not directly relevant to the civilian who is a victim of some manmade or natural disaster at
home, or to civilians exposed to war in their home. The second is a universally
relevant factor. Its importance was perhaps highlighted in the original definitions of PTSD which emphasised the existence of late-onset or delayed cases
of PTSD. This is seen as being less common today, with the evidence being
more for late presentation than late onset. For example, only two out of 120
non-combat PTSD cases were considered to be late onset (Burstein, 1985b),
and Solomon's study of alleged delayed onset cases in Israeli soldiers found that
only 10% were of true late onset (Solomon et al., 1989).

It is obvious why consideration of delayed onset PTSD should be examined
in relation to post-trauma experience. If some people do not develop PTSD
after trauma but do so later, then it is at least likely that some intervening factor
or factors play a part. In fact, the Israeli experience is that, although delayed
onset cases are actually uncommon, nevertheless they have fewer social
resources and also fewer post-trauma life events than acute onset cases
(Solomon, Mikulincer and Waysman, 1991).

Effects of homecoming experience

In a study of 40 Vietnam veterans (Butler et al., 1988), PTSD was found to be
associated with more negative homecoming experiences, and this was also the
case in another study (Foy et al., 1987). The same was found in British Falklands
veterans in whom PTI was associated with emotional difficulties in the immediate homecoming period (O'Brien and Hughes, 1991). This finding has been
repeatedly shown in case reports and is a generally accepted view.

Social support and PTI

There is a considerable body of research into the association between social support or perceived social support and PTI. Obviously there is a real problem with such research as it is almost inevitably retrospective. There is also an additional, somewhat related, problem in the question of whether social support affects PTI, or whether PTI affects perceived social support. This question is highlighted in the study of 45 Vietnam veterans, 15 with PTSD, 15 well combat controls, and 15 without a combat history (Keane, 1985). All three groups reported similar perceived social support in the three months prior to military service. However, those with PTSD reported that their social support had gradually and continuously fallen over time since Vietnam, while the healthy controls and non-combat group reported stable or increasing social support.

Vietnam and Israeli combat experience

In a Vietnam veterans questionnaire study with a less than 50% response rate, there was no relationship between social support and combat exposure, but high social support was associated with fewer PTI symptoms (Barrett and Mizes, 1988). An interesting study of Vietnam veterans still serving in 1982 (Stretch, 1986) not only showed that social support in the first year was related to a lower incidence of PTSD symptoms, but suggested that the prevalence of PTSD in soldiers still serving was lower than that in those who had left the service.

A number of the Israeli studies of combat stress reaction cases from the Lebanon War have shown that social support has a predictive relationship with PTSD (Solomon, Mikulincer and Avitzur, 1988) (Solomon and Mikulincer, 1990). In one of the studies (Solomon, Waysman and Mikulincer, 1990) loneliness was found to be the only direct antecedent of PTSD in the combat stress reaction group. Perceived social support was found to be relevant but was seen to be a feature of perceived loneliness.

Civilian experience

The civilian experience uniformly associates PTSD with low social support. However, the question of whether social support is perceived to be low due to distress or whether low social support causes distress is not definitely answered. For example, a comparison between residents exposed to a chemical spill and neighbours from a nearby town showed that the exposure group as a whole reported lower perceived social support and also more symptoms, but not neccesarily actual PTI (Bowler *et al.*, 1994).

Bodyhandlers have been found to be helped in coping if they have social support from colleagues and spouses (McCarroll *et al.*, 1993). In a highly selected group of battered women (Kemp *et al.*, 1995), perceived social support was predictive but was the least significant of the factors found to be of relevance.

In a community study of 2985 people, subjective impairment of social support was associated with chronic but not with acute PTSD (Davidson *et al.*, 1991). A study of 116 people following a tornado found 50 subjects to have mild or moderate PTSD, and 19 to have severe PTSD. Poor social support was associated with severe rather than mild or moderate PTSD.

Are there neuronal changes associated with PTSD?

The idea that PTI is associated with pathological changes in the brain is far from new. Initially it was thought that First World War shell shock was associated with a 'commotion' of the brain caused by rapid changes in pressure caused by the explosion of shells, and resulting in visible pathological changes. Clearly this is not the case. However, even before then there had been observation of autonomic nervous system dysfunction in 'Da Costa's syndrome' (Da Costa, 1871) and 'neurocirculatory asthenia' (Fraser and Wilson, 1918). Further strength to the association between these early cases of presumed PTSD and the sympathetic nervous system came with the discovery of improvement following bilateral surgical denervation of the adrenal glands (Crile, 1940).

Much of the theorising centred on sympathetic nervous system activity and PTSD is based upon the Second World War work of Kardiner (1941). Van der Kolk *et al.* (1985) have listed the five principal features of the condition described by Kardiner and now known as PTSD:

1. persistence of startle responses and irritability
2. proclivity to explosive reactions
3. atypical dream life
4. fixation on the trauma
5. constriction of the general level of personality functioning.

It can be seen that most of these correlate generally to the intrusive symptoms of PTSD, while the last could be compared with the withdrawal symptoms. Van der Kolk refers to the two groups as positive and negative symptom groups respectively.

Positive symptoms

These have been explained at two levels: a psychological explanation using conditioning, and a neuronal explanation. The two are not mutually exclusive and the one may underlie the other.

It is suggested that a process of classical conditioning explains the heightened autonomic reactivity of PTSD (Kolb, 1984). Unconditioned emotional, behavioural and physiological responses to a severe traumatic event become conditioned to otherwise neutral stimuli, both internal and external, so that these conditioned stimuli produce the same response with pronounced sympathetic nervous system activity (Murburg, McFall and Veith, 1990).

On the neuronal level Kolb (1987), like others, has suggested that overwhelming shock can cause such overstimulation that there is structural and potentially permanent neuronal change. He cites the changes in hearing following excessive noise exposure as an analogy. He suggests that there is then hypersensitivity of the cortex and a reduced capacity from habituation, so that lower brainstem structures escape from inhibitory control.

One of the structures implicated by a number of investigators is the locus coeruleus (LC). This is the major source of noradrenergic innervation of the limbic system and cortex. Electrical stimulation has been shown to induce states apparently equating to fear and alarm in animals (Krystal, 1990), while ablation in monkeys results in a loss of the normal fear response, and lesions in rats result in a failure of the normal rise in 3-methoxy-4-hydroxyphenylglycol (MPHG), an index of noradrenaline activity. This has led Krystal to suggest that the LC 'meets the criteria for a brain trauma centre'. It has been demonstrated that there can be long-term potentiation of neural circuits after intense exposure to an overwhelming stimulus. As the LC plays a role in the retrieval of memories, and in sleep control, it has been suggested that the intrusive phenomena, including vivid eidetic dreams, are related to long-term potentiation of the LC system.

Thus the classical conditioning model would be explained in neuropathological terms.

Negative symptoms

It is suggested that the best model for the negative symtoms of PTSD is that of inescapable shock or learned helplessness as induced experimentally in animals. Van der Kolk points out that animals which have been prevented from escaping from severe stress show:

1. reduced learning of escape strategies in new stressful situations
2. decrease in motivation for new learning and increased withdrawal
3. evidence of chronic subjective distress.

Stressors which produce no measurable change in naive mice produce noradrenaline depletion and the behavioural changes noted above in those previously exposed to inescapable shock. It seems that these negative symptoms are associated with noradrenaline and dopamine depletion in experimental animals and that this mechanism may operate in PTSD.

Positive and negative symptoms – a neurophysiological synthesis

At first glance it seems that the proposed mechanisms for positive and negative symptoms are contradictory. In explaining this, investigators have looked at the negative symptoms as being a tonic or background phenomenon, with a phasic or intermittent occurrence of the more obvious and dramatic positive symptoms. It is suggested that there is, as a result of neuronal change, a chronic depletion of noradrenaline and a resultant hypersensitivity of the adrenergic system. Thus transient stimulation by lesser stresses or associations leads to overactivity of noradrenaline-mediated behaviour presenting as the intrusive and overarousal symptoms of PTSD against the background of negative avoidance symptoms.

Are there hypothalamic–pituitary–adrenal axis changes?

The answer to this must surely be an unequivocal yes. The evidence for HPA changes in chronic stress conditions (Holsboer *et al.*, 1994) and PTSD has mounted gradually and is now overwhelming. However, like all the other observations, this does not mean that HPA axis abnormalities are the cause of PTSD. It may be that the cause of PTSD mediates its effect through the HPA, or that this is an associated or partial factor. One of the principal proponents of the theory of the importance of the HPA has been the team led by Yehuda. They have produced a large series of papers which have gradually developed the theory (Yehuda *et al.*, 1993a). One abnormality which is similar to that seen in a range of other psychiatric disorders is a blunting of the adrenocorticotrophic hormone response to corticotrophin-releasing hormone with a low but normal cortisol level (Smith *et al.*, 1989). However, although some of the HPA axis findings are similar to those in depression, anorexia etc., some are consistently different.

The basic theory is that there is enhanced negative feedback sensitivity of the HPA axis in PTSD. In one study (Yehuda *et al.*, 1993b) a low-dose dexamethasone suppression test was used in 21 male patients with PTSD and 12 controls. PTSD patients had greater cortisol suppression than controls, even when the patients also fulfilled diagnostic criteria for major depression. This confirms that the HPA abnormalities in PTSD are different from those in depression and are not explained by comorbid depression but are actually in the opposite direction (Yehuda *et al.*, 1991a). Others have also found that PTSD patients who had depression in addition did not show abnormal responses to the dexamethasone suppresion test (Halbreich *et al.*, 1989).

A study of 37 adolescent Armenian survivors of the 1988 earthquake (Goenjian *et al.*, 1996) looked at salivary cortisol and response to dexamethasone. Those with symptoms and closest to the epicentre had lower baseline cortisol and greater suppression. These HPA changes were specifically associated with the intrusive symptoms of PTSD. In addition, those with PTSD symptoms had a more rapid decline in 3-methoxy-4-hydroxyphenylglycol through the day. It is noted that this is congruent with previous studies and is used to support the contention that continued intrusive symptoms may, of themselves, not only cause distress, but evoke repeated physiological stress responses, which eventually alter HPA axis function.

In a study of 15 Vietnam veterans with PTSD and 11 controls, lymphocyte glucocorticoid receptors were measured diurnally (Yehuda *et al.*, 1991b). It was found that PTSD patients had levels of receptors 63% higher in the morning and 26% higher in the afternoon. This is in the opposite direction to findings in depression and supports the idea that there are specific HPA abnormalities in PTSD. It is consistent with the possibility of a chronic increased negative feedback sensitivity at some level in the axis.

Yehuda's team has produced a nice piece of support for their contention that enhanced negative feedback inhibition is the substrate of the HPA abnormalities in PTSD (Yehuda *et al.*, 1996). They used metyrapone to demonstrate the pituitary response directly by measuring ACTH response. Metyrapone caused a significantly greater increase of ACTH and 11–deoxycortisol in 11 veterans with PTSD than in 8 controls. They suggest that this finding should be taken in conjunction with the other abnormalities shown, lower basal cortisol levels, increased numbers of lymphocyte glucocorticoid receptors, and increased suppression of cortisol following dexamethasone compared with normals and depressed patients with major depression. Together with this evidence of increased pituitary action on direct stimulation without negative feedback, the findings provide clear support for the hypothesis of enhanced negative feedback of the HPA axis.

In comparison with both normal controls and with controls who have not developed PTSD but have been exposed to trauma, those with PTSD appear to have consistent differences in HPA function which are different from the classical simple response to stress. They have a tendency towards lower 24-hour urinary cortisol and plasma cortisol, increased cortisol regulation, increased numbers of lymphocyte glucocorticoid receptors, increased response to low-dose dexamethasone, increased response to metyrapone, and decreased or blunted response to corticotrophin-releasing factor. All these findings together suggest that PTSD can not only be differentiated from the normal response to trauma, but from other conditions. It is not surprising that the PTSD HPA findings are different from the usual response to stress as most people exposed to severe stressors do not develop PTSD. The majority, who do not have PTSD, have HPA responses expected after stress. It seems that the PTSD responses are a specific variant which requires stress for induction but is not a normal or inevitable response to stress. Those who develop PTSD may well also develop a sensitised HPA with enhanced negative feedback – responses qualitatively different from those seen in survivors who do not develop PTSD.

Are there other pathological changes?

There has been investigation of a massive range of possible biological markers or of indicators of pathology in PTI and PTSD. Most of the studies have used small samples, and repetition has not always produced replication, leading to questions about methodology and rigour of application as well as questioning the original findings.

Other hormonal changes

There has been some interest in thyroid hormones in PTSD. Clearly, there are associations with the previous section in that the release of thyroid hormones is controlled by a hypothalamic–pituitary–thyroid axis. Mason and others (1994) have studied thyroid hormones in great detail in 96 inpatient veterans with PTSD and 24 controls. They found raised levels of free and total tri-iodothyronine and of total thyroxine, but not of free thyroxine and thyroid-binding globulin. This confirmed previous studies and supports their belief that the abnormalities are not all explained by an increase in thyroid-binding globulin.

There is suggestion (Mason *et al.*, 1990) that serum testosterone levels in PTSD patients are higher than seen in depressed patients, even when symptoms of depression are present, and are closer to those in schizophrenic patients.

Evidence of pathological and morphological changes

There have been some findings of deficits in short-term memory in veterans with PTSD. This has led to increased interest in scanning techniques of the brain and measures of the hippocampus in particular. In a magnetic resonance imaging (MRI) scan study of 26 Vietnam combat veterans with PTSD and 22 carefully matched controls (Bremner *et al.*, 1995) the right-side hippocampal volume alone was significantly smaller (8%) in PTSD patients. In these patients the smaller hippocampal volume was associated with deficits in short-term verbal memory on the Wechsler Memory Scale.

A study was carried out of symptom provocation using script-driven imagery and positron emission tomography (Rauch *et al.*, 1996) in eight PTSD patients. The patients were used as their own controls by exposing them to both traumatic and neutral scripts sequentially while positron emission tomography was carried out and emotional state was recorded, along with heart rate. The traumatic scripts, but not the neutral scripts, resulted in increased blood flow in right-sided limbic, paralimbic and visual areas but decreased flow in left inferior frontal and middle temporal cortex.

Are there physiological changes?

In an interesting review article in 1990, Blanchard suggested that the consistent finding that Vietnam veterans had higher resting pulse rates and blood pressure might be indicative of a future increased rate of cardiovascular morbidity. An outpatient study of 32 Vietnam veterans with PTSD and 26 control veterans (Gerardi *et al.*, 1994) showed that baseline heart rate and systolic and diastolic blood pressures were higher in PTSD patients but temperature and respiration rates were not different.

There are a host of studies showing different physiological responses in PTSD patients in general and in Vietnam veteran patients in particular. The differences are seen from combat veteran controls, other controls, and other psychiatric patients.

Eleven Vietnam PTSD cases were compared with 11 controls (Blanchard *et al.*, 1982) with regard to their heart rate, blood pressure, forehead electro-myography (EMG), skin resistance level, and skin temperature changes in response to mental arithmetic tasks and to increasing volumes of combat sounds. There were differences found in heart rate, systolic blood pressure, and EMG. The best distinguishing measure was the heart rate response, which could be used to classify correctly 95.5% of the total sample.

A slightly larger study looked at a total of 40 veterans, including those with PTSD, comparable combat veterans without PTSD, veterans with other psychiatric disorders, and civilian phobics (Pallmeyer, Blanchard and Kolb, 1986). Mental arithmetic was again the neutral stimulus and combat sounds the relevant stimulus. The change in heart rate in response to low-intensity combat sounds effectively discriminated the PTSD cases from the other groups. This supports the idea of a conditioned emotional response in PTSD.

The interest in physiological responses as an indicator of PTSD has led to investigation of whether or not such responses can be dissimulated. In one study (Gerardi, Blanchard and Kolb, 1989) PTSD patients were unable to change their responses in the direction of normality but healthy controls could be trained to alter their responses in the direction of the PTSD response. However, even with intentional dissimulation on instruction the physiological responses were still a good means of differentiating the PTSD and control groups.

In a small study of four road traffic accident victims with PTSD (Blanchard, Hickling and Taylor, 1991), response to mental imagery of two scenes related to the accident was investigated. There were reliable heart rate responses to the images and some blood pressure changes.

Shalev and Rogel-Fuchs (1993) have reviewed the neurophysiological hypotheses of stress disorders, noting the important point that not only relevant external stimuli but also mental imagery can result in increased physiological responsiveness. This has led to study of the startle reflex and of habituation and stimulus discrimination in a search for understanding of the neurobiology of PTSD.

Is there a Grand Unified Theory which explains the observed changes and explains PTSD ?

It would be extremely helpful if a single sentence or equation could explain the cause of PTSD. This would negate all argument about validity and causation. However, the equation would need to explain not only who gets PTSD, but who does not. As of yet, it does not seem that we are really very near any such simple explanation of PTSD. There is a great deal that is known, but not enough to predict on a case by case basis who will get PTSD of what severity after which incidents. We know much about detectable abnormalities in sufferers, but not really about which, if any, of such abnormalities is the root cause. This section of the chapter will try to summarise what we know about causation of PTSD, although it will inevitably oversimplify.

• The first observation is that trauma is an essential element of causation of PTSD but does not explain it. Not everyone who is exposed to a particular trauma will develop PTSD. It has been suggested repeatedly now that events which might not be considered to be generally particularly traumatic may be followed by symptoms reminiscent of PTSD. There also seems little support for the view that the sort of trauma which can be followed by those symptoms associated with PTSD is of a particularly great degree of severity.

- The scale or severity of trauma is significant in predicting PTSD but insufficient. Studies of veterans with PTSD have shown that degree of exposure accounts for about 35% of the variance in PTSD at the most.
- A more comprehensive model using trauma and pre-traumatic characteristics was able to account for perhaps 60% of the variance of both PTSD and other PTI, with the trauma variables having more influence on PTSD than on other PTI. Importantly, this study confirmed the opinion that the various groups of potential factors investigated did tend to interact and the situation really is as complicated as it sometimes seems.
- Some of the pre-trauma factors which clearly seem to influence the occurrence of PTSD, at least after combat, include academic achievement, prior family problems, a history of abuse, combat exposure in the father, conduct disorder in childhood, and personal and family history of mental illness. Personality factors seem to play a part in both military and civilian PTSD.
- Post-trauma experience is also relevant. The uncommon, but very real, occurrence of delayed onset of PTSD seems to confirm this. Something must intervene. There is evidence that post-trauma experience, including social support and further life events, plays a part.
- There is evidence for a, as yet undefined, genetic influence, with higher concordance rates in monozygotic twins.
- PTSD can be seen as consisting of positive and negative symptoms, intrusive and arousal as opposed to avoidant. The positive symptoms can be seen in terms of classical conditioning which can be explained further on a neuroendocrine level as a potentiation of neural circuits after overwhelming stimulation. Learned helplessness has been used as a model of the negative symptoms and this, too, can fit in with a neuroendocrine hypothesis. It is suggested that there is a background tonic state of chronic noradrenaline depletion due to inescapable shock. Against this, positive symptoms intrude due to overactivity of noradrenaline with transient minor stimulation or reminders.
- This can be compared with the theory from neuroendocrine studies that there is enhanced negative feedback sensitivity through the hypothalamic–pituitary–adrenal axis demonstrated by consistent abnormalities unlike those in acute stress and unlike those in depression.

- Other hormonal abnormalities are consistent with dysfunction in this HPA axis.
- Consistent physiological responses to triggers and baseline alterations also give clinical confirmation of this neuroendocrine substrate of the disorder.
- The evidence is that there is clear support for a comprehensible neuroendocrine abnormality in PTSD with detectable evidence of pathology and physiological change. However, actual causation of the disorder remains a complex interaction of trauma type and severity, prior personal and family history, personality, pre-existing illness, and subsequent experience. The old idea that PTSD was entirely a consequence of trauma and that individual differences were essentially irrelevant is no longer tenable. Nevertheless, we have not, as of yet, returned to the idea that the normal or usual PTI is a brief affair, and that prolonged illnesses are a consequence of personal vulnerability. The truth is somewhere in between.

References

American Psychiatric Association (1994). *Diagnostic and Statistical Manual of Mental Disorders*, 4th edition. Washington: APA.

Astin, M.C., Ogland-Hand, S.M., Coleman, E.M. and Foy, D. (1995). Posttraumatic stress disorder and childhood abuse in battered women: Comparisons with maritally distressed women. *Journal of Consulting and Clinical Psychology*, **63**, 2: 308–12.

Atkinson, R.M., Henderson, R.G. Sparr, L.F. and Deale, S. (1982). Assessment of Viet Nam veterans for posttraumatic stress disorder in Veterans Administration disability claims. *American Journal of Psychiatry*, **139**, 9: 1118–21.

Barrett, T.W. and Mizes, J.S. (1988). Combat level and social support in the development of posttraumatic stress disorder in Vietnam veterans. *Behavior Modification*, **12**, 1: 100–15.

Behar D. (1984). Confirmation of concurrent illnesses in PTSD. *American Journal of Psychiatry*, **141**: 1310–11.

Blanchard, E.B. (1990). Elevated basal level of cardiovascular responses in Vietnam veterans with PTSD: A health problem in the making? *Journal of Anxiety Disorders*, **4**, 3: 233–7.

Blanchard, E.B., Hickling, E.J. and Taylor, A.E. (1991). The psychophysiology of motor vehicle accident related posttraumatic stress disorder. *Biofeedback and Self Regulation*, **16**, 4: 449–58.

Blanchard, E.B., Kolb, L.C., Pallmeyer, T.P. and Gerardi, R.J. (1982). A psychophysiological study of post traumatic stress disorder in Vietnam veterans. *Psychiatric Quarterly*, **54**, 4: 220–9.

Borus, J.F. (1974). Incidence of maladjustment in Vietnam returnees. *Archives of General Psychiatry*, **30**: 554–7.

Bowler, R.M., Mergler, D., Huel, G. and Cone, J.E. (1994). Aftermath of a chemical spill: psychological and physiological sequelae. *Neurotoxicology*, **15**, 3: 723–9.

Bownes, I.T., O'Gorman, E.C. and Sayers, A. (1991). Psychiatric symptoms, behavioural responses and post-traumatic stress disorder in rape victims. Division of Criminological and Legal Psychology First Annual Conference, 1991, Canterbury, England. *Issues in Criminological and Legal Psychology*, **1**, 17: 25–33.

Bremner, J.D., Randall, P., Scott, T.M., Bronen, R.A., Seibyl, J.P., Southwick, S.M., Delaney, R.C., McCarthy, G., Charney, D.S. and Innis, R.B. (1995). MRI-based measurement of hippocampal volume in patients with combat-related post-traumatic stress disorder. *American Journal of Psychiatry*, **152**, 7: 973–81.

Breslau, N. and Davis., G.C. (1987a). Posttraumatic stress disorder: The etiologic specificity of wartime stressors. 139th Annual Meeting of the American Psychiatric Association, 1986, Washington, DC. *American Journal of Psychiatry*, **144**, 5: 578–83.

Breslau, N. and Davis., G.C. (1987b). Posttraumatic stress disorder: The stressor criterion. *Journal of Nervous and Mental Disease*, **175**, 5: 255–64.

Brett, E.A. and Ostroff, R. (1985). Imagery and posttraumatic stress disorder: An overview. *American Journal of Psychiatry*, **142**, 4: 417–24.

Brill N.Q. and Beebe, G.W. (1955). *A Follow-up Study of War Neuroses*. Washington: Veterans Administration.

Bromet, E.J., Parkinson, D.K. and Schulberg, H.C. (1980). *Three Mile Island: Mental Health Findings*. Pittsburgh: University of Pittsburgh.

Bromet, E.J., Parkinson, D.K. and Schulberg, H.C. *et al.* (1982). Mental health of residents near the Three Mile Island reactor: a comparative study of selected groups. *Journal of Preventive Psychiatry*, **1**: 225–76.

Bunce, S.C., Larsen, R.J., and Peterson, C. (1995). Life after trauma: personality and daily life experiences of traumatized people. *Journal of Personality*, **63**, 2: 165–88.

Burstein, A. (1985a). Posttraumatic stress disorder. *Journal of Clinical Psychiatry*, **46**: 554.

Burstein, A. (1985b). How common is delayed posttraumatic stress disorder? *American Journal of Psychiatry*, **142**, 7: 887.

Butler, R.W., Foy, D.W., Snodgrass, L. and Hurwicz, M-L (1988). Combat-related post-traumatic stress disorder in a nonpsychiatric population. *Journal of Anxiety Disorders*, **2**, 2: 111–20.

Buydens-Branchey, L., Noumair, D. and Branchey, M. (1990). Duration and intensity of combat exposure and posttraumatic stress disorder in Vietnam veterans. *Journal of Nervous and Mental Disease*, **178**, 9: 582–7.

Card J.J. (1983). *Lives After Vietnam*. Lexington, Mass.: DC Heath.

Carmen, E.H. (1984). Victims of violence and psychiatric illness. *American Journal of Psychiatry*, **141**: 378–83.

Cavenar, J.O. and Nash, J.L. (1976). The effects of combat on the normal personality. *Comprehensive Psychiatry*, **17**: 647–53.

Centers for Disease Control Vietnam Experience Study (1988). Health status of Vietnam veterans. I: psychosocial characteristics. *Journal of the American Medical Association*, **259**, 18: 2701–8.

Chemtob, C.M., Bauer, G.B., Neller, G., Hamada R., Glisson, C. and Stevens, V. (1990). Post-traumatic stress disorder among Special Forces Vietnam veterans. *Military Medicine*, **155**, 1: 16–20.

Crile, G. (1940). Results in 152 denervations of the adrenal gland in treatment of neuro-circulatory asthenia. *Military Surgeon*, **87**: 509–13.

Da Costa, J.M. (1871). On irritable heart: a clinical study of a form of functional cardiac disorder and its consequences. *American Journal of Medical Science*, **61**: 17–52.

Davidson, J.R., Hughes, D., Blazer, D.G. and George, L.K. (1991). Post-traumatic stress disorder in the community: An epidemiological study. *Psychological Medicine*, **21**, 3: 713–21.

Davidson, J., Kudler, H. and Smith, R. (1987). Personality in chronic post-traumatic stress disorder: A study of the Eysenck inventory. *Journal of Anxiety Disorders*, **1**, 4: 295–300.

Davidson, J.R., Smith, R.D. and Kudler, H.S. (1989). Familial psychiatric illness in chronic posttraumatic stress disorder. *Comprehensive Psychiatry*, **30**, 4: 339–45.

Egendorf, A (1981). *Legacies of Vietnam: Comparative Adjustment of veterans and their peers*. House Committee Print No. 14. Washington: Government Printing Office.

Eisen, S.A. (1993). *Vietnam Experience Twin Study (VETS)*. Fedrip Database, National Technical Information Service (NTIS).

Emery, V.O, Emery, P.E., Shama, D.K. and Quiana, N.A.I. (1991). Predisposing variables in PTSD patients. *Journal of Traumatic Stress*, **4**, 3: 325–43.

Erlinger, C.P. (1983). Posttraumatic stress disorders, Vietnam veterans and the law. *Behavioral Sciences and the Law*, **142**: 90–93.

Figley C.R. (1978). Symptoms of delayed combat stress among a college sample of Vietnam veterans. *Military Medicine*, 143.

Figley C.R. and Leventman, S. (Eds.) (1980). *Strangers at Home: Vietnam Veterans Since the War*. New York: Praeger.

Fontana, A. and Rosenheck, R. (1993). A causal model of the etiology of war-related PTSD. *Journal of Traumatic Stress*, **6**, 4: 475–500.

Foy, D.W. and Card, J.J. (1987). Combat-related post-traumatic stress disorder etiology: Replicated findings in a national sample of Vietnam-era men. *Journal of Clinical Psychology*, **43**, 1: 28–31.

Foy, D.W., Resnick, H.S., Sipprelle, R.C. and Carroll, E.M. (1987). Premilitary, military, and postmilitary factors in the development of combat-related posttraumatic stress disorder. *Behavior Therapist*, **10**, 1: 3–9.

Foy, D.W., Sipprelle, R.C., Rueger, D.B. and Carroll, E.M. (1984). Etiology of post-traumatic stress disorder in Vietnam veterans: Analysis of premilitary, military, and combat exposure influences. *Journal of Consulting and Clinical Psychology*. **52**, 1: 79–87.

Fraser, F. and Wilson, R. (1918). The sympathetic nervous system and the 'irritable heart' of soldiers'. *British Medical Journal*, **2**: 27–9.

Gerardi, R.J., Blanchard, E.B. and Kolb, L.C. (1989). Ability of Vietnam veterans to dis-simulate a psychophysiological assessment or PTSD. *Behavior Therapy*, **20**, 1: 229–44.

Gerardi, R.J., Keane, T.M. Cahoon, B.J. and Klauminzer, G.W. (1994). An in vivo assess-ment of physiological arousal in posttraumatic stress disorder. *Journal of Abnormal Psychology*, **103**, 4: 825–7.

Ghods, S. (1992). The etiology of post-traumatic stress disorder among Iranian soldiers. *Dissertation Abstracts International*, **53**, 5–B: 25–9.

Goenjian, A.K., Yehuda, R., Pynoos, R.S., Steinberg, A.M., Tashjian, M., Yang, R.K., Najarian, L.M. and Fairbanks, L.A. (1996). Basal cortisol, dexamethasone suppres-sion of cortisol, and MHPG in adolescents after the 1988 earthquake in Armenia. *American Journal of Psychiatry*, **153**, 7: 929–34.

Goldberg, J., True, W.R., Eisen, S.A. and Henderson, W.G. (1990). A twin study of the effects of the Vietnam War on posttraumatic stress disorder. *Journal of the American Medical Association*, **263**, 9: 1227–32.

Green, B.L., Grace, M.C., Lindy, J.D., Gleser, G.C. and Leonard, A. (1990a). Risk factors for PTSD and other diagnoses in a general sample of Vietnam veterans. *American Journal of Psychiatry*, **147**, 6: 729–33.

Green, B.L., Grace, M.C., Lindy, J.D. and Leonard, A.C. (1990b). Race differences in response to combat stress. *Journal of Traumatic Stress*, **3**, 3: 379–93.

Green, B.L., Korol, M., Grace, M.C., Vary, M.G., Leonard, A.C, Gleser, G.C and Smitson, C.S. (1991). Children and disaster: Age, gender, and parental effects on PTSD symptoms. *Journal of the American Academy of Child and Adolescent Psychiatry*, **30**, 6: 945–51.

Greenwald, E. and Leitenberg, H. (1990). Posttraumatic stress disorder in a nonclinical and nonstudent sample of adult women sexually abused as children. *Journal of Interpersonal Violence*, **5**, 2: 217–28.

Halbreich, U., Olympia, J., Carson, S.W., Glogowski J., Yeh, C.M., Axelrod, S. and Desu, M.M. (1989). Hypothalamo–pituitary–adrenal activity in endogenously depressed post-traumatic stress disorder patients. *Psychoneuroendocrinology*, **14**, 5: 365–70.

Harkness, L.L. (1990). Children of war: A study of the offspring of Vietnam veterans with post traumatic stress disorder. *Dissertation Abstracts International*, **51**, 2–B: 657.

Hastings, T.J. (1991). The Stanford-Terman study revisited: Postwar emotional health of . World War II veterans. *Military Psychology*, **3**: 201–14.

Helzer, J.E. (1981). Methodological issues in the interpretations of the consequences of extreme situations. In *Stressful Life Events and Their Contexts*, pp. 108–29. Ed. B.S. Dohrwend and B.P. Dohrwend. New York: Prodist.

Helzer, J.E., Robins, L.N. and McEvoy, L. (1987). Post-traumatic stress disorder in the general population: Findings of the Epidemiologic Catchment Area survey. *New England Journal of Medicine*, **317**, 26: 1630–4.

Helzer, J.E., Robins, L.N., Wish, E. and Hesselbrock, M. (1979). Depression in Vietnam veterans and civilian controls. *American Journal of Psychiatry*, **136**: 526–9.

Henderson, S., Byrne, D.G. and Duncan-Jones, P. (1981). *Neurosis and the Social Environment*. Sydney: Academic Press.

Hendin, H., Haas, A.P., Singer, P., Gold, F. and Trigos, G.G. (1983). The influence of pre-combat personality on posttraumatic stress disorder. *Comprehensive Psychiatry*, **24**, 6: 530–4.

Hennessy, B. and Oei, T.P. (1991). The relationship between severity of combat exposure and army status on post-traumatic stress disorder among Australian Vietnam war veterans. Special issue: Research in anxiety and fear. *Behaviour Change*, **8**, 3: 136–44.

Holloway, H.C. and Ursano, R.J. (1984). The Vietnam veteran: Memory, social context, and metaphor. *Psychiatry*, **47**, 2: 103–8.

Holsboer, F., Grasser, A., Friess, E. and Wiedemann, K. (1994). Steroid effects on central neurons and implications for psychiatric and neurological disorders. *Annals of the New York Academy of Science*, **746**: 345–59.

Johnson, W. (1995). Narcissistic personality as a mediating variable in manifestations of post-traumatic stress disorder. *Military Medicine*, **160**, 1: 40–41.

Kardiner, A. (1941). *The Traumatic Neuroses of War*. New York: Jason Aaronson.

Keane, T.M. (1985). Social support in Vietnam veterans with posttraumatic stress disorder: A comparative analysis. *Journal of Consulting and Clinical Psychology*, **53**, 1: 95–102.

Kemp, A., Green, B.L., Hovanitz, C. and Rawlings, E.I. (1995). Incidence and correlates of PTSD in battered women: shelter and community samples. *Journal of Interpersonal Violence*, **10**: 1.

Kolb, L.C. (1984). The post-traumatic stress disorders of combat: A subgroup with a conditioned emotional response. *Military Medicine*, **149**, 5: 237–43.

Kolb, L.C. (1987). A neuropsychological hypothesis explaining posttraumatic stress disorders. *American Journal of Psychiatry*, **144**, 8: 989–95.

Krystal, J.H. (1990). Animal models for post traumatic stress disorder. In *Biological Assessment and Treatment of Posttraumatic Stress Disorder*, pp. 1–26. Ed. E.L. Giller Jr. Washington: American Psychiatric Press.

Kulka, R.A., Schlenger, W.E., Fairbank, J.A., Hough, R.L., Jordan, B.K., Marmar, C. and Weiss, D.S. (1990). Brunner Mazel Psychosocial Stress Series No. 18. *Trauma and the Vietnam War Generation: Report of Findings from the National Vietnam Veterans Readjustment Study*. New York: Brunner Mazel.

Lindy, J.D. and Titchener, J. (1983). 'Acts of God and man': character change in survivors of disasters and the law. *Behavioral Sciences and the Law*, **1**: 85–96.

Lopez-Ibor, J.J. Jr, Carras, S.F. and Rodriguez-Gamazo, M. (1985). Psychopathological aspects of the toxic oil syndrome catastrophe. *British Journal of Psychiatry* **147**: 352–65.

Lukasik, R.P. (1991). Posttraumatic stress disorder in Canadian aircraft accident survivors. *Dissertation Abstracts International*, **51**, 8–B: 40–58.

Lurie, S. and Geyer, P. (1994). Genetic and environmental influences of twins in post-traumatic stress. *Archives of General Psychiatry*, **51**, 10: 838.

Madakasira, S. and O'Brien, K.F. (1987). Acute posttraumatic stress disorder in victims of a natural disaster. *Journal of Nervous and Mental Disease*, **175**, 5: 286–90.

Malt, U. (1988). The long term psychiatric consequences of accidental injury: a longitudinal study of 107 adults. *British Journal of Psychiatry*, **153**: 810–18.

March, J.S. (1993). What constitutes a stressor? The 'criterion A' issue. In *PTSD – DSM-IV and Beyond*, pp. 37–56. Ed. J.R. Davidson and E.B. Foa. Washington: American Psychiatric Press.

Mason, J.W., Giller, E.L., Kosten, T.R. and Wahby, V.S. (1990). Serum testosterone levels in post-traumatic stress disorder inpatients. *Journal of Traumatic Stress*, **3**, 3: 449–57.

Mason, J., Southwick, S., Yehuda, R., Wang, S., Riney, S., Bremner, D., Johnson, D., Lubin, H., Blake, D. and Zhou, G. (1994). Elevation of serum free triiodothyronine, total triiodothyronine, thyroxine-binding globulin, and total thyroxine levels in combat-related posttraumatic stress disorder. *Archives of General Psychiatry*, **51**, 8: 629–41.

McCarroll, J., Ursano, R., Wright, K. and Fullerton, C. (1993). Handling bodies after violent death: strategies for coping. *American Journal of Orthopsychiatry*, **63**, 2: 209–14.

McFarlane, A.C. (1988). The aetiology of post-traumatic stress disorders following a natural disaster. *British Journal of Psychiatry*, **152**: 116–21.

McFarlane, A.C. (1989). The aetiology of post-traumatic morbidity: Predisposing, precipitating and perpetuating factors. *British Journal of Psychiatry*, **154**: 221–8.

McGorry, P.D., Chanen, A., McCarthy, E., Van Riel, R., McKenzie, B. and Singh, B.S. (1991). Posttraumatic stress disorder following recent-onset psychosis: An unrecognized postpsychotic syndrome. *Journal of Nervous and Mental Disease*, **179**, 5: 253–8.

Murburg, M.M., McFall, M.E. and Veith, R.C. (1990). Catecholamines, stress, and PTSD. In *Biological Assessment and Treatment of Posttraumatic Stress Disorder*, pp. 27–64. Ed. E.L. Giller Jr. Washington: American Psychiatric Press.

Murphy, S.A. (1984). After Mount St. Helens: disaster stress research. *Journal of Psychosocial Nursing and Mental Health Services*, **22**, 7: 9–18.

Muse, M. (1986). Stress-related, posttraumatic chronic pain syndrome: Behavioral treatment approach. *Pain*, **25**, 3: 389–94.

Nace, E.P., O'Brien, C.P., Mintz, J., Ream, N. and Meyers, A.L. (1978). Adjustment among Vietnam veteran drug users two years post service. In *Stress Disorders Among Vietnam Veterans:Theory, Research and Treatment*, pp. 71–128. Ed. C.R. Figley. New York: Brunner/Mazel.

O'Brien, L.S. and Hughes, S.J. (1991). Symptoms of post-traumatic stress disorder in Falklands veterans five years after the conflict. *British Journal of Psychiatry*, **159**: 135–41.

Pallmeyer, T.P., Blanchard, E.B. and Kolb, L.C. (1986). The psychophysiology of combat-induced post-traumatic stress disorder in Vietnam veterans. *Behaviour Research and Therapy*, **24**, 6: 645–52.

Pavlovsky, P. (1972). Occurrence and development of psychopathologic phenomena in burned persons and their relation to severity of burns, age and premorbid personality. *Acta Chirurgiae Plasticae*, **14**, 2: 112–19.

Penk, W.E., Robinowitz, R., Black, J., Dolan, M., Bell, W., Dorsett, D. and Ames, M.N.L. (1989). Ethnicity: PTSD differences among black, white and Hispanic veterans who differ in degrees of exposure to combat in Vietnam. *Journal of Clinical Psychology*, **45**, 5: 729–35.

Perry, S.W., Difede, J., Musngi, G. Frances, A.J. and Jacobsberg, A.L. (1992). Predictors of posttraumatic stress disorder after burn injury. *American Journal of Psychiatry*, **149**, 7: 931–5.

Rauch, S.L., van der Kolk, B.A., Fisler, R.E., Alpert, N.M., Orr, S.P., Savage, C.R., Fischman, A.J., Jenike, M.A. and Pitman, R.K. (1996). A symptom provocation study of posttraumatic stress disorder using positron emission tomography and script-driven imagery. *Archives of General Psychiatry*, **53**, 5: 380–87.

Reich, J.H. (1990). Personality disorders and PTSD. In *PTSD – Aetiology, Phenomenology and Treatment*. Ed. M.E. Wolf and A.D. Mosnaim. Washington: American Psychiatric Press.

Rosenheck, R. (1986). Impact of PTSD of World War II on the Next Generation. *Journal of Nervous and Mental Disease*, **174**, 6: 319–27.

Rosenheck, R. and Nathan, P. (1985). Secondary traumatization in children of Vietnam veterans. *Hospital and Community Psychiatry*, **36**, 5: 538–9.

Schnurr, P.P., Friedman, M.J. and Rosenberg, S.D. (1993). Premilitary MMPI scores as predictors of combat-related PTSD symptoms. *American Journal of Psychiatry*, **150**, 3: 479–83.

Schnurr, P.P., Friedman, M. and Rosenberg, S.D. (1994). Predicting postcombat PTSD by using premilitary MMPI scores: Reply. *American Journal of Psychiatry*, **151**, 1: 156–7.

Scott, M.J. and Stradling, S.G. (1994). Post-traumatic stress disorder without the trauma. *British Journal of Clinical Psychology*, **33**, 1: 71–4.

Shalev, A.Y. and Y. Rogel-Fuchs, S.G. (1993). Psychophysiology of the posttraumatic stress disorder: From sulfur fumes to behavioral genetics. *Psychosomatic Medicine*, **55**, 5: 413–23.

Shannon, M.P., Lonigan, C.J., Finch, A.J. and Taylor, C.M. (1994). Children exposed to disaster: I. Epidemiology of post-traumatic symptoms and symptom profiles. *Journal of the American Academy of Child and Adolescent Psychiatry*, **33**, 1: 80–93.

Sherwood, R.J., Funari, D.J. and Piekarski, A.M. (1990). Adapted character styles of Vietnam veterans with posttraumatic stress disorder. *Psychological Reports*, **66**, 2: 623–31.

Shore, J.H., Tatum, E.L. and Vollmer, W.M. (1986). Psychiatric reactions to disaster: The Mount St. Helens experience. *American Journal of Psychiatry*, **143**, 5: 590–595.

Shulman, E. (1994). Predicting postcombat PTSD by using premilitary MMPI scores. *American Journal of Psychiatry*, **151**, 1: 156.

Sierles, F.S., Chen, J.J., McFarland, R.E. and Taylor, M.A. (1983). Posttraumatic stress disorder and concurrent psychiatric illness: a preliminary report. *American Journal of Psychiatry*, **140**, 9: 1177–9.

Skre, I., Onstad, S., Torgersen, S., Lygren, S. and Kringlen, E. (1993). A twin study of DSM-III–R anxiety disorders. *Acta Psychiatrica Scandinavica*, **88**, 2: 85–92.

Smith, E.M., North, C.S., McCool, R.E. and Shea, J.M. (1990). Acute postdisaster psychiatric disorders: Identification of persons at risk. *American Journal of Psychiatry*, **147**, 2: 202–6.

Smith, E.M., Robins, L.N. and Przybeck, T.R. (1986). Psychosocial consequences of a disaster. In *Disaster Stress Studies: New Methods and Findings*. Ed. J.H. Shore. Washington: American Psychiatric Press.

Smith, M.A., Davidson, J., Ritchie, J.C., Kudler, H., Lipper, S., Chappell, P. and Nemeroff, C.B. (1989). The corticotropin-releasing hormone test in patients with posttraumatic stress disorder. *Biological Psychiatry*, **26**, 4: 349–55.

Solomon, S.D. and Canino, G.J. (1990). Appropriateness of DSM-III–R criteria for post-traumatic stress disorder. 5th Annual Meeting of the Society for Traumatic Stress Studies, 1989, San Francisco, California. *Comprehensive Psychiatry*, **31**, 3: 227–37.

Solomon, Z., Kotler, M., Shalev, A. and Lin, R. (1989). Delayed onset of PTSD among Israeli veterans of the 1982 Lebanon War. *Psychiatry Interpersonal and Biological Processes*, **52**, 4: 428–37.

Solomon, Z. and Mikulincer, M. (1990). Life events and combat-related posttraumatic stress disorder: The intervening role of locus of control and social support. *Military Psychology*, **2**, 4: 241–56.

Solomon, Z., Mikulincer, M. and Avitzur, E. (1988). Coping, locus of control, social support, and combat-related posttraumatic stress disorder: A prospective study. *Journal of Personality and Social Psychology*, **55**, 2: 279–85.

Solomon, Z., Mikulincer, M. and Waysman, M. (1991). Delayed and immediate onset posttraumatic stress disorder: The role of life events and social resources. *Journal of Community Psychology*. **19**, 3: 231–6.

Solomon, Z., Waysman, M. and Mikulincer, M. (1990). Family functioning, perceived societal support, and combat-related psychopathology: The moderating role of loneliness. *Journal of Social and Clinical Psychology*, **9**, 4: 456–72.

Spiro, A., Schnurr, P. and Aldwin, C. (1994). Combat-related posttraumatic stress disorder symptoms in older men. *Psychology of Aging*, **9**, 1: 17–26.

Stretch, R.H. (1986). Incidence and etiology of post-traumatic stress disorder among active duty Army personnel. Special issue: Applications of social psychology to military issues. *Journal of Applied Social Psychology*, **16**, 6: 464–81.

Sudak, H.S., Corradi, R.B., Martin, R.S. and Gold, F.S. (1984). Antecedent personality factors and the post-Vietnam syndrome: Case reports. *Military Medicine*, **149**, 10: 550–554.

Swank, R.L. (1949). Combat exhaustion: A descriptive and statistical analysis of causes, symptoms and signs. *Journal of Nervous and Mental Diseases*, **109**: 475–508.

Swett, C. (1990). Sexual and physical abuse histories and psychiatric symptoms among male psychiatric outpatients. *American Journal of Psychiatry*, **147**: 632–6.

Tarrier, N. (1995). Psychological morbidity in adult burns patients: Prevalence and treatment. *Journal of Mental Health*, **4**, 1: 51–62.

Titchener, J.L. and Kapp, F.T. (1976). Family and character change at Buffalo Creek. *American Journal of Psychiatry*, **133**: 295–9.

True, W.R., Goldberg, J. and Eisen, S.A. (1988). Stress symptomatology among Vietnam veterans: Analysis of the Veterans Administration Survey of Veterans II. *American Journal of Epidemiology*, **128**, 1: 85–92.

True, W.R., Rice, J., Eisen, S.A., Heath, A.C., Goldberg, J., Lyons, M.J. and Nowak, J. (1993). A twin study of genetic and environmental contributions to liability for posttraumatic stress symptoms. *Archives of General Psychiatry*, **50**, 4: 257–64.

True, W.R., Rice, J. and Heath, A.C. (1994). 'Genetic and environmental influences of twins in posttraumatic stress': Reply. *Archives of General Psychiatry*, **51**, 10: 838–9.

Tucker, P. (1987). Psychosocial problems among adult burn victims. *Burns*, **13**, 1: 7–14.

Van, der Kolk B., Greenberg, M., Boyd, H. and Krystal, J. (1985). Inescapable shock, neurotransmitters, and addiction to trauma: Toward a psychobiology of post traumatic stress. *Biological Psychiatry*, **20**, 3: 314–25.

Vinokur, A. (1987). Effects of recent and past stress on mental health: Coping with unemployment among Vietnam veterans and non-veterans. *Journal of Applied Social Psychology*, **17**: 710–30.

Weisaeth, L. (1989). The stressors and the post-traumatic stress syndrome after an industrial disaster. Special issue: Traumatic stress: empirical studies from Norway. *Acta Psychiatrica Scandinavica*, **80**, 355 (Suppl.): 25–37.

Wilson, J.P. (1978). *Identity, Ideology and Crisis: The Vietnam Veteran in Transition*, Vol. 2. Washington: Disabled American Veterans.

Wilson, J.P. (1985). Predicting post-traumatic stress disorders among Vietnam veterans. In *Post-Traumatic Stress Disorder and the War Veteran Patient*, pp. 102–47. Ed. W.E. Kelly. New York: Brunner Mazel.

World Health Organisation (1992). *International Classification of Diseases*, 10th edition, Geneva: WHO.

Worthington, E.R. (1977). Post-service adjustment and Vietnam era veterans. *Military Medicine*, **142**: 865–6.

Worthington, E.R. (1978). Demographic and pre-service variables as predictors of post-military service adjustment. In *Stress Disorders Among Vietnam Veterans*, pp. 173–87. Ed. C.R. Figley. New York: Brunner/Mazel.

Yehuda, R., Giller, E.L., Southwick, S.M., Lowy, M.T. and Mason, J.W. (1991a). Hypothalamic–pituitary–adrenal dysfunction in posttraumatic stress disorder. *Biological Psychiatry*, **30**, 10: 1031–48.

Yehuda, R., Levengood, R.A., Schmeidler, J., Wilson, S., Guo, L.S. and Gerber, D. (1996). Increased pituitary activation following metyrapone administration in post-traumatic stress disorder. *Psychoneuroendocrinology*, **21**, 1: 1–16.

Yehuda, R., Lowy, M.T., Southwick, S.M., Shaffer, D. and Giller, E.L. (1991b). Lymphocyte glucocorticoid receptor number in posttraumatic stress disorder. *American Journal of Psychiatry*, **148**, 4: 499–504.

Yehuda, R., Resnick, H., Kahana, B. and Giller, E.L. (1993a). Long-lasting hormonal alterations to extreme stress in humans: Normative or maladaptive? *Psychosomatic Medicine*, **55**, 3: 287–97.

Yehuda, R., Southwick, S.M., Krystal, J.H., Bremner, D., Charney, D.S. and Mason, A.W. (1993b). Enhanced suppression of cortisol following dexamethasone administration in posttraumatic stress disorder. *American Journal of Psychiatry*, **150**, 1: 83–6.

Zeiss, R.A. and Dickman, H.R. (1989). PTSD 40 years later: incidence and person–situation correlates in former POWs. *Journal of Clinical Psychology*, **45**, 1: 80–87.

CHAPTER 5

WHAT CONSTITUTES A STRESSOR?

By definition, post-traumatic illness follows some sort of trauma. It has been recognised for many years that illness can follow trauma. However, what constitutes trauma is far from clear. In particular the type or extent of trauma necessary to cause PTSD is an issue which has been argued fiercely since PTSD was defined in DSM-III.

The whole concept of PTI is that it would not have occurred if it were not for a preceding trauma. The evidence is that there certainly is an excess of mental illness following major traumatic events, and this suggestion is not generally challenged.

The concept of PTSD in particular, on the other hand, demands more than that it be an illness which occurs in response to traumatic events. In addition it has to be an illness which occurs only following certain particular classes or severity of traumata, and which does not ever occur in the absence of such events. Is this backed by empirical evidence?

This chapter will look at the standing of illness following trauma, will examine the evidence for post-traumatic mental health problems, and will examine in detail the stressors which cause PTSD and the evidence that there is a specific pattern of illness which follows major trauma but which does not occur in other situations. The significance and meaning of the concept of qualifying events will be discussed. The changing status and definition of the stressor criterion in DSM will be considered and examined, as well as compared with ICD. Finally, the argument for the abolition of the stressor criterion will be examined.

Trauma or stress and illness

There has long been an acceptance that illnesses of various types often follow traumatic events. For example, a retrospective study suggested that 80% of patients with thyroid disease reported some sort of traumatic event in the months preceding the onset of their illness.

Obviously there are real worries here about the search for meaning and the need to find a cause or explanation for events. However, although previous smaller scale studies have denied the association of life events and thyroid disease, a recent large-scale population case control study studied 95% of the new cases of Graves' disease in a population of more than one million, as well as 80% of the matched controls (Harris, Creed and Brugha, 1992). A postal questionnaire was used and showed a significantly higher rate of recent major life events or negative traumatic events in patients with thyroid disease (odds ratio 6.3). It might be thought that thyroid disease was a bad example of the effect of psychological trauma on physical illness given the demonstrated abnormalities in HPA axis and thyroid hormone levels in PTSD which are discussed in Chapter 4. However, it is not only in relation to thyroid disease that there has been suggestion of an effect of psychological trauma.

There is other empirical evidence for the occurrence of somatic illness, or even death, following trauma without physical injury, although the quality of the studies has varied (Falger et al., 1992; Carmel, Koren and Ilia, 1993; Blair, Blair and Rueckert, 1994; Lucas et al., 1995; Patti et al., 1995; Bowman and Markand, 1996). Studies have shown that widowers have an increased death rate from all causes within a year of their wives dying. This supports the adage of 'dying of a broken heart'. More recent studies of cardiac disease have shown an apparent increase in angina and in drug use in Israeli cardiac patients during the build-up to the Gulf War, and of exacerbation of pre-existing physical disease following negative life events in other studies.

These studies have mostly focused upon the immediate or early effects of trauma. However, there have also been studies into the complicated issue of the long-term effects of traumatic events on causation, course, or adjustment to, physical illness. For example there have been suggestions that women survivors of the Holocaust are less able to adjust to and cope with cancer (Baider, Peretz and Kaplan De Nour, 1992; Peretz et al., 1994). There is early indication that a history of childhood psychological trauma may predispose to chronic refractory lower back pain and to failed back surgery (Schofferman et al., 1993). There is a possible connection between sexual victimisation and irritable bowel syndrome (Walker et al., 1993), and sexual abuse has been connected with a wide range of problems in the long term, both physical and psychological.

Traditionally, trauma (or stresses) was generally considered to have a modifying rather than causative effect on illness, affecting the timing rather than the nature of illness, both physical and psychological. While it is widely, but not universally, accepted that 'stress' can affect peptic ulcer disease and coronary heart disease, it is not widely considered to cause them. It is generally felt that the nature of the disease suffered is determined by other factors, with stress or trauma having only a modifying effect. There is some research to support this view in infective disease, (Cassell 1976), and in pregnancy-related problems (Nuckells, Cassell and Kaplan, 1972). Indeed, this was a major impetus to the development of the concept of PTSD. In both DSM-I and DSM-II, psychological responses to trauma were considered to be brief and essentially self-limiting. Chronic illness was considered to represent pre-existing conditions or predisposition. This was all changed by the idea that there was a specific and distinct form of illness which only occurred after trauma and which could be chronic.

Life event work

The idea that major stresses can have a modifying effect on illness has been the focus of much life event research. This will not be reviewed in detail here, except to look at the theories surrounding and following Holmes and Rahe's work (1967). Their work with the Social Readjustment Rating Scale had two specific aspects relevant to the topic under discussion.

They considered stresses to be of measurable magnitude and therefore produced a score sheet of the amount of readjustment the average person required to assimilate a range of stressful, traumatic or change events, not all of which are generally considered to be negative. This involves an explicit assumption that the order of effect of a particular class of event, say divorce, bereavement, loss of job, birth of a child etc., is equivalent for people in general and for an individual.

When looked at now this suggestion does not really seem to have face validity. The amount of readjustment required after the death of a parent, for example, would seem logically to vary widely depending upon circumstances. Even ignoring, without any good justification, internal variation in subjects, the effects upon a child of terminal illness and death in a parent and the effects of the sudden death from natural causes of the parent of a 60 year old would appear to be very different. What justification is there for suggesting that divorce, or a move of house, or the death of a parent, will require an equivalent amount of readjustment from a range of different people? It seems glaringly obvious that the amount of readjustment required depends upon what the event means to the person experiencing it.

This work already raises two of the most difficult questions in the study of the relationship of trauma to illness:

* what exactly is trauma?
* can it be reliably measured?

Another explicit assumption of the Social Readjustment Scale was that stressors were cumulative or, more specifically, additive. Whether or not it was intended by the authors, many came to consider that two events worth 10 points on the scale had equivalent effect to one event worth 20 points. It was common to sum events requiring readjustment over a specific period of time and use the additive score to make statements about the risk of psychological problems in the short term.

Again, this idea does not necessarily seem to have face validity. It might well be argued that if something happened twice or if there were a series of events, then the risk of illness would increase proportionately. However, it could equally be argued that coping with a previous event would have a protective or hardening effect, rendering the subject permanently or temporarily less susceptible to the effects of life events. Conversely it could be argued that events might have a sensitising effect, rendering the subject more vulnerable and likely to develop illness following a lesser stressor than if he or she had suffered either stressor alone.

Trauma and PTI

There is no problem with the concept that mental illness in general is more common after trauma. There is no need to specify a specific quality or severity of stressor, and no need to propose a specific sort of symptomatology or nature of illness following trauma. If trauma can be followed by mental illness generally, then is there a need for PTSD?

In fact there is clear evidence for an increased rate of mental illness following traumatic events in many studies, both in association with PTSD as a co-morbid illness, and independent of the incidence of PTSD.

For example, the Epidemiological Catchment Area Study (Helzer, Robins and McEvoy, 1987), showed that a lifetime diagnosis of PTSD was associated with an increased risk of some other psychiatric diagnosis, particularly obsessive compulsive disorder and affective disorders, but not schizophrenia or anorexia nervosa. Davidson's similar North Carolina study (Davidson *et al.*, 1991), again found more other PTI with PTSD, but different conditions were over-represented, with PTSD patients being found to be 20 times as likely to have had a diagnosis of schizophrenia but not to have an increase of some affective disorders and substance abuse.

That PTI can occur independent of PTSD is demonstrated in some of the other studies which have found different results when looking at PTSD and other PTI in populations exposed to traumatic events. Shore (Shore, Tatum and Vollmer, 1986; Shore, Vollmer and Tatum, 1989) found that the lifetime rate of PTSD in the population exposed to the Mount St Helens disaster was a little higher than that in controls, whereas generalised anxiety disorder and depression were much more increased and occurred in many people in the absence of PTSD. This differential effect was also found in the study of earthquakes in Chile and California. In both areas the prevalence of depression was increased nearly threefold, while the California group had no significant rise in PTSD and the Chile group had a sevenfold increase (Durkin 1993). Similarly, Abenhaim's study of survivors of terrorist incidents in France (Abenhaim, Dab and Salmi, 1992) showed PTSD rates varying between 8% and 30% depending upon degree of injury, while the rate of depression was constant across all groups at 13%.

These findings suggest a complicated, if not contradictory, association of trauma with psychiatric illness.

1. All studies show increased mental illness after trauma.
2. Those who develop PTSD are more likely to have a comorbid illness; the nature of the co-morbid illness varies between studies.
3. Some subjects develop other illnesses in the absence of PTSD.
4. Some studies show what appears to be a different effect upon PTSD from the effect upon other illnesses.
   a) This suggests that there is a different relationship between PTSD and trauma and between other PTI and trauma, thus giving support to the concept of PTSD.
   b) The data from Chile/California and from France are at least suggestive that there is a qualitative yes or no relationship between trauma and depression, but a possible threshold or dose-related relationship between PTSD and trauma.

Trauma and PTSD

The concept of illness following catastrophic events long precedes DSM-III and PTSD. However, it was previously accepted, at least in classificatory terms, that the response to such overwhelming stressors was essentially brief. Some, like Kardiner (1941), had described what appeared to be a specific pattern of response to such events, but the received wisdom was still that chronic illness after trauma involved the precipitation, bringing forward in time, or exacerbation of constitutional mental illness rather than a separate syndrome.

DSM-III changed all that in its definition of PTSD. It made two main changes:

- PTSD was associated with a unique 'nature' of stressor.
- PTSD was described as a unique pattern of illness only found in response to such stressors.

There has been much debate and disagreement about not only the importance but also the very meaning, of the stressor criterion in DSM-III. In what way were the stressors indicated by DSM-III as being capable of causing PTSD unique and different from stressors which could also cause or precipitate PTI but could not cause PTSD? At its simplest the argument was between whether the magnitude of the stressor or its specific nature or type was what differentiated between a stressor which could and could not produce PTSD. Could any sort of stressor cause PTSD if it were big enough or severe enough, or are there only certain sorts of PTSD-invoking events?

The stressor criterion evolves in DSM

Before looking at the questions of size or nature of trauma needed to cause PTSD, it is important to recognise that the definition of the traumatic event causing PTSD has not remained constant but has evolved. Major factors affecting such evolution have been empirical observation, but also political and social concerns.

The definition of criterion A in DSM-IV, and the description of the stressor in ICD-10 differ from the definition in DSM-III. The nature, cause and meaning of the changes are of great significance in the research and clinical study of the disorder. It is also important to remember that in addition to the listed diagnostic criteria there are comments and aids to practice contained in the text of the classification systems which must be taken into account in practice and which help in the understanding of the logic behind the criteria.

In summary, there has been a significant change in the position and significance of the stressor criterion in the development from DSM-III to DSM-IV and ICD-10. The different forms of the criterion can be seen and compared in Table 5.1.

Table 5.1. *The stressor criterion*

DSM – III	The existence of a recognisable stressor that would evoke significant symptoms of distress in almost anyone
DSM – IIIR	Experience of an event that is outside the range of usual human experience and that would be markedly distressing to almost anyone, e.g. serious threat to one's life or physical integrity; serious threat or harm to one's children, spouse or other close relative or friends; sudden destruction of one's home or community; or seeing someone who has recently been, or is being, seriously injured or killed as the result of an accident or physical violence
ICD – 10	Exposure to an exceptionally threatening or catastrophic stressor, either brief or prolonged
DSM – IV	Experienced, witnessed, or been confronted with an event or events which involved actual or threatened death or serious injury, or a threat to the physical integrity of self or others . . . and response involved intense fear, helplessness, or horror

In essence, the progression in DSM has been a relaxing of the stringency of the criterion. Initially PTSD was only considered to be a possibility following extreme or disastrous stressors. 'Normal' or expected stressors which were not considered to be able to cause PTSD were originally listed. In addition, the stressor had to be 'outside the range of normal human experience' in DSM-IIIR. Gradually, as DSM has progressed, the range of 'qualifying' stressors has been widened and there has even been suggestion that the stressor criterion should be abandoned completely as a wider and wider range of events has been demonstrated to be followed, on occasions, by PTSD symptoms.

The focus of the stressor criterion has moved away from the nature of the stressor to the nature of the perception of the victim, so that the current DSM-IV criterion requires two elements. The sufferer must have 'experienced', 'witnessed', or 'been confronted by' a threat to 'physical integrity' or worse. They must also have responded with 'intense fear, helplessness, or horror'. There is no need for the trauma to be of an unusual, dramatic, or catastrophic type. An increasingly wide range of events has been accepted as being causal of PTSD.

ICD-10 has bucked this trend by insisting upon 'catastrophic' stressors and moving back towards the stressor criterion as it was originally described in DSM-III. It requires the traumatic event to be 'of an exceptionally threatening or catastrophic nature, which is likely to cause pervasive distress in almost anyone', and goes on to give a list of examples.

ICD-10, however, has much wider symptomatological criterion boundaries than DSM-IV, with very few symptoms being actually required for the diagnosis. Some survivors who would not be diagnosed as having PTSD under DSM-IV because of the lack of appropriate symptoms might well be so diagnosed under ICD-10 if the trauma fitted. On the other hand, some who would be diagnosed as having PTSD under DSM-IV would fail to pass the stressor test in ICD-10 because the event was not exceptional or catastrophic, and they would therefore not have ICD-10 PTSD.

Is PTSD caused by unique stressors?

What is the evidence that certain stressors can cause PTSD and others cannot? If the idea of only a certain type of stressor holds true, then it should be fairly easy to prove. Either only stressors above a certain level of magnitude will be followed by PTSD or it will only follow stressors of particular types.

Much of the debate on this subject has been fuelled and shaped by a 1987 paper by Breslau and Davis entitled 'The Stressor Criterion'. Although this paper was written before DSM-IIIR and DSM-IV, it is still a good starting point for discussing the relevance and nature of the stressor criterion as it was seen by many as playing 'Devil's Advocate' and focusing discussion and critical thinking.

In the paper Breslau and Davis suggested that the concept of PTSD was based primarily upon: 'the clinical, but untested, impressions of clinicians, specifically the impression that a characteristic configuration of symptoms can be traced to an extraordinary traumatic event'.

They suggested that at the time of writing the unique nature of neither the symptomatology nor the stressor had yet been empirically demonstrated.

Big stressors or unusual stressors?

Breslau and Davis point out that in addition to PTSD, DSM-III also includes the diagnostic category of adjustment reaction. This is 'a maladaptive reaction to an identifiable psychosocial stressor'. Two differences between it and PTSD are that it is not supposed usually to last more than six months, and it does not have a specific clearly defined set of symptoms, rather being a sort of 'catch-all' for problems which do not fulfil diagnostic criteria for other Axis I conditions and being excluded from diagnosis in addition to another Axis I diagnosis. The range of stressors accepted as being likely to cause adjustment reactions includes many which are so common as to be considered a normal part of life experience and which could certainly not be called catastrophic. According to DSM-III, such stressors would not qualify as causative agents for PTSD.

The DSM-III PTSD stressor was required to be 'generally outside the range of usual human experience' and to be such that it 'would evoke significant symptoms of distress in almost anyone'. This is clearly quite a different level of stressor from that which is required to cause adjustment reactions.

What, exactly, does 'outside the range of usual human experience' mean? Is it a qualitative or a quantitative matter? DSM-III does not give any operational definition for qualifying stressors. It does suggest that the clinician's decision as to whether or not an event qualifies has to be 'based on the clinician's assessment of the stress an "average" person in similar circumstances and with similar sociocultural values would experience'. The only other help that DSM-III really gives is to provide a short list of qualifying and non-qualifying events.

Obviously this means that determining whether or not a stressor is a qualifying one may be very difficult. This is of great importance in considering how to diagnose PTSD. It would be quite wrong to apply post hoc arguments and suggest that stressors followed by the occurrence of the cluster of PTSD symptoms were qualifying stressors. This is unacceptable if the qualifying stressor itself forms part of the operational definition. If you define qualifying stressors as those which are followed by PTSD symptomatology, then there is no need for the stressor to form part of the definition.

It is suggested by some that the definition of qualifying criteria in DSM-III implicitly includes the patient's subjective perception of the event in the decision as to whether or not a stressor qualifies. However, it seems more likely that the subjective perception of the clinician is used, as it is the clinician who is required to consider the effect of the event upon an average person in similar circumstances. The list of examples given specifically excludes certain events, apparently simply because they are common, and without taking note of the subject's perceptions. Thus chronic illness, whatever its nature, did not qualify in DSM-III despite subsequent report of symptoms of PTSD following it, whereas natural disasters such as floods or earthquakes did qualify.

Apparently the DSM-III stressor criterion did not take into account the perception of the event or the reality of the threat, the proximity, or the degree of exposure. This seems to be fairly obviously inappropriate.

It is perfectly possible that someone who is involved in an earthquake but suffers no physical injury, loss or bereavement, may see himself as lucky and not perceive himself to have been exposed to a stressor outside the usual range of human experience. On the other hand, a person who unexpectedly develops a potentially fatal long-term illness may perceive himself to have suffered, or be suffering from, a major source of stress.

The question of whether qualifying stressors are tested in terms of magnitude or nature is not simply of academic interest. Throughout DSM-III there is a separate axis, Axis-IV, for measuring the severity of current stressors having an effect upon an illness or upon an Axis-I diagnosis. The unstated assumption is again that stressors may affect the course and intensity of any illness rather than its specific nature. With PTSD, however, this Axis-IV measurement is instead brought into the definition of the disorder. It explicitly moves away from the non-specific to the specific, with the clear statement that a specific stressor causes a specific configuration of illness. Some time after Breslau's paper, McFarlane (1991) suggested in his review of PTSD that 'the threshold and quality of the stressor required to trigger the onset of the characteristic symptoms is one of the major issues needing clarification'.

Breslau and Davis suggest that the rules in DSM-III are arbitrary. They contest that DSM-III adopts the classical stress paradigm in which the focus is only on the magnitude of the stressor, ignoring the much more difficult to measure psychological–clinical paradigm, which sees the meaning and content of the stress as more important than the quantity.

However, it might also be thought that this criticism seems unfounded. When DSM-III talks of events outside the range of normal human experience and *also* being capable of causing significant distress in almost anyone, then it seems that there is some attempt to consider the psychological–clinical approach, even if it appears to be based upon the perception of 'the average man' rather than that of the subject. It seems that the definition of the stressor criterion is based neither solely upon magnitude nor upon the type of stressor.

Ursano (1987) wrote one of a series of criticisms of the work of Breslau and Davis. He said that they had wrongly suggested that the PTSD stressor criterion referred to a particular class of stressors when, in fact, it was associated with the quantity of the stress, being so defined in DSM-III. Other writers criticised the work of Breslau and Davis and used it as a platform to further the debate about whether it is the quantity or the nature of stressor which qualifies for PTSD, and whether subjective perception is involved. This argument has yet to be definitively resolved. For some stressors at least, there is a positive relationship between magnitude and rate of PTSD. In addition, there seems to be evidence that some sorts of stressors such as violent crime and combat are more likely to cause PTSD.

Despite the intense debate upon the subject, it is actually quite clear that debate alone cannot answer the question of what can and cannot cause PTSD. In a diagnosed case of PTSD, the stressor which caused it is a qualifying stressor by definition. It has already been suggested, however, that this is an unreasonable and inaccurate way of approaching the problem. It means that the stressor criterion becomes superfluous and is no longer part of the definition set for PTSD. Although this idea has latterly been attractive to some, it has been resisted firmly by the American Psychiatric Association in DSM-IV. They have moved firmly towards perception and individual response to traumatic events but have shunned the idea that the stressor is unnecessary and can be defined by retrospection after identification of symptom profiles.

What we need to do in order to examine the qualifying stressor question is first of all to determine whether the clinical criteria for PTSD are unique, and then, if they are, find out which stressors, under which circumstances, do lead to PTSD. It is necessary first to ensure that there is a specific sort of illness which follows trauma before we can identify causative traumata.

Is the response to traumatic stressors unique?

It has already been pointed out that other illnesses can follow any and all of the traumatic stresses which are also believed to be capable of causing PTSD. A number of investigators have found an excess of a range of mental illnesses following trauma (Tierney and Baisden, 1979; Ursano, 1981a, 1981b; Escobar *et al.*, 1983; Sierles *et al.*, 1983; Behar, 1984; Davidson *et al.*, 1985). This does not interfere with our study of the stressor in PTSD as long as PTSD has a clinical profile which is distinguishable from other illnesses and specific to PTSD.

So are there clinical phenomena which are specific to PTSD? At this stage there are certainly no biochemical, physiological or pathological measures which can confidently separate all cases of PTSD from all other illnesses. In addition, by no means all of the symptoms of PTSD are specific to that condition. As Breslau and Davies have pointed out, the only symptom group from PTSD which is not included in the diagnostic criteria for any other disorder (ignoring the catch-all adjustment reaction) is the intrusive re-experiencing symptom group.

Logically, therefore, if we look at events which are followed by re-experiencing symptoms this will establish the limit of the stressor which is capable of causing PTSD. We must not forget, however, that not everyone with re-experiencing symptoms has PTSD because this is only one of the diagnostic criteria and because the majority of people who are exposed to traumatic events show immediate effects but do not develop long-term disability.

In fact studies (Horowitz, 1979), including those of industrial accidents (Schottenfeld and Cullen, 1985), have shown that re-experiencing phenomena are sometimes suffered even following events which would not be reasonably considered to be any of: catastrophic, outside the range of normal human experience, or distressing to almost anyone. In addition to obviously catastrophic events, re-experiencing symptoms have been noted after such diverse events as childbirth, loss of job, injury, marital difficulties, and a range of natural illnesses. It seems that simple measures of class or magnitude of stressor are insufficient to define stressors which can cause the symptom cluster which is PTSD.

Back to 'big stressors or unusual stressors?'

Following Breslau and Davis and the series of commentaries there was further research. In DSM-IIIR the stressor criterion was modified as detailed above. It was remembered that some time before, Krystal (1971) had emphasised that we 'cannot translate the intensity of the stimulus to its traumatogenic potential'. Even if it is possible to measure the severity of a stressor, this alone does not tell us whether or not it will cause PTSD.

Ursano had expressed the opinion that a number of papers (Glass, 1957; Egendorf, 1981; Ursano, 1981a, 1981b; Belenky, Tyner and Sodet, 1983; Shore, Tatum and Vollmer, 1986) had already demonstrated a clear relationship between PTSD and the quantity of stress rather than the quality. This certainly seems to be the case with war stressors, but the evidence is less clear for almost all other traumatic situations.

In 1989, Weisaeth reported a study of 246 employees of a paint factory which had exploded, leading to threatening fires. Half of the sample had not been present in the factory at the time, and of those who were present about half were placed in a high-stress group because they were nearest to the explosion and at most risk, while the rest constituted a medium-stress group. Perhaps surprisingly, he found that two-thirds or more of all the subjects reported at least one previous episode of significant threat to their life and of witnessing the severe injury or death of others. He did find a relationship between severity of stressor and PTSD symptoms as measured by the PTSS-30 symptom scale. However, he also found a significant, though lower, rate of symptoms in the group who were not present at the time. It does not seem likely that this group would be considered in DSM-IIIR terms to have been exposed to a qualifying stressor. This study could be seen as lending relatively more weight to the quantity rather than quality argument. It suggests that increased exposure renders people more likely to get PTSD. However, it also shows that people can suffer PTSD symptoms in the absence of a qualifying stressor. Even though those not at the site were not in any physical danger, they were exposed to a stressful and traumatic experience in that they presumably realised that if the fire had happened during the opposite shift, then they would have been caught up in it. Their perceptions may have been similar to those near the fire but less severe.

It is also somewhat disturbing in that it suggests that the majority of the population had already experienced at least one event outside the range of normal human experience. Epidemiological studies have also found a high life-time prevalence of traumatic events which might qualify as the stressor in PTSD. If they are so frequent, how can these events not be normal?

There is also, however, significant support for the idea that it is not only the intensity of the stressor which is important, but that particular sorts of stressors, or particular elements of stressors, influence PTSD incidence. In civilian disasters (Green *et al.*, 1990) it has been suggested repeatedly that certain elements of stressors increase the likelihood of long-lasting PTI rather than immediate distress followed by readjustment. In Vietnam veterans also, specific stressors or aspects of stress have been identified as being of importance, particularly exposure to, or participation in, abusive violence, and also physical injury.

Relevant factors that have been identified as being associated with higher risk of PTSD following civilian disasters have been:

- violent loss (Gleser, Green and Winget, 1981; Shore, Tatum and Vollmer, 1986)
- physical injury (Green, Grace and Gleser, 1985)
- exposure to grotesque death (Taylor and Frazer, 1982)
- life threat (Gleser, Green and Winget, 1981; Green, Grace and Gleser, 1985).

It can be observed that in the case of civilian traumata, PTSD is generally less common than it is in combat if representative samples are studied. The one exception to this observation is in the area of violent crime. One stress which has also consistently been found to be associated with very high rates of PTSD has been rape (Kilpatrick *et al.*, 1989). Putting to one side the questions about the source of subjects and the 'set' of the studies which have led to suggestions that the rates are perhaps exaggerated, nevertheless there does seem to be a very high rate of PTSD after rape. It would generally be accepted that this is not surprising because a priori reasoning suggests that rape is a very specific stressor which involves an extreme threat to the person, an invasion, a loss of control, and a feeling of helplessness. An excess of PTSD after rape, however, is not necessarily an argument for the specific nature of the stressor hypothesis. Rape is clearly a stressor of great magnitude. Even if there is not an overt threat of violence, the extent of personal invasion, helplessness and assault is great. Even in rape there has been shown to be an association between degree of threat and violence and PTSD. Study of rape lends weight to both the magnitude and the quality arguments.

The National Institute of Mental Health DSM-IIIR criteria study

A National Institute of Mental Health (NIMH) study (Solomon and Canino, 1990) of the appropriateness of DSM-IIIR criteria for PTSD was described as the first study specifically to examine the sequelae of ordinary and extraordinary stressors. It was quite a complicated prospective study on two sites, based on the fact that unrelated epidemiological studies happened to have been underway in the two areas of St Louis and Puerto Rico before traumatic incidents occurred in the two localities. In each site there were four groups:

previous study respondents exposed to trauma
previous study respondents not so exposed
new subjects exposed to trauma
new subjects not exposed.

The study was conducted by face-to-face interview using the DIS with disaster supplement. At St Louis there were 543 subjects, 452 of whom had been seen before, and in Puerto Rico there were 912, of whom 375 had been seen previously. At one year after the trauma, 84% of the St Louis study were re-interviewed, and 87% of the Puerto Rico sample at two years. Results for the two areas were reported separately.

The *St Louis* study looked at a group who were forced out of their homes by a flood in which five died. Then part of the group found that during the flood their homes had been exposed to more then 300 times the allowed limit of the poison dioxin so they could not return. The American government bought out the area and this subgroup were all re-housed.

While controlling for lifetime pre-disaster PTSD, the extraordinary (disaster) stressors and also the ordinary (such as job, family, money, illness problems etc.) stressors were entered as predictors in a statistical analysis of co-variance (ANCOVA). This model accounted for 21% of the total variance of PTSD symptoms.

Disaster exposure just failed to predict level of PTSD symptoms (p=0.0513), while move of house (p=0.0001), household illness (p=0.0363), and a catchall group of other 'upsetting' events, were predictive.

Obviously the allegedly non-disaster events were actually likely to have been increased by the consequences of the disaster, but this observation that 'secondary disasters' were more important in predicting PTSD than the actual trauma had been reported earlier (Erikson, 1976). Interestingly, this earlier report had also been in association with the consequences of a flood. The observations tend to support a magnitude rather than quality of stressor argument, although this may be complicated by the idea that some of the additional stressors found to be predictive could be seen as potentially secondary to the original stressor and a consequence of it. It harks back to the social readjustment work and the idea that stresses may be cumulative. However, unlike the earlier work, this study did seem to show that the defined symptoms of PTSD were related to quantity of stressor. More importantly, it suggested that PTSD was not associated only with a specific class or severity of event but could perhaps follow an accumulation of 'normal' events.

In *Puerto Rico* the relevant stressor for the exposed group was a tropical storm which killed 180, made 4000 homeless, and caused significant material loss to 19 000. When the same model was entered into an ANCOVA, it explained only 11% of the variance.

The results were different. This stressor of similar nature but apparently greater severity was of predictive value for PTSD symptoms (p=0.0011). So too were a break-up of relationship with best friend (p=0.0001), having to take someone into one's home (p=0.004), and other 'upsetting events' (p=0.0001). Unlike in St Louis, these other stressors were not all overtly related to the initial stressor and were not necessarily 'secondary'. It seemed that the 'less traumatic' events also played a part in predicting PTSD. This apparently greater primary stressor had a much closer relationship to PTSD than the flood stressor in St Louis.

It is important to point out that the follow-up studies were not done at the same relative time and this may have affected outcome because of the natural course of symptoms. However, the study does suggest that PTSD symptomatology was related more to the size of the stressor than to its nature. It does not support the idea that PTSD follows only certain classes of events. At least in the early stages, PTSD following lesser trauma was more associated with the subsequent consequences of the trauma and related events, whereas with a stressor of greater magnitude it was associated either with the index stressor or with possibly unrelated occurrences. This needs repetition and confirmation. What is also very interesting is the confirmation that relatively little of the variance was explained by events.

Field trials for DSM-IV

As with many other categories, field trials were designed and carried out prior to the publication of DSM-IV. One of the hypotheses studied was the suggestion that the 'outside the range of normal human experience' etc. statement in DSM-IIIR was vague and unreliable. It was far from clear what normal human experience actually was. In field trials in five sites, a total of 400 help-seekers and 128 random community subjects were examined using different definitions of the stressor criterion. Whatever the definition used for the stressor, similar rates of PTSD symptomatology were found. It might be suggested that the stressor criterion is redundant in that it does not materially help to define cases.

Of major interest, and confirmed elsewhere, was that a surprisingly high proportion of subjects had suffered stressors considered to be traumatic at some point in their life, again raising the question of what is normal. Clearly, the events sometimes followed by PTSD symptomatology are by no means always 'outside the range of normal human experience' in a statistical sense. This observation has been confirmed in other epidemiological studies which have shown that up to 70% of population samples will have experienced at least one DSM-IV qualifying stressor at some time.

'Lesser' stressors shown to be followed by PTSD

There have been a number of studies of the complete range of PTSD symptomatology apparently occurring in the absence of stressors which would appear to fit the operational definition of the stressor criterion. A number of these have been mentioned elsewhere and include psychotic illness, loss of job or protracted trouble at work, bereavement, interpersonal relationship problems, and physical illness. It has been seen to occur occasionally after apparently minor stresses or potential 'near misses' such as minor car accidents, or not being on duty at the time of an incident.

This apparently definite occurrence of the clinical picture of PTSD in the absence of a catastrophic stressor causes further confusion. Loss of job, for example, cannot be considered to be either 'outside the range of normal human experience' or 'such as to be markedly distressing to almost anyone'. Yet the characteristic symptom profile of PTSD can occur. This raises, or brings us back to, two interesting questions.

1. Is the existence of the PTSD symptom profile necessarily an indicator of morbidity?
2. What is the significance of perception in measuring stressor magnitude?

Do symptoms after stressors equal disability?

It has been suggested (O'Donohue and Elliott, 1992) that there is an inherent possible contradiction in the 'markedly distressing to almost anyone' statement in DSM. The question, at its simplest, is whether PTSD is an expected response to trauma, or whether it deviates from the normal or expected response. If it is the expected response then there is an argument that it is not abnormal and is not an illness or pathological response. This argument has been debated at length in Chapter 3.

In the case of rape, for example, logic would suggest that intrusive phenomena, avoidance of reminders, arousal, and a persistence of problems for four weeks, would be expected or normal. Is it therefore reasonable to say that PTSD is 'normal' after rape but 'abnormal' after more common and apparently less severe stresses such as road traffic accidents which one would not 'logically' expect to produce such symptoms? Kilpatrick has, as a result of such observations, suggested that PTSD should not be considered as an Axis-I diagnosis, but as a 'condition not attributable to a mental disorder' (Kilpatrick *et al.*, 1989).

Horowitz, too (Horowitz, Weiss and Marmar, 1987), has spoken of the danger of misdiagnosis of PTSD in those with 'normal rather than pathological responses'. His words are emphasised by a study of Falklands veterans who were clearly exposed to severe stressors which showed high rates of reported PTSD symptoms on direct questioning, but no evidence of demonstrable associated disability (O'Brien and Hughes, 1991).

Does perception of the stressor matter?

The question of the relevance of perception to the traumatic nature of a stressor is a very important one. It seems to be minimised in the earlier editions of DSM which described traumata as being likely to be distressing to almost anyone. Indeed, in much of the early research centring on Vietnam veterans and their war experience it was clearly felt that what mattered was the amount of exposure of an individual to what was, by definition, a traumatic and potentially pathogenic situation. Subsequent experience with other traumatic events and review of previous such experience have led to serious questioning of this idea. It becomes inescapable that an individual's perception and experience of events are of considerable significance and an objective scaling of stressors cannot be done.

In DSM-IV, the idea of individual perception is given centre stage as one of the two parts of the stressor criterion. The new definition markedly reduces the magnitude and quality hurdle for qualifying events, but brings in a new requirement of perception of the event. The definition of the event is much more loose and encompassing, but there is a clear demand for a specific range of emotional response. Thus the victim must suffer intense fear or helplessness for the event to be a qualifying one.

Within certain very wide boundaries it is not the nature or magnitude of the stressor which is seen as important, but the perception of the victim. This is a long way away from DSM-III PTSD and from the original idea of a catastrophic stress.

There seems little doubt that cases do occur in which all of the criteria for DSM-IV PTSD are fulfilled, including the disability criterion, but which would clearly have failed to pass the stressor criterion tests of either DSM-IIIR or DSM-III. Examples are many. There have been reports of PTSD apparently occurring in 15% of a series of cases of chronic unexplained facial pain (Aghabeigi, Feinmann and Harris, 1992), and in more than 40% of cases of recent onset psychotic illness (McGorry *et al.*, 1991). There have been cases reported after childbirth (Ballard, Stanley and Brockington, 1995). In each of these cases it is suggested that the medical condition was the relevant stressor even though none of them would seem to fulfil DSM-III or DSM-IIIR definitions for Criterion A.

Even more interesting examples of a challenge to the stressor criterion come from two studies of what could be termed unintentional, rather than natural, disasters. Following the Herald of Free Enterprise disaster in which a car ferry rolled over and capsized, killing 193 people, 14 cases of PTSD in people who were not involved in the incident as victims, rescuers or witnesses were referred to mental health services (Dixon, Rehling and Shiwach, 1993). These patients were all employed by ferry companies working from the local ports and strongly identified with the victims. Not all of them knew people who were killed, and not all of them worked for the ferry company involved. Some of them had what would be described as severe re-experiencing symptoms such as stereotyped nightmares of the event of a ferry capsize. However, as they had not been there and these were actually not memories but imagination, it is difficult to be clear how they could be categorised. That these people were suffering disability seems indisputable. They had no legal or financial imperative for complaining and were actually seeking medical intervention for distress. Except that the experiences that were causing intrusive, avoidance and arousal phenomena had not actually happened to them, they seemed to have PTSD.

In another study a plane crashed into a hotel and the surviving staff members were investigated (Smith *et al.*, 1990). Although rates were lower than for those actually present, a proportion of the staff not on duty and not present also developed apparent PTSD in a similar way. This did not include simply those people who, for example, should have been on duty but did not turn up. Most of them were not at the hotel because they were not supposed to be there. Admittedly this study showed that the best predictor of disability was previous mental health history, but it did seem that people who were not exposed to the trauma seemed to suffer the sequelae that might be expected if they had been so exposed.

This seems to represent very strong support for the contention that perception of stress and perception of danger or near miss may be very important in determining which individuals are exposed to a qualifying stressor. Even though none of these people was actually exposed to risk, they were confronted by the risk that they ran and reminded that their escape from the trauma was one which they were helpless to control. In actual fact they were not at risk on the specific occasions studied but they were at equal risk in the past and the future as those who were involved and perceived themselves as having been put in danger.

As a result of such studies, and of clinical observation, an argument has been presented that the concept of a 'qualifying' stressor should be dropped as it is restrictive and unhelpful. It is suggested that what is important is not what happens, but what the victim perceives or feels.

Do we need a stressor criterion at all?

In his study of the stressor criterion prior to the publication of DSM-IV, March (1993) considers the extreme 'broad' and 'narrow' views of the stressor criterion in PTSD. He points out that the very narrow definition which restricts qualifying events to those which can truly be described as catastrophic has the potential for very high specificity. If we accept that PTSD symptoms are not pathognomonic, then a narrow or strict definition of the stressor criterion will allow only the most definite cases to be diagnosed. A broad definition, however, at its broadest would say that the stressor criterion could effectively be abolished. Stressors could be defined in the way previously described as wrong or dangerous. In other words, the focus of the intrusive and avoidant symptoms would be teleologically defined as a qualifying stressor. If an event were followed by PTSD symptomatology then it would be a qualifying stressor. There is some logic in this. The only symptoms specific to PTSD are the re-experiencing ones. If an event is capable of producing re-experiencing symptoms, then it is traumatic! This would be more sensitive but would appear to be potentially less specific, although as there is no permanent gold-standard definition of PTSD it is difficult to press the sensitivity–specificity argument.

If we alter the stressor criterion we are not changing diagnostic sensitivity or specificity – we are changing the definition of the condition and what actually is and is not PTSD!

One of the arguments which March gives against the broadest definition is that it relies greatly upon the B, C and D criteria for PTSD – the intrusive (B), avoidant (C) and physiological arousal (D) symptoms. He complains that the C and D (avoidant and physiological) criteria are far from uniformly applied, apparently because not everyone accepts PTSD as a stressor-driven anxiety disorder (March, 1990). He suggests that many people see intrusive symptomatology as synonymous with PTSD and have a tendency, conscious or otherwise, to see the other symptoms as superfluous. The most obvious support for this complaint is seen in the diagnostic guidelines of ICD-10 which only require intrusive symptomatology and describe the other symptom groups as being commonly present. This might well mean wide variation in diagnosis, with forensic and political consequences. At its most basic, anyone who has distressing intrusive memories of any phenomenon has PTSD, and the thing that they remember is a qualifying traumatic event! March comes to the conclusion that the two-stage stressor criterion as actually adopted by DSM-IV is the best option.

Others have nevertheless suggested that there is no need for the stressor criterion. They point out the presence of PTSD symptoms following a wide range of stressors. McFarlane and Yehuda (Yehuda and McFarlane, 1995) have pointed out the important fact that PTSD is not the 'normal' response to even the most traumatic stresses. It is always the minority of people who develop PTSD. Scott and Stradling (1994), in their provocatively titled 'PTSD without the trauma' describe a series of cases in which all of the other criteria of PTSD have been demonstrated in the absence of a single major traumatic event but following repeated or chronic minor stresses. Scott points out that this and other work demonstrates that a major traumatic event is neither a necessary nor a sufficient cause of PTSD. His own work shows that it is not necessary to have a major stressor to have PTSD symptomatology. A very large number of studies show that the majority of those exposed to catastrophic stresses do not develop PTSD. Therefore, why should we retain the stressor criterion?

What is the current status of the stressor criterion?

As noted above, DSM-IV has substantially modified, but not done away with, the stressor criterion for PTSD. ICD-10, on the other hand, has joined the arena only recently, and has stuck to the narrow definition of stressor (while leaving the other criteria more vague).

It is not surprising that the DSM-IV committee did not move to the very broad definition and effectively dispose of the stressor criterion by describing it retrospectively as the event which was the focus of the other symptoms.

Despite the lack of empirical evidence first pointed out by Breslau and Davis, there is still an adherence to the view that PTSD is a specific syndrome which only occurs after stressors and then only after stressors of a certain magnitude or intensity. The view remains with many that PTSD is something different and that it is the specific possible consequence of severe trauma. This view is held despite the evidence that:

- the only symptom group specific to PTSD (re-experiencing or intrusive symptoms) occurs after traumata which are not catastrophic or severe
- no matter how severe the stressor PTSD is not the normative response
- traumatic events can also be followed by other psychiatric illnesses.

In addition to this dogmatic point of view, there are major political reasons why the stressor criterion in PTSD will not be dropped. PTSD was defined in order to explain specific problems of those exposed to extreme stress, to legitimise these problems, and to draw attention to them. As a consequence, a whole range of medical and social changes was instigated, particularly, but not exclusively in the USA. Services were provided to a previously ignored group considered to be disadvantaged. The condition was publicly, and loudly, used in legal circles to explain or even excuse certain behaviours, and as a means by which victims could gain compensation for loss. Even the general public came to recognise and accept the concept of PTSD. Not only did this serve to help sufferers, but it also provided an acceptable, and less stigmatised, face of psychiatric illness itself.

Even if logic suggested that there was no need for a specific stressor criterion it would currently still be sociopolitically unacceptable to do away with it. Its position has changed considerably since the first definition of PTSD in DSM-III, but it still holds an important position which is unlikely to be relinquished. There has been a shift away from 'objective' definitions of qualifying stressors, and towards the meaning of events to the subject. This seems to make sense, particularly as it has been demonstrated that there are no particular events which can, with any degree of confidence, be predicted to cause PTSD in a specific individual. Despite the complaints of some, the current situation is that in order to qualify as a stressor the event must involve significant threat or injury to someone, and be accompanied in the subject by feelings of terror or helplessness.

Summary

The current situation can therefore be summarised as follows.

- Stressors can affect the onset and course of a range of physical and mental illnesses.
- PTSD symptoms do not only follow extreme stressors.
- PTSD symptoms are not the usual consequence of extreme stressors, except as relatively transient phenomena.
- Stressors are not sufficient to explain the occurrence of PTSD, with no specific quality or magnitude of stressor predictably causing PTSD in an individual.
- Other psychological symptoms and illnesses can follow extreme, and other 'normal', stressors.
- PTSD is more likely to follow certain classes of stressor such as combat, grotesque or abusive violence, or violent crime. However, it can follow other stressors.
- PTSD frequency increases with magnitude of stressor in combat and probably in some other stressful situations.
- It has not been convincingly demonstrated that there is a lower level or dose of stressor below which PTSD cannot occur.
- It has not been convincingly demonstrated that there are certain classes of perceived stressful events following which PTSD cannot occur.
- Although there appears to be a dose-related incidence of PTSD following trauma, the same does not appear to have been demonstrated for other PTI, with apparently equivalent increases in, for example, depression, following events of similar nature but differing intensity.
- As PTSD is currently defined, changing the definition of the stressor criterion does not alter the specificity or sensitivity of diagnosis. Rather it alters the incidence and prevalence of the disease by changing its definition.
- The true relationship between trauma or stressor and PTSD is not going to be worked out until we have some other, independent, means of identifying PTSD, such as a blood test.

References

Abenhaim, L., Dab, W. and Salmi, L.R. (1992). Study of civilian victims of terrorist attacks (France 1982, 1987). *Journal of Clinical Epidemiology*, **45**, 2: 103–9.

Aghabeigi, B., Feinmann, C. and Harris, M. (1992). Prevalence of postraumatic stress disorder in patients with chronic idiopathic facial pain. *British Journal of Oral Maxillofacial Surgery*, **30**, 6: 360–64.

Baider, L., Peretz, T. and Kaplan De Nour, A. (1992). Effect of the Holocaust on coping with cancer. *Social Sciences Medicine*, **34**, 1: 11–16.

Ballard, C. G., Stanley, A.K. and Brockington, I.F. (1995). Post traumatic stress disorder (PTSD) after childbirth. *British Journal of Psychiatry*, **166**: 525–8.

Behar, D. (1984). Confirmation of concurrent illnesses in PTSD. *American Journal of Psychiatry*, **141**: 1310–11.

Belenky, G., Tyner, C. and Sodet F. (1983). Israeli Battleshock Casualties: 1982 and 1983. *Report NP-83–4*. Washington DC: Division of Neuropsychiatry, Walter Reed Army Institute of Research.

Blair, J. A., Blair, R.S. and Rueckert, P. (1994). Pre-injury emotional trauma and chronic back pain. An unexpected finding. *Spine*, **19**, 10: 1144–6.

Bowman, E. S. and Markand, O.N. (1996). Psychodynamics and psychiatric diagnoses of pseudoseizure subjects. *American Journal of Psychiatry*, **153**, 1: 57–63.

Breslau, N. and Davis, G.C. (1987). Posttraumatic stress disorder: The stressor criterion. *Journal of Nervous and Mental Disease*, **175**, 5: 255–64.

Carmel, S., Koren, I. and Ilia, R. (1993). Coping with the Gulf war: subculture differences among ischemic heart disease patients in Israel. *Social Sciences and Medicine*, **37**, 12: 1481–8.

Cassell, J. (1976). The contribution of the social environment to host resistance. *American Journal of Epidemiology*, **104**: 107–23.

Davidson, J.R., Hughes, D., Blazer, D.G. and George, L.K. (1991). Post-traumatic stress disorder in the community: An epidemiological study. *Psychological Medicine*, **21**, 3: 713–21.

Davidson, J., Swartz, M., Storck, M., Krishnan, R.R. and Hammett, E. (1985). A diagnostic and family study of posttraumatic stress disorder. *American Journal of Psychiatry*, **142**, 1: 90–93.

Dixon, P., Rehling, G. and Shiwach, R. (1993). Peripheral victims of the Herald of Free Enterprise disaster. *British Journal of Medical Psychology*, **66**, 2: 193–202.

Durkin, M.E. (1993). Major depression and post traumatic stress disorder following the Coalinga and Chile Earthquakes: a cross cultural comparison. *Journal of Social Behavior and Personality*, **8**: 5.

Egendorf, A. (1981). Legacies of Vietnam: Comparative Adjustment of Veterans and their Peers. *House Committee Print No. 14. Washington: Government Printing Office*.

Erikson, K.T. (1976). *Everything in its Path – Destruction of a Community in the Buffalo Creek Flood*. New York: Simon & Schuster .

Escobar, J.I., Randolph, E.T., Puente, G., Spiwak, F., Asamen, J.K., Hill, M. and Hough, R.L. (1983). Post-traumatic stress disorder in Hispanic Vietnam veterans. Clinical phenomenology and sociocultural characteristics. *Journal of Nervous and Mental Disease*, **171**, 10: 585–96.

Falger, P.R., Op den Velde, W., Hovens, J.E., Schouten, E.G., De Groen, J.H. and Van Duijn, H. (1992). Current posttraumatic stress disorder and cardiovascular disease risk factors in Dutch Resistance veterans from World War II. *Psychotherapy and Psychosomatics*, **57**, 4: 164–71.

Glass, A. (1957). *Observations upon the Epidemiology of Mental Illness in Troops during Warfare. Symposium on Preventive and Social Psychiatry*. Washington DC: Walter Reed Army Institute of Research.

Gleser, G., Green, B. and Winget, C. (1981). *Prolonged Psychosocial Effects of Disaster: A Study of Buffalo Creek*. New York: Academic Press.

Green, B, Grace M. and Gleser, G. (1985). Identifying survivors at risk: Longterm impairment following the Beverly Hills Supper Club Fire. *Journal of Consulting and Clinical Psychology*, **53**: 672–8.

Green, B.L., Grace, M.C., Lindy, J.D. and Gleser, G.C. (1990). War stressors and symptom persistence in posttraumatic stress disorder. *Journal of Anxiety Disorders*, **4**, 1: 31–9.

Harris, T., Creed, F. and Brugha, T.S. (1992). Stressful life events and Graves' disease. *British Journal of Psychiatry*, **161**: 535–41.

Helzer, J.E., Robins, L.N. and McEvoy, L. (1987). Post-traumatic stress disorder in the general population: Findings of the Epidemiologic Catchment Area survey. *New England Journal of Medicine*, **317**, 26: 1630–34.

Holmes, T. and Rahe, R. (1967). The social readjustment rating scale. *Journal of Psychiatric Research*, **11**: 213–18.

Horowitz, M.J. (1979). Brief therapy of the stress response syndrome. *Psychiatric Clinics of North America*, **2**, 2: 365–77.

Horowitz, M.J., Weiss, D.S. and Marmar, C. (1987). Diagnosis of posttraumatic stress disorder. *Journal of Nervous and Mental Disease*, **175**, 5: 267–8.

Kardiner, A. (1941). *The Traumatic Neuroses of War*. New York: Jason Aaronson.

Kilpatrick, D.G., Saunders, B.E., Amick-McMullan, A. and Best, C.L. (1989). Victim and crime factors associated with the development of crime-related post-traumatic stress disorder. *Behavior Therapy*, **20**, 2: 199–214.

Krystal, H. (1971). Trauma: considerations of its intensity and chronicity. *International Psychiatry Clinics*, **8**, 1: 11–28.

Lucas, P.A., Leaker, B.R., Murphy, M. and Neild, G.H. (1995). Loin pain and haematuria syndrome: a somatoform disorder. *Quarterly Journal of Medicine*, **88**, 10: 703–9.

March, JS. (1990). The nosology of posttraumatic stress disorder. *Journal of Anxiety Disorders*, **4**, 1: 61–82.

March, J.S. (1993). What constitutes a stressor? The 'criterion A' issue. In *PTSD – DSM – IV and Beyond*, pp. 37–56. Ed. J.R. Davidson and E.B. Foa. Washington: American Psychiatric Press.

McFarlane, A.C. (1991). Post-traumatic stress disorder. *International Review of Psychiatry*, **3**, 2: 203–13.

McGorry, P.D., Chanen, A., McCarthy, E., Van, R.R., McKenzie, D. and Singh, B. (1991). Posttraumatic stress disorder following recent onset psychosis: an unrecognized postpsychotic syndrome. *Journal of Nervous and Mental Disease*, **179**, 5: 253–9.

Nuckells, K., Cassell J. and Kaplan, B. (1972). Psychosocial assets, life crisis and the prognosis of pregnancy. *American Journal of Epidemiology*, **95**: 431–46.

O'Brien, L.S., and Hughes, S.J. (1991). Symptoms of post-traumatic stress disorder in Falklands veterans five years after the conflict. *British Journal of Psychiatry*, **159**: 135–41.

O'Donohue, W., and Elliott, A. (1992). The current status of post-traumatic stress disorder as a diagnostic category: Problems and proposals. *Journal of Traumatic Stress*, **5**, 3: 421–39.

Patti, G., Pignalberi, C., Chimenti, C., Cianflone, D. and Maseri, A. (1995). Psychological stress as precipitating factor of the acute manifestations of ischemic cardiopathy. *Cardiologia*, **40**, 4: 229–34.

Peretz, T., Baider, L., Ever Hadani, P. and De Nour, A.K. (1994). Psychological distress in female cancer patients with Holocaust experience. *General Hospital Psychiatry*, **16**, 6: 413–18.

Schofferman, J., Anderson, D., Hines, R., Smith, G. and Keane, G. (1993). Childhood psychological trauma and chronic refractory low-back pain. *Clinical Journal of Pain*, **9**, 4: 260–65.

Schottenfeld, R.S., and Cullen, M.R. (1985). Occupation-induced posttraumatic stress disorders. *American Journal of Psychiatry*, **142**, 2: 198–202.

Scott, M.J. and Stradling, S.G. (1994). Post-traumatic stress disorder without the trauma. *British Journal of Clinical Psychology*, **33**, 1: 71–4.

Shore, J.H., Tatum, E.L. and Vollmer, W.M. (1986). Psychiatric reactions to disaster: The Mount St. Helens experience. *American Journal of Psychiatry*, **143**, 5: 590–95.

Shore, J.H., Vollmer, W.M. and Tatum, E.L. (1989). Community patterns of post-traumatic stress disorders. *Journal of Nervous and Mental Disease*, **177**, 11: 681–5.

Sierles, F.S., Chen, J.J., McFarland, R.E. and Taylor, M.A. (1983). Posttraumatic stress disorder and concurrent psychiatric illness: a preliminary report. *American Journal of Psychiatry*, **140**, 9: 1177–9.

Smith, E.M., North, C.S., McCool, R.E. and Shea, J.M. (1990). Acute postdisaster psychiatric disorders: Identification of persons at risk. *American Journal of Psychiatry*, **147**, 2: 202–6.

Solomon, S.D. and Canino, G.J. (1990). Appropriateness of DSM-III-R criteria for posttraumatic stress disorder. 5th Annual Meeting of the Society for Traumatic Stress Studies, 1989, San Francisco, California. *Comprehensive Psychiatry*, **31**, 3: 227–37.

Taylor, A.J. and Frazer, A.G. (1982). The stress of post-disaster body handling and victim identification work. *Journal of Human Stress*, **8**, 4: 4–12.

Tierney, K. and Baisden, B. (1979). Crisis Intervention Programmes for Disaster Victims: A Source Book and Manual for Small Communities. *DHEW Publication No. (ADM) 79–675*. Washington: Department of Health, Education and Welfare.

Ursano, R. (1981a). The Vietnam era prisoner of war: Precaptivity personality and the development of psychiatric illness. *American Journal of Psychiatry*, **138**: 315–18.

Ursano, R. (1981b). Psychiatric illness in US Air Force Vietnam prisoners of war: A five year follow up. *American Journal of Psychiatry*, **138**: 310–14.

Ursano, R.J. (1987). Posttraumatic stress disorder: The stressor criterion. *Journal of Nervous and Mental Disease*, **175**, 5: 273–5.

Walker, E.A., Katon, W.J., Roy Byrne, P.P., Jemelka, R.P. and Russo, J. (1993). Histories of sexual victimization in patients with irritable bowel syndrome or inflammatory bowel disease. *American Journal of Psychiatry*, **150**, 10: 1502–6.

Weisaeth, L. (1989). The stressors and the post-traumatic stress syndrome after an industrial disaster. Special issue: Traumatic stress: empirical studies from Norway. *Acta Psychiatrica Scandinavica*, **80**, 355 (Suppl.): 25–37.

Yehuda, R. and McFarlane, A.C. (1995). Conflict between current knowledge about PTSD and its original conceptual basis. *American Journal of Psychiatry*, **152**: 1705–13.

CHAPTER 6

POST-TRAUMATIC ILLNESS OTHER THAN POST-TRAUMATIC STRESS DISORDER

It is the author's contention that this chapter is of great importance. With no apologies for repetition, it is emphasised that:

> not everyone who is exposed to trauma develops post-traumatic illness
> not all post-traumatic illness is post-traumatic stress disorder.

Although the term PTSD was put forward only in the late seventies and confirmed in 1980, there is no suggestion that the concept that exposure to major trauma can cause mental illness is new. It has long been recognised that trauma can be followed by mental illness. In an editorial addressing a different aspect of controversy surrounding PTSD, Andreasen (1995) reminds us that there was recognition of PTI in DSM-I but that at that time it was 'conceptualised and defined psychologically', that it was seen as being 'by definition acute and reversible' as it was included in 'transient situational personality disorders', and that no characteristic symptoms were specified. She sees the creation of PTSD as being required to meet the need of a generation of Vietnam veterans, many of whom had severe stress syndromes, and as it being a 'general name' because of the similarity of the syndrome across various stressors.

Essentially, DSM-I recognised that trauma could produce acute illness and implicitly indicated psychological causation. However, it did not describe a specific syndrome and saw chronic illness as representing precipitation or aggravation of a constitutional or potential disorder rather than a specific response to trauma. One of the dangers of the concept of PTSD as defined in DSM-III and modified by later editions is that it is perceived, albeit incorrectly, as a generic term for PTI and synonymous with it. There has been relatively little interest in other forms of PTI. Cases or series of cases described or diagnosed in the decades and even centuries before DSM-III are now described as having been cases of PTSD in retrospect. This may or may not be accurate, but such opinions must inevitably only be based on belief or dogma rather than on specific knowledge.

There are a number of relevant issues surrounding other PTI and PTSD. These include:

- the status of other mental illnesses defined as being specifically post-traumatic
- the occurrence of mental illnesses after trauma which also occur in the absence of trauma
- the co-existence of PTSD and other conditions in a single subject.

The three areas will be addressed individually.

Other stress disorders

The two principal classificatory systems have taken somewhat different attitudes to the location of PTSD and stress disorders within their classification system.

ICD-10 (World Health Organisation, 1992) includes within the major group of 'neurotic, stress-related, and somatoform disorders', the grouping 'F43 Reaction to severe stress, and adjustment disorders'. It suggests that this group of disorders differs from others in that they are identifiable 'not only on grounds of symptomatology and course', but because of their relationship with either 'exceptionally stressful life events' or 'significant life change'. Such events are seen as being 'the primary and overriding causal factor', in the absence of which the condition would not have occurred. It is thus that the conditions are separated from others which may be precipitated or aggravated by stressful events.

The conditions listed are:

F43.0	acute stress reaction
F43.1	post-traumatic stress disorder
F43.2	adjustment disorders
F43.20	brief depressive reaction
F43.21	prolonged depressive reaction
F43.22	mixed anxiety and depressive reaction
F43.23	with predominant disturbance of other emotions
F43.24	with predominant disturbance of conduct

F43.25   with mixed disturbance of emotions and conduct
F43.28   with other specified predominant symptoms
F43.8   other reactions to severe stress
F43.9   reaction to severe stress, unspecified.

DSM-IV (American Psychiatric Association, 1994) does not have a separate group of stress-related disorders but squarely places the defined post-traumatic illnesses within the group described as anxiety disorders, as:

309.81 post-traumatic stress disorder
       specify if: acute or chronic
       specify if: delayed onset
308.3 acute stress disorder.

Adjustment disorders are classified separately near the end of Axis-I.

The positioning of PTSD and other PTI in DSM-IV has not been without debate or controversy. Brett (1993) has reviewed the argument about whether PTSD should be considered an anxiety or dissociative disorder. The article also describes the debate about whether DSM-IV should have taken the opportunity to establish a separate category of stress-related disorders as in ICD-10.

An integral part of this debate was the suggestion that a new disorder be defined in DSM-IV to represent changes following repeated trauma which differed from those seen in PTSD. The suggested name was disorders of extreme stress not otherwise specified, or DESNOS. Although the title seems to suggest a hotch-potch of left-over cases, the researchers suggested that there was a particular syndrome with specific stressors being causal (Worzel, 1992). Herman (1992) has described the specifics of the trauma as being repetitive and prolonged exposure associated with a subordinate or abused role where the victim is somehow in the power of, or at the mercy of, the stress or its perpetrator. Zlotnick has particularly drawn the parallel between sexual abuse and this pattern of traumatic exposure, because of the obvious features of repetition and powerlessness in the position of the victim of sexual abuse (Zlotnick et al., 1996). A syndrome is described which, in addition to anxiety and dissociative symptoms, includes hostility, alexithymia, social dysfunction, maladaptive and self-destructive behaviour, and adult victimisation. Clearly there is marked overlap with PTSD, although some behavioural and interpersonal changes seem more apparent.

However, DESNOS was not accepted into DSM-IV and the only new addition was acute stress disorder.

Acute stress disorder

Acute stress disorder was a new addition to DSM-IV and was introduced to ICD-10 as acute stress reaction at the same time as PTSD. The rationale behind its addition to DSM-IV was given by Davis *et al.* (1993) in a review of the use of the MacArthur data sets to consider proposed new diagnostic categories for DSM-IV.

Davis *et al.*, pointed out that until then there was no condition which could be used to describe a transient disturbance suffered only by victims of trauma. Two factors strongly supported the definition of such a condition. A pragmatic one was that it would appear in ICD-10, with which DSM would generally be compatible. More empirically, there was evidence that there was a consistent pattern of the existence of a mixture of dissociative and anxiety symptoms after trauma. The seven data sets used were of varying sizes and had been obtained at various times from different countries and situations. The older data looked at about a thousand patients from the Lebanon War, MacFarlane's 469 fire-fighters, and much smaller groups from the Piper Alpha oil rig and the Hyatt–Regency hotel collapse. The more recent groups were from a firestorm and an earthquake and a very small group of journalists who witnessed an execution, all from America.

The evidence was supportive of the concept of acute stress disorder in that:

1. the postulated symptoms, including anxiety symptoms and dissociative symptoms, were intercorrelated
2. such symptoms were associated with impairment or disability
3. they were associated with degree of exposure
4. numbers with symptoms fell significantly by four months post-incident
5. symptom presence in the aftermath was associated with increased risk of later morbidity, including PTSD.

As elsewhere in ICD-10, the diagnostic guidelines for acute stress reaction are much less prescriptive or less clear than those for acute stress disorder in DSM-IV.

The description of *acute stress reaction* says that the onset of symptoms is 'within a few minutes' if not immediate and in association with 'an exceptional stressor'. A 'mixed and usually changing' clinical picture is described in which 'no one symptom type predominates for long'. It is expected that the symptoms will resolve within a few hours of removal from the stressor but, even if the stressor continues, will be minimal within three days.

This extremely swift onset and brief duration are at variance with the

DSM-IV concept which has an onset within four weeks, a minimum duration of two days, and a maximum duration of four weeks. The symptom complex defined as *acute stress disorder* follows exposure to a stressor defined in the same way as that for PTSD. There must be a re-experiencing phenomenon, marked avoidance, and increased anxiety or arousal. In addition there must be three of five dissociative phenomena present, although it may be considered difficult to tease out five separate and independent phenomena from: subjective numbing or detachment, reduced awareness of surroundings, derealisation, depersonalisation, and dissociative amnesia. As is the case for PTSD, there is a requirement for 'clinically significant distress or impairment' and in addition the phenomena must not be better explained by some pre-existing problem.

As yet, there remains a real shortage of empirical studies into acute stress disorder, its prevalence, and its longitudinal course. Although it seems quite clear that acute reactions do occur and that they are to some extent predictive of outcome, it is probably not justified to extrapolate from the results of battle shock experiences to all other traumatic events. While acute reactions appear to be a sensitive predictor of PTSD, they are not necessarily so specific. Shalev *et al.* (1996) conducted one small-scale study of 51 patients injured in traumatic events. They found that the Impact of Events Scale score at one week was 92% sensitive and 34% specific at predicting the 25% of patients with PTSD at six months. Thus most who developed PTSD had an acute reaction but most who had an acute reaction did not develop PTSD.

A number of studies have now suggested that, of the acute symptoms, the dissociative symptoms in particular immediately following an incident are to some extent predictive of PTSD. This work has included retrospective studies of veterans (Marmar *et al.*, 1994) and prospective studies of emergency workers (Koopman, Classen and Spiegel, 1994) and victims (Feinstein, 1989; Cardena and Spiegel, 1993). Koopman (Koopman *et al.*, 1995) has reviewed the concept of acute stress disorder and particularly the relevance of dissociative symptoms.

Enduring personality change after catastrophic experience

Despite the work concerning DESNOS, the only specific long-term disorder listed in DSM-IV as being caused by traumatic events is PTSD. The situation is, however, somewhat different in ICD-10. As stated, ICD contains a specific stress-related section, F43. In that section it suggests that although the course of PTSD is fluctuating, recovery can be expected in the majority of cases. It is suggested that 'in a small proportion of patients' there may be a chronic course over many years and a transition to 'an enduring personality change'. Readers are referred to section F62 in the Disorders of Adult Personality and Behaviour, to 'Enduring personality changes not attributable to brain damage and disease'. This section includes F62.0, Enduring Personality Change after Catastrophic Experience.

The section is intended to describe cases in which there is 'evidence of a definite and enduring change in a person's pattern of perceiving, relating to, or thinking about the environment and the self'. There should be 'inflexible and maladaptive behaviour' not present before the stressor. It is suggested that there may be difficulty in differentiating between such a change following a catastrophic stressor and the unmasking, by such a stressor, of underlying pre-existing personality disorder.

For *enduring personality change after catastrophic experience* there is a need for exposure to such a catastrophic stressor as prolonged captivity in a hostage situation, concentration camp, torture or disaster. The experience may or may not be followed by PTSD before the enduring change. Specifically, the diagnostic guidelines call for additional features not present before the trauma such as:

a hostile or mistrustful attitude towards the world
social withdrawal
feelings of emptiness or hopelessness
a chronic feeling of being on edge or threatened
estrangement.

All of this should be present for at least two years and should preferably be confirmed by a key informant.

Although most of these features are similar to diagnostic symptoms in DSM-IV post-traumatic stress disorder, ICD-10 states that this disorder excludes PTSD.

Interestingly, the clinical description section states that such changes following 'short-term exposure to a life-threatening experience such as a car accident' should not be included as recent research, which is not referenced, indicates that such a development depends on pre-existing psychological vulnerability. This seems to be an important matter. If this 'enduring personality change' is different from PTSD and is a consequence of innate or acquired vulnerability when it occurs after a single or individual traumatic event but is caused by trauma when it occurs after prolonged trauma or disaster, then it should be a useful way of investigating both the dimensions of trauma and the nature of vulnerability. However, there is an almost total absence of empirical evidence concerning this category other than the vaguely comparable work on DESNOS which focuses on the effects of prolonged or repeated trauma.

an 'enduring personality change'. There is a clear perception, albeit little backed by empirical rather than anecdotal evidence, that treatment is more likely to be effective if started relatively early rather than late. However, this diagnostic category seems to suggest that if symptoms are present at two years and are accompanied by the attitudes listed above, then the change can be seen as enduring. Obviously not everybody who has PTSD or PTI symptoms two years after trauma demonstrates the mistrusting, hostile, and markedly avoidant behaviours listed, but if such changes are enduring and seen as a definite change in personality, then it seems important to study the incidence of such states and their onset and presentation in order to investigate whether, in this particular subgroup at least, there may be a preventive role for some form of early intervention.

Adjustment disorders

Although they place adjustment disorders in different sections of the classifications, both ICD-10 and DSM-IV have similar attitudes to these diagnoses.

In ICD-10 adjustment disorders are grouped with the reactions to severe stress, but in DSM-IV they are grouped separately at the end of the Axis I classification.

There are some differences but essentially both classifications see adjustment disorders as arising in relation to an identifiable stressor or life change without specifying the severity of the event causing the condition. In both classifications, the range of observed symptoms is required to be such that it does not meet diagnostic criteria for any other Axis-I diagnosis. It is in this way that adjustment disorders seem to be a sort of 'catch all' for those who seem to have some significant problem, have had something happen in their life, but who cannot be diagnosed as suffering from any other formal psychiatric disorder. It seems inevitable, therefore, that this is a very heterogeneous group of patients with a wide range of symptoms and a wide range of severity of symptoms.

ICD-10 suggests that symptoms should commence within one month, and DSM-IV three months, of the onset of the stressor. Both agree that symptoms should settle within six months or at least within six months of cessation of the stressor. Both have a number of subdivisions of the condition depending upon the emphasis of the presenting symptoms, but none of the symptoms is specific to adjustment disorder.

ICD-10, unlike the supposedly atheoretical DSM-IV, comments upon the major part played by 'predisposition or vulnerability' in the genesis of adjustment disorders compared with that in PTSD and acute stress reaction.

Adjustment disorders have been considered in a number of empirical studies. In an epidemiological study of 201 refugees from Vietnam (Hinton *et al.*, 1993), there was a current prevalence of any psychiatric disorder of 18.4%, with adjustment disorders being the most common conditions represented, at 8.5%. In 111 Iranian refugees arriving in Canada after the revolution and actively seeking psychiatric consultation, about 10% had PTSD while 60% had adjustment disorders. A study of 65 burns unit patients referred for clinical psychiatric evaluation found that 8% had PTSD while 62% had an adjustment disorder. What is most interesting is that the two groups of adjustment disorder and PTSD patients could not be differentiated on the basis of either type or severity of burn injury, so that traumatic exposure did not seem to predict who got PTSD and who had an adjustment disorder.

Adjustment disorders have also been found to be common in various other groups exposed to stressful events, including police officers and children who have been maltreated (Saathoff and Buckman, 1990).

Many studies have not directly addressed adjustment disorders for various reasons including, for example, the time limitation applied to any such diagnosis. Those that have done so have tended to find adjustment disorders to be more common than PTSD. While some studies of small, very specific groups exposed to specific stressors have found PTSD to be more common than adjustment disorder, logic would suggest that, particularly when a large group is exposed to trauma, there will be varying degrees of exposure and perceived threat and therefore some will de facto be exposed to 'qualifying' stressors for PTSD and others not. Therefore, adjustment disorders might be expected to be more common. However, it is very difficult to demonstrate this because of the way in which adjustment disorders have been defined in the classificatory systems. By definition, if it is possible to make another Axis 1 diagnosis, then a diagnosis of adjustment disorder cannot be made. The same is not true for many other diagnoses. For example, there is no reason why PTSD, obsessive compulsive disorder or major depression, and substance misuse disorder could not be diagnosed in the same person at the same time. The same is not true for adjustment disorders.

Other mental disorders after trauma

Obviously any other mental disorder can occur in somebody who just happens to have been exposed to trauma, and there is no reason to believe that all subsequent mental disability, any more than all subsequent physical disability, is a consequence of a single event or series of events in a person's history. The simple fact that a condition either started or was diagnosed at some point after a traumatic event does not prove causation or even aggravation. However, it is true that almost all conditions have, at some point, been associated in some way with trauma as a predisposing, precipitating or aggravating factor. There is a very large body of work about life events which to some extent precedes and is comparable with, but separate from, the work on PTI.

Long before the definition of PTSD and beside the diagnosis of gross stress reaction in DSM-I, clinicians had considered on clinical grounds that various illnesses were in some way related to stress. The difficulty with such diagnoses compared with those considered above is that they do not represent specific symptom complexes or syndromal patterns consistently associated with trauma plus or minus prior vulnerability, but are conditions which are regularly and usually diagnosed without any reference to trauma or to stressors. If they can also be associated with such stressors, then there is a need to be able to differentiate between onset, exacerbation or recurrence of a disorder in a person who just happens to have been exposed to trauma, and cases in which the two are related.

Coincidence or causation?

There are a number of possible pointers that mental disorders are in some way related to the trauma:

> temporal link
> course
> content.

Temporal link

It is not pathognomonic, but if a mental disorder starts *de novo* within a few weeks of a major stressor, then it is reasonable to have a high degree of suspicion that there is a link. In general, the further away in time the onset, the less likely that there is a causal link.

As an example, a person who develops a first episode hypomanic illness less than ten days after his wife and children are all killed in a road traffic accident probably has an underlying propensity or vulnerability to an affective disorder, but it is equally probable that he would not have suffered that illness at that time if it were not for the trauma.

The situation is less straightforward for pre-existing or previous illnesses. There must be a greater suspicion that recurrence of a previous illness or exacerbation of a pre-existing illness is part of the underlying disease process rather than a response to trauma. However, there must nevertheless be a considerable suspicion that if a previous illness recurs immediately after a traumatic event, then the episode was at least 'brought forward' by the incident. Similarly, if a current mental illness deteriorates significantly immediately after trauma, there is at least suspicion that the deterioration is a consequence of the incident, either as a specific response or a general response to stress or a life event.

There is a significant body of literature concerning the concept of delayed onset of PTSD. Indeed, DSM-IV actually contains a specifier for delayed onset of PTSD. Most workers in the field have seen Second World War veterans who appear to have functioned very well for 40 or 50 years without significant disability but then present with apparent late onset of new symptomatology, usually following a change in life circumstances or loss of support structures such as retirement from work, death of a spouse, or physical illness (Pomerantz, 1991; Herrmann and Eryavec, 1994). There are occasional case histories of similar delayed onset following civilian trauma (Lim, 1991). The 14-year follow-up of Buffalo Creek survivors (Green *et al.*, 1990b) found a general reduction in disability over time but a small group with delayed onset of problems, not just PTSD. A specific study of late-onset PTSD in Israeli soldiers with late presentation of PTSD found that only 10% of so-called late-onset cases represented true late onset of symptoms rather than delayed presentation or help seeking (Solomon *et al.*, 1989), while a study of 76 underground train drivers under whose trains people had killed themselves found a reduction in symptomatology over time and no late-onset cases (Tranah and Farmer, 1994). Thus the incidence of delayed-onset PTI has only been substantially demonstrated for PTSD and while it does exist it seems likely that the majority of cases of delayed onset probably represent delayed help-seeking or the additional effect of loss of support structures. In general, PTSD and PTI, like many disorders, tend to decrease in severity of symptomatology as the time since the traumatic event extends.

Course

The course of the illness may be a pointer to a relation to trauma. In addition to the occurrence of an exacerbation following trauma, there may be clear anniversary reactions. There is general acceptance that anniversary reactions can occur. If the man mentioned above who had his first episode of hypomanic illness within a few days of the death of his whole family in a road traffic accident then has his second and third episodes each within a week of the first and second anniversaries of their deaths, then this is strong circumstantial evidence of a connection. Even the lay press accepts the concept of anniversary reactions as being logical, and the *Sunday Times* (Hinde, 1994) reported a marked increase in those being cared for by the Ex-services Mental Welfare Organisation, Combat Stress, at the time of the fiftieth anniversary of the D-day landings, attributing the response to the general 'hype' and promotion of memories. One empirical study of a very different group looked at young mothers over the ten years following the Three Mile Island nuclear accident. It found two patterns of psychological response which were not confined to PTSD or its equivalent. One group had a constant low level of insignificant symptomatology; the other had a raised and clinically significant level of symptoms which increased significantly at the time of the restarting of the reactor and at the tenth anniversary of the incident.

Another significance of course of illness may not be in the subsequent course of the illness in the years following a traumatic event but in a change in the course immediately following the incident. For example, if a person with bipolar disorder has a history of a number of episodes of illness but none for many years and then has an episode following trauma, then this seems suggestive of a relationship. Similarly, in illnesses such as bipolar disorder the 'normal' pattern of episodes or recurrences may be disrupted by a traumatic event. For example, if a person has had a depressive episode once each year in February and March for three years and then has an additional episode in September following a major incident in August, then this is suggestive of a relationship.

This effect upon course may also be seen with severity or duration of episode. Again, this is most readily demonstrated with recurrent affective disorders. If the person above has moderate episodes of depression lasting one month each year but then has a severe episode lasting six months within a month of a traumatic incident, then it is likely that the trauma has had an effect. If a person has previously had a number of brief episodes of depression but following an accident at work in which they narrowly escaped with their life they develop a severe illness which continues without recovery for three years, then it is likely that this is a PTI.

Content

The content of the illness may also be an indicator of PTI. For example, if in the months following a road traffic accident a subject develops a specific phobia, then the fact that the phobia is one of driving or of travelling by car (Hickling and Blanchard, 1992; Blanchard *et al.*, 1994; Bryant and Harvey, 1995) is highly indicative that this is post-traumatic illness.

There is also the possibility that a person may develop obsessive compulsive disorder following trauma. If the content of the ruminations centres around the trauma or the rituals are intended to fend off a recurrence of the event, then it is likely that this is a PTI. Depression following trauma may also involve pre-occupation with thoughts of the incident as a prominent feature, and this too is suggestive of PTI.

Substance-related disorders

Substance misuse has long been associated with post-traumatic problems. It was particularly highlighted in Vietnam veterans that there was an association of drug and alcohol abuse with 'readjustment problems' and then with PTSD. The association of the two disorders is complicated and it is not possible to state clearly that one is causal of the other. Substance abuse has been seen as comorbidity with PTSD, comorbidly with other PTI or concurrent illnesses, and also in isolation following trauma. (Jelinek and Williams, 1984), when reviewing problems in Vietnam veterans, summed up the issues nicely when they said 'substance abuse may suppress, exacerbate or perpetuate PTSD'. In addition, it can appear after trauma in the absence of PTSD (Hyer *et al.*, 1991). That it is by no means clear whether substance abuse is a response to PTI or an attempt to cope with it is shown by the fact that, unlike certain other possible comorbid diagnoses, the mean time of onset of substance abuse after trauma in Vietnam veterans is not later than that of PTSD. If the two conditions start at the same time it is hard to say that either one is a consequence of the other. It is not impossible, however, that heavy drinking is a very early coping strategy for those with PTSD or is a method of coping which is used before they are even aware of symptoms.

There can be no doubt that, as with a range of other physical and psychological problems, some sufferers with PTSD may use substances such as alcohol and illicit drugs as a form of self-medication to help them to cope with the symptoms of PTSD. The disinhibiting and mood-altering effects of drugs may also aggravate PTSD symptoms such as irritability, impaired interaction with others, and physiological arousal symptoms. The chronic effects of drug and alcohol abuse, including withdrawal and tolerance effects and recurrent effects of intoxication, may interfere with the resolution of post-traumatic issues and with treatment.

It is not only following combat that substance abuse has been associated with exposure to trauma. There is evidence that incest survivors (Graziano, 1992), battered women (Smith and Gittelman, 1994) and adults who were severely abused as children (Hanson, 1990) have higher rates of substance-related problems separate from PTSD or other specific trauma-related illness. A study of 73 survivors of the Herald of Free Enterprise sinking (Joseph *et al.*, 1993) showed a general increase in consumption of alcohol, cigarettes, sleeping tablets, and prescribed antidepressants at six months. There was a reduction in consumption at 30 months but levels had not yet fallen to baseline. In general, most studies which have considered substance misuse after trauma have shown an increase whether the investigators have associated it with PTSD or have seen it as a separate response or PTI (Zweben, Clark and Smith, 1994).

When comorbid PTSD and substance abuse are considered, there is often a debate as to which problem should be tackled first, with a danger of therapists suggesting that the alcohol or drug problem will not come under control until the PTSD is treated or that attempts to treat PTSD are wasted in the face of substance misuse. There is no evidence that either argument has any great validity. Logic alone would suggest that there is a need to look at both problems in their own right. The usual treatment strategies for each are not likely to interfere with the other. It seems appropriate either to tackle both concurrently or, if necessary, to deal initially with the one which is causing greatest disability at the time.

Psychotic disorders

The relationship between psychotic disorders and trauma is interesting and was concisely reviewed in the lay press by Wesseley (Can Life Really Drive You Mad? Body and Mind, 1994) recently. He reported a personal injury case in which it was claimed that following an injurious incident a plaintiff suffered psychotic illness caused or triggered by the relevant trauma. The case was hotly argued and the judge accepted that although a significant number of people with psychotic illnesses reported some form of life event in the fortnight before the onset of illness, such events as were reported were commonly minor or recurring events which happened to many other people in the same time period and were not proven to be triggers or causative factors. He did not accept that it had been demonstrated that life events had been proven to cause or trigger psychotic illnesses. It seems clear that people who develop such severe mental illnesses will naturally seek some cause and will latch on to remembered events, retrospectively attaching attribution. The sort of events usually recalled are not of the nature or severity of those seen as 'qualifying' events for PTSD or other PTI. The judge held that such events occur frequently and even if they are precipitating events they must only bring illness onset forward by a couple of weeks. Obviously a high court judge's opinion is not put forward as the definitive scientific word on this subject but it does accord with consensus opinion (Marchevsky and Baram, 1992) that there is no clear evidence that major traumatic events cause or significantly bring forward psychotic illness. One dissenting opinion from the nursing press (Yaktin and Labban, 1992) suggests that throughout the 12 years of the Lebanon War, both immediately after heavy fighting and some months after such episodes, there was an increased incidence of schizophrenia in men. On the other hand, in a group of 65 burned patients referred for clinical psychiatric opinion (Perez *et al.*, 1994) only one had schizophrenia even though about 10% had self-inflicted burns. A study of 426 ex prisoners of war showed the expected excess of PTSD and some other disorders but no increase in rates of schizophrenia (Eberly and Engdahl, 1991).

One interesting anomaly is a paper (Gurian, Wexler and Baker, 1992) detailing a very small subgroup of women with late-onset paraphrenia who differ from other cases in clinical features, and who tend to have a history of both primary infertility and severe trauma in early life. This does not seem to have been reported elsewhere.

A number of papers, particularly those written before the definition of PTSD, refer to the high rate of diagnosis or misdiagnosis of schizophrenia in veterans. In his series of case reports, Van Putten (Van Putten and Emory, 1973) talks of a high rate of misdiagnosis of schizophrenia, and 54% of Zarcone's treatment sample of Vietnam veterans had been diagnosed as suffering from schizophrenia. It has been suggested that what was defined a hundred years ago as 'hysterical psychosis' (Van der Hart, Witztum and Friedman, 1993) is really a form of PTSD presenting with predominantly florid dissociative symptoms as a form of 'reactive dissociative psychosis'.

Following the definition of PTSD work centred upon the comorbidity of psychosis with PTSD. There has been no convincing demonstration of an increased rate of schizophrenia in combination with PTSD. Indeed, Hryvniak's paper (Hryvniak and Rosse, 1989), while showing a very high rate of comorbidity in veterans with PTSD, demonstrated a wide range of comorbid diagnoses but no excess of schizophrenia in comparison with patients without PTSD. This has been the general finding and was supported in the Epidemiological Catchment Area Study and most others, with the notable exception that one single study found a much increased risk of schizophrenia in those with PTSD which has not been supported elsewhere. In general, psychotic illnesses are amongst the few psychiatric disorders which, like mental impairment, are not over-represented in those exposed to traumatic incidents.

More recently interest has centred upon the role of schizophrenia or other psychoses as a traumatic incident. It is suggested that the experience of a psychotic illness is so traumatic that such an illness can be considered a qualifying event for PTSD. This has led to a whole series of individual cases and series as written by McGorry and others (Shaner and Eth, 1989; McGorry *et al,*. 1991, 1994; McGorry, 1991, 1993; Lundy, 1992; Williams-Keeler, Milliken and Jones, 1994).

Mood disorders

There is a general acceptance that depression can be at least triggered by external events. At one time the terms 'reactive depression' and 'endogenous depression' were widely used as classificatory terms to differentiate between depression caused by 'internal' factors and depression which was a consequence of external events. In fact, this dichotomy does not, of course, fit with observed facts and it is clear that external events may generally have an influence. Long before the definition of PTSD, diagnoses of depression were made in people who had been exposed to traumatic events, with the implicit or explicit acknowledgement that the illness would not have occurred or would not have occurred at that time if it were not for the trauma. Such recognition was most explicitly acknowledged in civil litigation cases where 'clinical depression' was often the diagnosis used to define nervous shock suffered as a result of trauma.

There is empirical evidence that those exposed to trauma may suffer from affective disorders. A possible complicating factor is the significance of loss or bereavement as part of the trauma. For example, in a study of 146 friends of adolescent suicide victims (Brent *et al.*, 1993, 1994), 29% developed depressive illnesses with a mean duration of eight months. Many traumatic incidents involve loss, and the relationship between loss and depression has been recognised for many years, perhaps epitomised by Freud's *Mourning and Melancholia*.

In a study of psychiatric outpatient attendees the group of 76 who reported significant trauma experience in the past two years had a higher rate of affective symptoms than the group of 443 who did not report such experiences (Brom and Witztum, 1992).

Although the majority of recent studies have naturally focused on PTSD, those which have looked at affective disorders specifically or as alternative or comorbid diagnoses have consistently found high rates of depression. The depressive illnesses have been seen both as comorbid diagnoses and as separate diagnoses. Major depression has been shown to be significantly more common in inpatient Vietnam veterans with PTSD than in inpatients without PTSD (Hryvniak and Rosse, 1989). When the Buffalo Creek flood disaster survivors were followed up 14 years later (Green *et al.*, 1992) major depression was still closely related to PTSD symptomatology, and 53% of road traffic accident victims with PTSD also had major depression (Blanchard *et al.*, 1995).

Major depression is not, however, only related to PTSD or necessarily a consequence of it. While MacFarlane's 469 fire-fighters (McFarlane and Papay, 1992) and a group of Vietnam veterans (Mellman *et al.*, 1992) had major depression as the second most common diagnosis after PTSD, a number of other studies have found depression to be more common. In a small group of 38 young Afghan refugees (Mghir *et al.*, 1995) major depression was twice as common as PTSD. Battered women (Gleason, 1993), Vietnamese refugees (Hinton *et al.*, 1993), and survivors of a rural earthquake in India (Sharan *et al.*, 1996) have shown rates of depression at least as high as, if not higher than, rates of PTSD. When the effects of earthquakes in Chile and California were compared (Durkin, 1993), it was found that although the rate of PTSD increased dramatically in the Chilean subjects and not the Californians, both groups had a 2.7 times increase in rates of major depression not seen in a control area.

Reports of onset of hypomanic episodes following major trauma rather than life events in general tend to be anecdotal and there is no empirical evidence of increased rates.

Anxiety disorders

It would hardly be surprising if there were an excess of anxiety disorders after trauma. DSM-IV actually includes the specific PTIs in the group of anxiety disorders. Despite the arguments as to whether PTSD is an anxiety or a dissociative disorder (Brett, 1993) there is clear evidence of anxiety symptoms in the syndromal descriptions of both post-traumatic stress disorder and acute stress reaction. One might expect, therefore, an excess of other anxiety disorders after trauma, both as comorbid disorders and also as stand-alone diagnoses.

There certainly is good evidence of an excess of a range of other anxiety disorders.

Those exposed to a wide range of traumatic events have been shown to have an increased prevalence of generalised anxiety disorder (GAD). When MacFarlane looked at 147 of the fire-fighters at highest risk some 42 months after the Ash Wednesday fires (Spurrell and McFarlane, 1993), 46% had GAD, about the same number as for PTSD. Following the Exxon Valdez oil spills, a group of 599 subjects were assessed at one year (Palinkas *et al.*, 1993) and rates of 20.2% for GAD and 9.4% for PTSD were found. High exposure to the disaster increased the rate of GAD 3.6 times and that of PTSD 2.9 times in comparison with those who had not had such exposure. In the long-term follow-up of the Mount St Helens victims, rates for GAD continued to be raised (Shore, Vollmer and Tatum, 1989), and a group of 101 Sri Lankan civilians exposed to war trauma had a GAD prevalence of 26%.

Specific phobias are likely to follow trauma and this is also far from unexpected. Learning theory would easily explain the fact that underground train drivers have an increased rate of phobic states of driving trains after they have been involved in an incident in which someone has killed themselves under their train (Farmer *et al.*, 1992). Avoidance symptoms amounting to specific phobia in such circumstances and similar problems following road traffic accidents seem entirely logical. In a small group of 33 road traffic accident victims seeking help at a pain clinic, the rate of phobia was increased 3.2 times (Kuch *et al.*, 1991), while in a group referred specifically for private psychiatric help in such circumstances 13 of 20 had PTSD and 12 of these had a phobia of driving (Hickling and Blanchard, 1992). A review of the effects of road traffic accidents confirms the importance of phobic symptoms, while another study of 55 help-seekers found a rate of phobia near 40% and two and a half times that of PTSD.

Obsessive compulsive disorder has been reported to occur frequently in Vietnam veterans as, for example, in a community study of 2985 veterans who also showed higher rates of social phobia as well as GAD (Davidson *et al.*, 1991). There are case reports of obsessive compulsive disorder in Vietnam veterans (Pitman, 1993) and the condition is more common in battered women (Gleason, 1993) and the adult survivors of child rape. The 391 subjects in this latter study (Saunders *et al.*, 1992) also had higher rates of social phobia and agoraphobia. A study of 200 Vietnam veterans indicated that lifelong prevalence of panic disorder was predicted by war experience (Green *et al.*, 1990a). Social phobia has been more commonly reported than specific phobia in Vietnam veterans (Orsillo *et al.*, 1996).

Thus, although there may be differences between rates of conditions depending upon the nature or intensity of trauma, the evidence is that a wide range of anxiety disorders can be considered to be a post-traumatic illness at times.

Somatoform disorders

The somatoform disorders as defined in DSM-IV include somatic or physical symptom presentations (Hryvniak and Rosse 1989) in various patterns that are not fully explained by any general medical condition and are not intentionally or consciously produced. They do not require a psychological explanation or causation of symptoms. Only in conversion disorder or what has for many years been known as conversion hysteria is it explicitly stated that psychological factors are judged to be relevant and that there are expected to be preceding psychological conflicts or stressors. A similar or comparable classification is used in ICD-10.

The presentation of somatisation symptoms or frank conversion hysteria has been associated for many years with major trauma. It was perhaps best epitomised in the particular conditions of the First World War when there were many cases of hysterical blindness, mutism or paralysis. Photographs of long lines of unseeing soldiers being led by each placing a hand on the shoulder of the man in front have been widely seen but it is clear that in some of those cases at least some of the men had not actually been exposed to gas attack but rather to the terror of the possibility of it. The UK base hospitals had wards full of service personnel with hysterical paralyses and mutism, fictional descriptions of which have been recently drawn from original records by Pat Barker in her *Regeneration* trilogy including the Booker Prize winning, *Ghost Road*. The various contemporary accounts by poets such as Sassoon and Blunden give vivid descriptions of traumatic hysteria.

Frank hysterical presentations seem less common today, although there are some case histories presented (De Mol, Retif and Aerens, 1981; Rothbaum and Foa, 1991). There seems to be a lack of accord about the presentation of somatic symptoms in those exposed to severe trauma. For example, a group of 311 Vietnam veterans with PTSD did not have an excess of somatisation (Orsillo *et al.*, 1996), while in a community study of 2985 veterans somatisation was associated with chronic rather than acute PTSD (Davidson *et al.*, 1991). Although a French study suggested that somatisation was common in trauma victims (Darves *et al.*, 1995), road traffic accident patients presenting at pain clinics were said not to have an increased rate of somatoform pain disorder (Kuch *et al.*, 1991).

In studies of patients not initially presenting with PTI there has been seen to be some association between somatisation and trauma. For example, when 28 patients with irritable bowel syndrome were compared with 19 with demonstrable inflammatory bowel disease, 32% of the former compared with none of the latter had a history of severe sexual trauma (Walker *et al.*, 1993). In a larger study of anxiety disorders 654 subjects were involved. Of these, 5.5% had a lifetime history of somatoform disorder which is probably about ten times the usually expected rate. This group with a history of somatisation were also more likely to have had a history of PTSD (Rogers *et al.*, 1996). In addition, GAD was associated with higher rates of somatisation than other disorders.

Schottenfeld has written a number of papers looking at the psychological effects of occupational trauma on workers, particularly of chemical exposure. He has suggested that those with PTSD can be differentiated from those with somatoform disorders (Schottenfeld and Cullen, 1986). However, although he suggests that PTSD patients may recover and somatisers tend not to do so, he also indicates that there is an atypical form of PTSD which presents with somatisation (Schottenfeld and Cullen, 1985).

A potentially contentious area centres around cultural or racial issues and somatisation and PTI. This is not the place to explore the arguments about whether psychological problems present more commonly with physical rather than emotional or affective symptoms in some cultures which use models of health and health care other than a Western bio-medical model. However, a number of investigators have implied or stated that physical presentations of PTI occur more often in other cultures. For example, in a study of South East Asian refugees in America it was stated (Mattson, 1993) that PTSD presented itself in physical complaints 'because of a cultural tradition of somatisation of mental problems'. Similar suggestions have been made for a wide range of other nationalities. For example, it has been stated that in Nicaraguan survivors of a low intensity war the rates of psychological 'caseness' (albeit only as measured by the GHQ) were 62% for men and 91% for women, with somatisation being predominant. In Central American refugees coming to America for reasons other than financial migration (Cervantes, Salgado and Padilla, 1989), somatisation was strongly correlated with PTSD. Sri Lankan civilians showed a rate of somatisation of 41% (Somasundaram and Sivayokan, 1994), higher than that for PTSD.

Dissociative disorders

The dissociative disorders form a specific group in DSM-IV and also in ICD-10 which includes essentially the same diagnostic categories of dissociative amnesia, dissociative fugue, depersonalisation disorder, and dissociative identity disorder. The first two were known in DSM-III as psychogenic states, and dissociative identity disorder was known as multiple personality disorder

(MPD). This last is a diagnosis which is not accepted in all parts of the world. Indeed, ICD-10 is more than a little sceptical, suggesting that it may be a factitious or iatrogenic disorder. It is generally not accepted in Britain and there has been little work done in Europe with the notable exception of a study of 71 multiple personality disorder patients in the Netherlands (Boon and Draijer, 1993), over 80% of whom were said to have PTSD. Proponents of dissociative identity disorder/multiple personality disorder have strongly refuted the 'sociocognitive' explanation which denies that this is a genuine significant disorder (Gleaves, 1996) and have strongly connected it with trauma. A Rorschach test investigation of 14 MPD patients (Armstrong, 1991) has suggested that there are lots of trauma-related features in MPD but that it can be separated from PTSD. However, many papers have linked MPD with PTSD, even suggesting that the one is a form of the other (Passen, 1993; Murray, 1994).

There is a large number of papers considering dissociative symptoms in general and MPD in particular as a sequel of sexual abuse and assault (Young *et al.*, 1991; McElroy, 1992; LaPorta, 1992).

Consideration of the symptomatology of the specific PTIs of PTSD and acute stress disorder will show that each includes dissociative symptoms in the diagnostic criteria. Psychogenic or dissociative amnesia is one such symptom, and flashbacks are clearly dissociative states which can even involve complicated behaviours which could be described as dissociative fugues, as in the criminal case described by Bisson in the UK (Bisson, 1993). However, it should be noted that his report emphasises the view that such episodes may be over-emphasised or over-reported and are probably rare.

The presence of dissociative symptoms in the diagnostic criteria for PTSD means that it is hardly surprising that there is a general association of trauma and PTSD with dissociative symptoms (Classen, Koopman and Spiegel, 1993; Atchison and McFarlane, 1994). A large number of papers have reported either cases or series supporting the view that there is an excess of dissociative symptoms in Vietnam veterans, particularly those with chronic PTSD, and suggesting that both PTSD and MPD are post-traumatic illnesses (Spiegel, 1984; Brende, 1987; Young, 1987; McDougle and Southwick, 1990; Branscomb, 1991).

While it is clear that some of the symptoms described as dissociative are common after trauma, it is again pointed out that multiple personality disorder or dissociative identity disorder is not a concept or diagnosis in general use in Britain and many other parts of the world. If it is really as common after trauma as some of the American literature suggests, then this is hard to explain. It is not merely that another name is used, but the symptomatology is not seen even though many patients with PTSD, and many survivors of child sexual abuse, are seen.

Comorbidity

Before considering comorbidity or the concurrent occurrence of two or more mental disorders which can be described as post-traumatic illnesses in the same person, it is necessary to consider the concept of comorbidity in general.

DSM-IV, like DSM-III before it, is said to be atheoretical and free from a hierarchical structure. This is different from the approach in the older ICD-9 in which a hierarchical model was obvious and it was accepted that in the process of diagnosis one would attempt to give a single diagnosis as high up the hierarchy as was appropriate and, importantly, that it was possible for symptoms from a condition lower in the hierarchy to be present in addition. Thus additional 'neurotic' symptoms were considered consistent with a psychotic diagnosis but not vice versa. The DSM-III and DSM-IV atheoretical approach was different, without a hierarchical structure, and without any pressure to seek a single diagnosis to explain a patient's problems. With some specific exceptions, it was explicitly stated that it was appropriate to make multiple diagnoses at the same time, without a need to consider some diagnoses to be subordinate or secondary to another. A concept of multiple diagnoses has therefore become accepted and has been shown to be appropriate in many studies.

The Epidemiological Catchment Area studies have confirmed earlier beliefs (Boyd, 1984) that for a wide range of psychiatric disorders there is an increased risk of the presence of some other, co-existing, disorder. The ECA studies have shown that for all of the specific psychiatric disorders studied, sufferers are more likely to have some other psychiatric diagnosis in addition. The same is true for PTSD, and in general people with PTSD were twice as likely to have some other diagnosis as people without PTSD. The increased risk was present for a range of disorders, with obsessive-compulsive disorder being the most over-represented, followed by affective disorders, then anxiety disorders and antisocial personality, and then substance misuse disorders. Rates for schizophrenia, eating disorders, and cognitive impairment were not increased. Nearly 80% of those with full-blown PTSD had some other diagnosis.

This finding is not an isolated one. There is a large body of research into comorbidity with PTSD. There are a number of reviews (Davidson and Foa, 1991; Davidson *et al.*, 1991) and that of Keane (Keane and Wolfe, 1990) points out the importance of the diffuse nature of the PTSD constellation and the tendency for PTSD sufferers to endorse a wide range of symptoms.

There is evidence that children have increased rates of comorbid disorders with PTSD, usually being those generally recognised to be of onset in childhood (Goenjian *et al.*, 1995).

The 14-year follow up of Buffalo Creek survivors confirmed a high rate of comorbidity with PTSD (Green *et al.*, 1992), as seen with Vietnam veterans (Sierles *et al.*, 1986), but showed proportionately less dysthymia, substance abuse and antisocial personality disorder in this civilian disaster group.

Generally, schizophrenia has not been found to be more common as a comorbid diagnosis in those with PTSD than in patients with other psychiatric diagnoses (Hryvniak and Rosse 1989) and is not over-represented (Roszell, McFall and Malas, 1991).

Most relevant studies have associated substance abuse with PTSD, particularly in Vietnam veterans (Boudewyns *et al.*, 1991; Brady *et al.*, 1994; Brown and Wolfe, 1994; Polles and Smith, 1995).

Summary

The majority of those exposed to trauma will make a good recovery and, while they will inevitably be affected by their experience, will not develop significant mental disorder. Of those who do, by no means all will have PTSD and it is important that the appropriate diagnosis is made if help is to be offered appropriately. It should not be assumed that just because somebody has suffered a catastrophic stressor all of their problems in the immediate or distant future should be attributed to it. At the same time it is important that the possible significance of such events should not be ignored, any more than other relevant features of the history.

A relatively new diagnostic category in both classificatory systems is acute stress disorder. The importance of this is probably as much in its indication of the possibility of future problems as in its own presentation. A significant number of people will suffer a mixture of anxiety and dissociative symptoms in the immediate aftermath of trauma. Some of these will request, and/or benefit from, brief interventions. Most will then recover, but some will go on to develop chronic PTI. Acute stress disorder is a sensitive but not very specific indicator of future PTI.

DSM-IV did not include the new category of DESNOS whereas ICD-10 did include enduring personality change. It does seem that a small number of people go on to have permanent personality change following major trauma. However, there is a virtual absence of empirical research and this should be a future focus as, if such people can be identified in advance, this may tell a great deal about the effects of stress and about vulnerabilities. The disadvantage of such a diagnosis is the possible associated therapeutic nihilism.

Adjustment disorders differ from defined PTI in that they can follow a much wider range of life events without specific intensity or meaning. They tend to be a sort of catch-all for those who have some form of psychological disorder which is not clearly defined and are therefore likely to be a heterogeneous group.

When defining the role of a traumatic event in causation of illness, useful factors include timing, course and content of the disorder. In addition, it is possible that trauma may not specifically cause an illness but may bring it forward, may aggravate it, or may extend it.

Substance misuse has been repeatedly associated with trauma. Many people use depressant substances, in particular in self-medication, for painful psychological symptoms. There is also suggestion that those with a history of substance misuse are more likely to develop PTI and, of course, those with substance misuse problems may arguably be considered to be more likely to be exposed to potentially dangerous or traumatic incidents. Substance misuse is a common comorbid diagnosis.

There is no reliable evidence that schizophrenia can be considered to be a post-traumatic illness or that it is a common comorbid diagnosis with PTSD. There is interest, however, in the idea that this traumatic illness in itself can be a qualifying stressor for PTSD.

The link between affective disorders and trauma is strong, and clearly predates the definition of PTSD. The role of bereavement and grief should not be ignored. Affective disorders are also common comorbid diagnoses with PTSD as well as representing PTI in themselves.

As PTSD and acute stress disorder are classified in DSM-IV as anxiety disorders, it is hardly surprising that almost all anxiety disorders are seen as being common sequelae of trauma and that there is significant comorbidity.

Somatoform disorders have been found to be more common in some groups of victims of trauma than in others. In previous widespread traumatic events such as the stresses of the First World War, frank hysterical presentations were common, but this has been much less so in recent conflicts. Some papers show apparent excess of somatisation problems in survivors from groups who use traditional systems other than those of Western biomedicine.

Dissociative disorders, like anxiety symptoms, are included in the diagnostic criteria for PTSD. An overlap or association is therefore to be expected. However, the very commonly reported association of extremely high rates of PTSD in patients with dissociative identity disorder are inevitably at variance with observations in Britain, where the latter is generally not accepted as a valid concept.

It is accepted that the majority of those with PTSD will have at least one other, comorbid, diagnosis. This is an interesting concept. While it is accepted that in the atheoretical approach of DSM-IV multiple diagnoses are common, the rates in PTSD are very high indeed. It may be that there is more work yet to be done about the boundaries of PTSD and about the overlap of symptoms which can be present in this and in other disorders. This links in with some of the work suggesting that PTSD sufferers endorse a wide range of symptoms and have high scores on clinical scales of instruments such as the MMPI.

References

American Psychiatric Association (1994). *Diagnostic and Statistical Manual of Mental Disorders*, 4th edition. Washington: APA.

Andreasen, N. (1995). Posttraumatic stress disorder: psychology, biology, and the manichaean warfare between false dichotomies. Editorial. *American Journal of Psychiatry*, **152**, 7: 963–5.

Armstrong, J. (1991). The psychological organization of multiple personality disordered patients as revealed in psychological testing. *Psychiatric Clinics of North America*, **14**, 3: 533–46.

Atchison, M. and McFarlane, A.C. (1994). A review of dissociation and dissociative disorders. *Australian and New Zealand Journal of Psychiatry*, **28**, 4: 591–9.

Bisson, J.I. (1993). Automatism and post-traumatic stress disorder. *British Journal of Psychiatry*, **163**: 830–32.

Blanchard, E.B., Hickling, E.J., Taylor, A.E. and Loos, W. (1995). Psychiatric morbidity associated with motor vehicle accidents. *Journal of Nervous and Mental Disease*, **183**, 8: 495–504.

Blanchard, E.B., Hickling, E.J., Taylor, A.E., Loos, W.R. and Gerardi, R.J. (1994). Psychological morbidity associated with motor vehicle accidents. *Behaviour Research and Therapy*. **32**, 3: 283–90.

Boon, S. and Draijer, N. (1993). Multiple personality disorder in the Netherlands: A clinical investigation of 71 patients. *American Journal of Psychiatry*, **150**, 3: 489–94.

Boudewyns, P.A., Woods, M.G., Hyer, L. and Albrecht, J.W. (1991). Chronic combat-related PTSD and concurrent substance abuse: Implications for treatment of this frequent 'dual diagnosis'. *Journal of Traumatic Stress*, **4**, 4: 549–60.

Boyd, J.H. (1984). Exclusion criteria of DSM-III: a study of co-occurrence of hierarchy-free syndromes. *Archives of General Psychiatry*, **41**: 983–9.

Brady, K.T., Killeen, T., Saladin, M.E., Dansky, B. and Saunders, B.E. (1994). Comorbid substance abuse and posttraumatic stress disorder: Characteristics of women in treatment. *American Journal on Addictions*, **3**, 2: 160–64.

Branscomb, L.P. (1991). Dissociation in combat-related post-traumatic stress disorder. *Dissociation: Progress in the Dissociative Disorders*, **4**, 1: 13–20.

Brende, J.O. (1987). Dissociative disorders in Vietnam combat veterans. *Journal of Contemporary Psychotherapy*, **17**, 2: 77–86.

Brent, D.A.C.R., Perper, J., Moritz, G., Allman, C., Liotus, L.S.J.R.C. and Balach, L. (1993). Bereavement or depression? The impact of the loss of a friend to suicide. *Journal of the American Academy of Child and Adolescent Psychiatry*, **32**, 6: 1189–98.

Brent, D.A., Perper, J.A., Moritz, G., Liotus, L., Schweers, J. and Canobbio, R. (1994). Major depression or uncomplicated bereavement? A follow up of youth exposed to suicide. *Journal of the American Academy of Child and Adolescent Psychiatry*, **33**, 2: 231–40.

Brett, E. A. (1993). Classification of PTSD in DSM-IV: anxiety disorder, dissociative disorder, or stress disorder. *In PTSD: DSM-IV and Beyond*, pp. 191–206. Ed. J. R. Davidson and E. B. Foa. Washington: American Psychiatric Press.

Brom, D. and Witztum, E. (1992). Recent trauma in psychiatric outpatients. *American Journal of Orthopsychiatry*, **62**, 4: 545–51.

Brown, P.J. and Wolfe, J. (1994). Substance abuse and post-traumatic stress disorder comorbidity. *Drug and Alcohol Dependence*, **35**, 1: 51–9.

Bryant, R.A. and Harvey, A.G. (1995). Processing threatening information in post-traumatic stress disorder. *Journal of Abnormal Psychology*, **104**, 3: 537–41.

Can life really drive you mad? Body and mind. (1994). *The Times*, London. 13 April.

Cardena, E. and Spiegel, D. (1993). Dissociative reactions to the San Francisco Bay Area earthquake of 1989. *American Journal of Psychiatry*, **150**, 3: 474–8.

Cervantes, R.C., Salgado, de S.V.N. and Padilla, A.M. (1989). Posttraumatic stress in immigrants from Central America and Mexico. *Hospital and Community Psychiatry*, **40**, 6: 615–19.

Classen, C., Koopman, C. and Spiegel, D. (1993). Trauma and dissociation. *Bulletin of the Menninger Clinic*, **57**, 2: 178–94.

Darves, B.J.M., Benhamou, A.P., Degiovanni, A. and Lepine, J.P.G.P. (1995). Psychological trauma and mental disorders. *Annales Medico-Psychologiques*, **153**, 1: 77–81.

Davidson, J.R. and Foa, E.B. (1991). Diagnostic issues in posttraumatic stress disorder: Considerations for the DSM-IV. Special issue: Diagnoses, dimensions, and DSM-IV: The science of classification. *Journal of Abnormal Psychology*, **100**, 3: 346–55.

Davidson, J.R., Hughes, D., Blazer, D.G. and George, L.K. (1991). Post-traumatic stress disorder in the community: An epidemiological study. *Psychological Medicine*, **21**, 3: 713–21.

Davis, W., Bauer, M., Severno, S. and Spiegel, D. (1993). DSM-IV in progress. MacArthur Data Reanalyses: Examples from the 2nd Stage of Empirical Review. *Hospital and Community Psychiatry*, **44** (5): 432–4.

De Mol, J., Retif, J. and Aerens, C. (1981). Post-traumatic conversion hysteria. A case report of hysterical paraplegia. *Acta Psychiatrica Belgica*, **81**, 1: 46–56.

Durkin, M.E. (1993). Major depression and post traumatic stress disorder following the Coalinga and Chile Earthquakes; a cross cultural comparison. *Journal of Social Behavior and Personality*, **8**: 5.

Eberly, R.E. and Engdahl, B.E. (1991). Prevalence of somatic and psychiatric disorders among former prisoners of war. *Hospital and Community Psychiatry*, **42**, 8: 807–13.

Farmer, R., Tranah, T., O. Donnell I. and Catalan, J. (1992). Railway suicide: the psychological effects on drivers. *Psychological Medicine*, **22**, 2: 407–14.

Feinstein, A. (1989). Posttraumatic stress disorder: A descriptive study supporting DSM-III–R criteria. *American Journal of Psychiatry*, **146**, 5: 665–6.

Gleason, W.J. (1993). Mental disorders in battered women: An empirical study. *Violence and Victims*, **8**, 1: 53–68.

Gleaves, D.H. (1996). The sociocognitive model of dissociative identity disorder: a reexamination of the evidence. [Review]. *Psychological Bulletin*, **120**, 1: 42–59.

Goenjian, A.K., Pynoos, R.S., Steinberg, A.M., Najarian, L.M., Asarnow, J.R., Karayan, I., Ghurabi, M. and Fairbanks, L.A. (1995). Psychiatric comorbidity in children after the 1988 earthquake in Armenia. *Journal of the American Academy of Child and Adolescent Psychiatry*, **34**, 9: 1174–84.

Graziano, R. (1992). Treating women incest survivors: A bridge between 'cumulative trauma' and 'post-traumatic stress,'. *Social Work in Health Care*, **17**, 1: 69–85.

Green, B.L., Grace, M.C., Lindy, J.D., Gleser, G.C. and Leonard, A. (1990a). Risk factors for PTSD and other diagnoses in a general sample of Vietnam veterans. *American Journal of Psychiatry*, **147**, 6: 729–33.

Green, B.L., Lindy, J.D., Grace, M.C., Gleser, G.C., Leonard, A.C., Korol, M. and Winget, C.l. (1990b). Buffalo Creek survivors in the second decade: Stability of stress symptoms. *American Journal of Orthopsychiatry*, **60**, 1: 43–54.

Green, B.L., Lindy, J.D., Grace, M.C. and Leonard, A.C. (1992). Chronic posttraumatic stress disorder and diagnostic comorbidity in a disaster sample. *Journal of Nervous and Mental Disease*. **180**, 12: 760–66.

Gurian, B.S., Wexler, D. and Baker, E.H. (1992). Late life paranoia: possible association with early trauma and infertility. *International Journal of Geriatric Psychiatry*, **7**, 4: 277–84.

Hanson, R.K. (1990). The psychological impact of sexual assault on women and children: A review. *Annals of Sex Research*, **3**, 2: 187–232.

Herman, J.L. (1992). Complex PTSD syndrome in survivors of prolonged and repeated trauma. *Journal of Traumatic Stress*, **5**: 3.

Herrmann, N. and Eryavec, G. (1994). Delayed onset PTSD in World War II veterans. *Canadian Journal of Psychiatry*, **39**, 7: 439–41.

Hickling, E.J. and Blanchard, E.B. (1992). Post-traumatic stress disorder and motor vehicle accidents. *Journal of Anxiety Disorders*, **6**, 3: 285–91.

Hinde, S. (1994). Old soldiers crack after D Day hype. (Anxiety disorder in D Day veterans). *The Sunday Times*, 6 November.

Hinton, W.L., Chen, Y.J., Du, N. and Tran, C.G. (1993). DSM-III–R disorders in Vietnamese refugees: Prevalence and correlates. *Journal of Nervous and Mental Disease*, **181**, 2: 113–22.

Hryvniak, M.R. and Rosse, R.B. (1989). Concurrent psychiatric illness in inpatients with post-traumatic stress disorder. *Military Medicine*, **154**, 8: 399–401.

Hyer, L., Leach, P., Boudewyns, P. and Davis, H. (1991). Hidden PTSD in substance abuse inpatients among Vietnam veterans. *Journal of Substance Abuse Treatment*, **8**, 4: 213–19.

Jelinek, J.M. and Williams, T. (1984). Post-traumatic stress disorder and substance abuse in Vietnam combat veterans: Treatment problems, strategies and recommendations. *Journal of Substance Abuse Treatment*, **1**, 2: 87–97.

Joseph, S., Yule, W., Williams, R. and Hodgkinson, P. (1993). Increased substance use in survivors of the Herald of Free Enterprise disaster. *British Journal of Medical Psychology*, **66**, 2: 185–91.

Keane, T.M. and Wolfe, J. (1990). Comorbidity in post-traumatic stress disorder: An analysis of community and clinical studies. Special issues: Traumatic stress: New perspectives in theory, measurement, and research: II. Research findings. *Journal of Applied Social Psychology*, **20**: 1776–88.

Koopman, C., Classen, C., Cardena, E. and Spiegel, D. (1995). When disaster strikes, acute stress disorder may follow. *Journal of Traumatic Stress*, **8**, 1: 29–46.

Koopman, C., Classen, C. and Spiegel, D.A. (1994). Predictors of posttraumatic stress symptoms among survivors of the Oakland/Berkeley, California, firestorm. *American Journal of Psychiatry*, **151**, 6: 888–94.

Kuch, K., Evans, R.J., Watson, P.C. and Bubela, C. (1991). Road vehicle accidents and phobias in 60 patients with fibromyalgia. *Journal of Anxiety Disorders*, **5**, 3: 273–80.

LaPorta, L. (1992). Childhood trauma and multiple personality disorder: the case of a 9-year-old girl. *Child Abuse and Neglect*, **16**, 4: 615–20.

Lim, L. (1991). Delayed emergence of post-traumatic stress disorder. *Singapore Medical Journal*, **32**, 1: 92–3.

Lundy, M.S. (1992). Psychosis-induced posttraumatic stress disorder. *American Journal of Psychotherapy*, **46**, 3: 485–91.

Marchevsky, S. and Baram, E. (1992). Is a diagnosis of occupational post-traumatic schizophrenia possible? *Medicine and Law*, **11**, 1–2: 127–36.

Marmar, C.R., Weiss, D.S., Schlenger, W.E., Fairbank, J.A., Jordan, B.K., Kulka, R.A. and Hough, R.L. (1994). Peritraumatic dissociation and posttraumatic stress in male Vietnam theater veterans. *American Journal of Psychiatry*, **151**, 6: 902–7.

Mattson, S. (1993). Mental health of Southeast Asian refugee women: An overview. *Health Care for Women International*, **14**, 2: 155–65.

McDougle, C.J. and Southwick, S.M. (1990). Emergence of an alternate personality in combat-related posttraumatic stress disorder. *Hospital and Community Psychiatry*, **41**, 5: 554–6.

McElroy, L.P. (1992). Early indicators of pathological dissociation in sexually abused children. *Child Abuse and Neglect*, **16**, 6: 833–46.

McFarlane, A.C. and Papay, P. (1992). Multiple diagnoses in posttraumatic stress disorder in the victims of a natural disaster. *Journal of Nervous and Mental Disease*, **180**, 8: 498–504.

McGorry, P.D. (1991). Negative symptoms and PTSD. *Australian and New Zealand Journal of Psychiatry*, **25**, 1: 9–13.

McGorry, P.D. (1993). Posttraumatic stress disorder postpsychosis. *Journal of Nervous and Mental Disease*, **181**, 12: 766.

McGorry, P.D., Chanen, A., McCarthy, E., Van, R.R., McKenzie, D. and Singh, B. (1991). Posttraumatic stress disorder following recent onset psychosis: an unrecognized postpsychotic syndrome. *Journal of Nervous and Mental Disease*, **179**, 5: 253–9.

McGorry, P.D., McFarlane, C., Mihalopoulos, C., Henry, L., Harrigan, S., McKenzie, D., Cooper, J. and Herrmann, H.E. (1994). Post traumatic stress disorder following first episode psychosis: Prevalence and relationship to early negative symptomatology. *Schizophrenia Research*, **11**, 2: 185.

Mellman, T.A., Randolph, C.A., Brawman-Mintzer, O. and Flores, L.P. (1992). Phenomenology and course of psychiatric disorders associated with combat-related posttraumatic stress disorder. *American Journal of Psychiatry*, **149**, 11: 1568–74.

Mghir, R., Freed, W., Raskin, A. and Katon, W. (1995). Depression and posttraumatic stress disorder among a community sample of adolescent and young adult Afghan refugees. *Journal of Nervous and Mental Disease*, **183**, 1: 24–30.

Murray, J.B. (1994). Dimensions of multiple personality disorder. *Journal of Genetic Psychology*, **155**, 2: 233–47.

Orsillo, S.M., Weathers, F.W., Litz, B.T., Steinberg, H.R., Huska, J.A. and Keane, T.M. (1996). Current and lifetime psychiatric disorders among veterans with war zone-related posttraumatic stress disorder. *Journal of Nervous and Mental Disease*, **184**, 5: 307–13.

Palinkas, L., Petterson, J., Russell, J. and Downs, M. (1993). Community patterns of psychiatric disorders after the Exxon Valdez oil spill. *American Journal of Psychiatry*, **150**, 10: 1517–23.

Passen, C. (1993). PTSD, dissociative disorders, multiple personality disorders: diagnosis and treatment. *Journal of the American Institute of Homeopathy*, **86**, 2: 81–91.

Perez, J.J., Gomez, B.G., Lopez, C.J., Salvador-Robert, M. and Garcia, T.V. (1994). Psychiatric consultation and post-traumatic stress disorder in burned patients. *Burns*, **20**, 6: 532–36.

Pitman, R.K. (1993). Posttraumatic obsessive-compulsive disorder: A case study. *Comprehensive Psychiatry*, **34**, 2: 102–7.

Polles, A.G. and Smith, P.O. (1995). Treatment of coexisting substance dependence and posttramatic stress disorder. *Psychiatric Services*, **46**, 7: 729–30.

Pomerantz, A.S. (1991). Delayed onset of PTSD: delayed recognition or latent disorder? *American Journal of Psychiatry*, **149**, 11: 1609.

Rogers, M.P., Weinshenker, N.J., Warshaw, M.G., Goisman, R.M., Rodriguez-Villa, F.J., Fierman, E.J. and Keller, M.B. (1996). Prevalence of somatoform disorders in a large sample of patients with anxiety disorders. *Psychosomatics*, **37**, 1: 17–22.

Roszell, D.K., McFall, M.E. and Malas, K.L. (1991). Frequency of symptoms and concurrent psychiatric disorder in Vietnam veterans with chronic PTSD. *Hospital and Community Psychiatry*, **42**, 3: 293–6.

Rothbaum, B.O. and Foa, E.B. (1991). Exposure treatment of PTSD concomitant with conversion mutism: A case study. *Behavior Therapy*, **22**, 3: 449–56.

Saathoff, G.B. and Buckman, J. (1990). Diagnostic results of psychiatric evaluations of state police officers. *Hospital and Community Psychiatry*, **41**, 4: 429–32.

Saunders, B.E., Villeponteaux, L.A., Lipovsky, J. and Kilpatrick, D.G. (1992). Child sexual assault as a risk factor for mental disorders among women: A community survey. *Journal of Interpersonal Violence*, **7**, 2: 189–204.

Schottenfeld, R.S. and Cullen, M.R. (1985). Occupation-induced posttraumatic stress disorders. *American Journal of Psychiatry*, **142**, 2: 198–202.

Schottenfeld, R.S. and Cullen, M.R. (1986). Recognition of occupation induced post-traumatic stress disorders. *Journal of Occupational Medicine*, **28**, 5: 365–9.

Shalev, A.Y., Peri, T., Canetti, L. and Schreiber, S. (1996). Predictors of PTSD in injured trauma survivors: a prospective study. *American Journal of Psychiatry*, **153**, 2: 219–25.

Shaner, A. and Eth, S. (1989). Can schizophrenia cause posttraumatic stress disorder? *American Journal of Psychotherapy*, **43**, 4: 588–97.

Sharan, P., Chaudhary, G., Kavathekar, S.A. and Saxena, S. (1996). Preliminary report of psychiatric disorders in survivors of a severe earthquake. *American Journal of Psychiatry*, **153**, 4: 556–8.

Shore, J.H., Vollmer, W.M. and Tatum, E.L. (1989). Community patterns of post-traumatic stress disorders. *Journal of Nervous and Mental Disease*, **177**, 11: 681–5.

Sierles, F.S., Chen, J., Messing, M., Besyner, J. and Taylor M.B. (1986). Concurrent psychiatric illness in non-Hispanic outpatients diagnosed as having posttraumatic stress disorder. *Journal of Nervous and Mental Disease*, **174**, 3: 171–3.

Smith, P. and Gittelman, D. (1994). Psychological consequences of battering. Implications for women's health and medical practice. *North Carolina Medical Journal*, **55**, 9: 434–9.

Solomon, Z., Kotler, M., Shalev, A. and Lin, R. (1989). Delayed onset of PTSD among Israeli veterans of the 1982 Lebanon War. *Psychiatry Interpersonal and Biological Processes*, **52**, 4: 428–37.

Somasundaram, D.J. and Sivayokan, S. (1994). War trauma in a civilian population. *British Journal of Psychiatry*, **165**: 524–7.

Spiegel, D. (1984). Multiple personality as a post-traumatic stress disorder. *Psychiatric Clinics of North America*, **7**, 1: 101–10.

Spurrell, M.T. and McFarlane, A.C. (1993). Post-traumatic stress disorder and coping after a natural disaster. *Social Psychiatry and Psychiatric Epidemiology*, **28**, 4: 194–200.

Tranah, T. and Farmer, R.D. (1994). Psychological reactions of drivers to railway suicide. *Social Sciences Medicine*, **38**, 3: 459–69.

Van der Hart, O., Witztum, E. and Friedman, B. (1993). From hysterical psychosis to reactive dissociative psychosis. *Journal of Traumatic Stress*, **6**, 1: 43–64.

Van Putten, T. and Emory, W.H. (1973). Traumatic neuroses in Vietnam returnees. A forgotten diagnosis? *Archives of General Psychiatry*, **29**, 5: 695–8.

Walker, E.A., Katon, W.J., Roy Byrne, P.P., Jemelka, R.P. and Russo, J. (1993). Histories of sexual victimization in patients with irritable bowel syndrome or inflammatory bowel disease. *American Journal of Psychiatry*, **150**, 10: 1502–6.

Williams-Keeler, L., Milliken, H. and Jones, B. (1994). Psychosis as precipitating trauma for PTSD: A treatment strategy. *American Journal of Orthopsychiatry*, **64**, 3: 493–8.

World Health Organisation (1992). *International Classification of Diseases*, 10th edition. Geneva: WHO.

Worzel, M.A. (1992). Pilot study to validate criteria for proposed new DSM IV category: Disorders of extreme stress not otherwise specified (DESNOS). *Dissertation Abstracts International*, **52**, 9–B: 4991–2.

Yaktin, U., and Labban, S. (1992). Traumatic war. Stress and schizophrenia. *Journal of Psychosocial Nursing and Mental Health Services*, **30**, 6: 29–33.

Young, W.C. (1987). Emergence of a multiple personality in a posttraumatic stress disorder of adulthood. *American Journal of Clinical Hypnosis*, **29**, 4: 249–54.

Young, W.C., Sachs, R.G., Braun, B.G. and Watkins, R.T. (1991). Patients reporting ritual abuse in childhood: a clinical syndrome. Report of 37 cases. *Child Abuse and Neglect*, **15**, 3: 181–90.

Zlotnick, C., Zakriski, A.L., Shea, M.T., Costello, E., Begin, A., Pearlstein, T. and Simpson, E. (1996). The long-term sequelae of sexual abuse: support for a complex posttraumatic stress disorder. *Journal of Traumatic Stress*, **9**, 2: 195–205.

Zweben, J.E., Clark, H.W. and Smith, D.E. (1994). Traumatic experiences and substance abuse: Mapping the territory. *Journal of Psychoactive Drugs*, **26**, 4: 327–44.

CHAPTER 7

DIAGNOSIS AND ASSESSMENT

What is the purpose of diagnosis?

It is important to consider the reason for making a diagnosis. For many mental disorders the reasons for making a diagnosis are quite transparent. Diagnosis can be considered to serve three main purposes:

- to ease communication by allowing a shorthand way of describing a particular sort of problem or set of clinical findings
- to allow predictions to be made about likely course
- to allow rational treatment, management and allocation of services.

Even when the primary focus of concern is not service allocation, the making of a diagnosis usually has the same significance. For example, in a forensic psychiatric setting, the diagnosis of schizophrenia says something about the condition, the likely course, and the likely response to treatment. It does not, per se, say anything about responsibility for the particular act or omission under consideration or about the cause of the illness.

This is not the case in PTSD. The diagnosis itself defines aetiology. By the nature of the aetiologically significant events, this also usually identifies a person or organisation which is allegedly responsible for causing, or failing to prevent, the disorder. The diagnosis of PTSD not only provides a useful shorthand, makes predictions about course, and suggests likely management options, but it also acts as a key.

This key can provide access to a variety of doors and resources.

- It may allow previously denied access to treatment services, for example through the Veterans Administration system in the USA and elsewhere, or through access to Ministry of Defence medical services in the UK.

- It may allow access to financial and social support such as that provided for veterans in the USA. There has been suggestion over the years that the Veterans Administration system is such that there is a positive pressure for veterans to be diagnosed as sick because they are then entitled to a range of social and financial benefits.
- It may confirm that an illness state is attributable to employment and therefore give access to enhanced pension rights and benefits.
- It may be used as the evidence for nervous shock and therefore damages leading to compensation at law.
- It may be used as mitigation, or even occasionally to excuse, behaviours frowned upon by society.

It is suggested that these additional common features of a diagnosis of PTI or PTSD in particular mean that there may be particular pitfalls in making the diagnosis of PTSD which are associated with the potential patient's positive motivation to receive a diagnosis. It is an unusual situation, but it is certainly possible that patients presenting may actually want to be diagnosed as having PTSD when it is perhaps uncommon for them to want to be diagnosed as having some other psychiatric illness.

It is therefore more than usually important that diagnoses of PTI be reliable.

What are the dangers of an incorrect diagnosis?

There are three possible ways to fail in the diagnostic process:

1. to fail to make a diagnosis when a condition is present
2. to make a diagnosis when no condition is present
3. to make the wrong diagnosis.

Failure to diagnose

Obviously, if a health professional fails to uncover a significant clinical condition of any sort, the potential patient will probably suffer and may be in danger of their life.

This is by no means specific to mental health, but there is a long history of suggestions that mental health problems are underdiagnosed. There are a number of reasons for this.

- Sufferers may simply fail to notice that anything is wrong.
- They may not realise that what is wrong is an illness or a health matter.
- By reason of public opinion, stigma, guilt, or shame:
  - they may not decide to seek help
  - they may not actually present their problems to a professional
  - the professional may not recognise or seek the relevant signs and symptoms
  - the sufferer may consciously conceal symptoms or actively avoid help.

There is a considerable literature looking at the dangers of missing a diagnosis of PTSD or of underdiagnosis. It is suggested that by its very nature, PTSD is likely to be underdiagnosed. The hypothesis is that in addition to all the factors which interfere with recognition of other mental health problems, one of the particular constellations of PTSD symptoms – in fact the only specific group, that of avoidance phenomena – may actively prevent help-seeking or even admission of problems.

Of course it is important to use a degree of common sense in this area. The sort of question to which any sort of answer has the same meaning must be avoided. In the throes of therapeutic vigour, there is a possibility that it might be suggested that all those who admit to PTSD symptoms have PTSD, while all those who do not are either in denial or their avoidant symptoms are overwhelming! For example, if a person has no clear memory of a theoretically traumatic event 20 years ago, is this necessarily evidence of psychogenic amnesia, an avoidance symptom, or is it just possible that they have forgotten because they are well and the trauma is just something in the past?

Blank (1994) produced a long review article on the detection and differential diagnosis of PTSD in 1994. It is written from the basic assumption that PTSD will be underdiagnosed and under-reported, so that it is necessary to search for and detect symptoms which will not be volunteered. He gives great detail about techniques and skills needed to make sufferers report their symptoms, but makes no reference at all to the possibility that some may actually manufacture or exaggerate problems. He gives a detailed account of differentiation between PTSD and other mental health diagnoses. However, in the main this looks at ways in which PTSD may be misdiagnosed as something else rather than at the possibility that something else may be misdiagnosed as PTSD.

Some of the factors which are listed as possibly interfering with diagnosis include:

- level of clinician empathy and rapport
- pain felt by the clinician on discussing horrific incidents

- psychodynamic, psychopathological, and defence features in the patient such as:
  - repression
  - dissociation
  - isolation of affect
  - partial amnesia
  - disguised dreams
  - holding in of traumatic memories
  - conflicts and impacted affects in the unconscious over time
  - symbolic expression of anxiety
  - identification with the aggressor
- patient embarrassment or shame
- the waxing and waning of symptoms over time
- latency before onset of symptoms
- fear of increased intensity of symptoms
- rational or irrational fear of reprisal or retribution.

Saunders *et al.* (Saunders, Arata and Kilpatrick, 1990) also believe that PTSD is underdiagnosed and have suggested that one of the reasons is that without specific enquiry, subjects are unlikely to report a history of being a victim of violent crime, and that the rate of such report doubles with use of a simple screening instrument. This last is probably important. It seems a reasonable addition to the normal psychiatric assessment interview to ask whether the patient has ever been exposed to any significant traumatic event and if any such event is an ongoing cause of concern.

Weisaeth has produced a series of papers looking at the employees of a factory which was severely damaged by fire (Weisaeth, 1989a, 1989b 1989c). He has suggested that those with greatest exposure are most resistant to enquiry about their status and also most likely to be ill. This means that response rates are important in obtaining true prevalence rates. This may well be true, but in clinical terms a refusal or reluctance to take part in a research project may not necessarily have bearing upon a decision about whether or not to seek help for distress or disability.

Making a diagnosis in the absence of disability or illness

Not surprisingly, this concept has been little studied. The search for people who have been diagnosed as suffering from PTSD when they do not actually have the condition is not an area likely to appeal to those interested in PTSD.

The dangers of making a diagnosis of PTSD when none exists are not as obvious as those of failing to make the diagnosis. The potential loss to third parties or society can be fairly easily recognised when one considers the possibility of motivated faking of PTSD. However, there may be potential damage to the alleged sufferer as well. A diagnosis of PTSD may bring with it the idea that the problem does not belong to the subject but is outwith his control. Clinical observation suggests that in some cases such a diagnosis may serve the purpose of excusing as well as explaining a subject's life difficulties in a way which does not lead him to feel that he has responsibility for change. It is somebody else's fault, outside his control, and not his responsibility. It is not suggested that this response is common, but it is possible that an erroneous diagnosis of PTSD may actually do harm rather than good.

There have been anecdotal references to the issue of incorrect diagnosis. Neal (Lillywhite and Neal, 1993) commented upon a case report by Spector (Spector and Huthwaite, 1993), and pointed out the need to ensure that the traumatic event was a qualifying one before making a diagnosis of PTSD. In the face of the spread of the application of the diagnosis of PTSD to the consequences of an ever-wider range of events, the need only to apply a diagnosis of PTSD to people following major trauma has been reinforced elsewhere (Lees-Haley, 1986)

LaGuardia et al. (1983) suggested that the 'set' or attitude and expectation of investigators might influence the rate of diagnosis of PTI in studies, while it was suggested that a positive rate of 86% in survivors of the Aleutian Enterprise sinking who sought compensation (Rosen, 1995) represented 'advice' from their legal representatives and symptom sharing.

A number of authors have referred to the observation that the courts' reliance on PTSD as being virtually equivalent to nervous shock has led to problems of 'stretching' the clinical criteria of PTSD markedly to make subjects fit the picture demanded by the courts, and to inappropriate diagnoses being made (Sparr, 1995).

More interest has been shown in the issue of malingering or factitious PTSD, and the incorrect allocation of a diagnosis of PTSD following active effort by the subject.

The general assumption of clinicians is that patients will honestly represent their problems because they have come along to seek help. Certainly, illness and preconceptions may interfere with the process, but the expectation is that the patient will not attempt to deceive. This is probably generally the case, but, as has already been noted, there may be additional consequences of a diagnosis of PTSD which can influence the patient. This is obviously more significant when the diagnosis is to be made in a legal or non-clinical setting. It is important to remember that there is no pathognomonic test for PTSD, and that *none* of the tests used was developed or initially validated in an adversarial setting.

There have been individual case reports (Salloway, Southwick and Sadowsky, 1990; Neal and Rose, 1995) of people simulating PTSD for gain such as hospitalisation, opiates or compensation. In addition, there have been one or two short series of cases of such presentations(Sparr and Pankratz, 1983), including one of seven help-seeking veterans who had not been to Vietnam (Lynn and Belza, 1984).

Perhaps most disturbingly, there is evidence from an admittedly very small number of cases that factitious PTSD may be used, perhaps successfully, as a defence against the charge of murder. Two cases (Sparr and Atkinson, 1986) highlight the need for verification of facts in such circumstances.

Applying the wrong diagnosis

It is hopefully clear from earlier chapters that not only is it true that the majority of people exposed to trauma do not develop PTI, but that not all PTI is PTSD. It has already been pointed out that there is a danger that in the legal setting there is potential pressure to make the diagnosis of PTSD fit. However, in addition, there may be a tendency for clinicians to make the assumption that mental illness following trauma is necessarily PTSD. This is not the case.

There is no systematic study of the possibility of diagnosing another condition as PTSD. As noted above, what emphasis there has been is in the other direction, looking at the possibility of diagnosing PTSD as almost any other psychiatric condition.

DSM permits, if not encourages, the application of as many diagnoses as are appropriate, and this seems helpful. If a person develops a specific phobia following trauma but is diagnosed as PTSD, then they may not receive appropriate treatment. On the other hand, if they are diagnosed as having both PTSD and specific phobia, then they will presumably receive treatment appropriate for the specific phobia. It is therefore of concern that some authors such as Blank (1994) counsel against multiple diagnoses and urge clinicians to consider whether other symptoms might be explained by PTSD.

In addition to the possibility that diagnosis of PTSD rather than some other PTI or unrelated mental disorder may interfere with the provision of treatment, there is another, less obvious, danger.

Patients often search for meaning in illness and this is well recognised. If an illness is explained as PTSD rather than some other diagnosis, it may have an effect upon the patient which is specific to this condition. PTSD is seen as a direct consequence of abnormal events, a condition which can occur in normal individuals, and something outside the individual's control. In many instances it is someone else's fault.

This can have an effect on those diagnosed of 'justifying' their disability and also setting it up as something outside for which they should not take responsibility. This can interfere with the patient's effort at recovery and reinforce disability. Obviously, this is particularly unfortunate if the diagnosis is not PTSD, as not only may the patient's motivation to recover and to take responsibility for their health be affected, but they may not receive the most appropriate treatment.

Diagnostic methods

Obviously the methods used to make a diagnosis will vary according to the situation. Different techniques will be used in community studies, in clinical situations, in diagnostic and aetiological research, in clinical research, in benefit assessments, in civil medicolegal situations, and in forensic cases.

Some possible methods include:

- symptom recognition instruments
- clinical diagnostic interview
- structured interview
- psychometric tests
- pathological tests
- physiological tests
- multimodal assessments.

Diagnosis of PTI other than PTSD

There is no intention to detail the diagnostic methodology for the wide range of mental disorders which can sometimes present as PTI. Readers are referred to texts on the individual conditions.

The method of diagnosing PTSD will be considered in detail because of the special significance of this diagnosis. A diagnosis of PTSD not only defines the disorder present, but also identifies the cause.

For other PTI, the diagnosis is a two-stage procedure. The condition will be identified using the diagnostic process generally adopted in clinical or research practice as appropriate. Some, but by no means all of the diagnostic procedures will be the same as those used in PTSD. However, the identification of a diagnosis in a person who has been exposed to trauma does not mean that a PTI is present, or that the condition diagnosed is a PTI. In recent years, studies have repeatedly shown that a history of trauma is common in community samples as well as help-seeking patients. Mental disorders are also common. It is likely that the two will co-exist without necessarily having a causal relationship in a significant number of cases.

There is no single pathognomonic feature which indicates that a condition constitutes a PTI other than PTSD.

Indicators which can be considered include:

- content of symptoms
- timing of symptoms
- varying intensity of symptoms
- patient perception.

No single factor is definitively indicative of PTI and it is necessary to come to an overall clinical opinion.

Content of symptoms

Symptoms may be coloured by the relevant traumatic event. For example, following a significant road traffic accident, a specific phobia of driving is likely to represent a PTI. Ruminations may be about the trauma. Depressive thought processes or psychotic delusional phenomena may refer to the event.

Timing of symptoms

If a person has never suffered psychological symptoms before and then develops problems in the immediate aftermath, there is at least a prima facie case that the one is related to the other. This is much less the case if a disorder develops or presents years later with no obvious further trigger or repetition.

Some patients develop anniversary reactions, as described in Chapter 6 where the recognition that mental disorders may be post-traumatic is discussed.

Not everybody with a PTI will have been free of previous mental disorder, which is possible, for example, for a person who suffers from a recurrent major depressive disorder which is attributable to trauma. One indicator of this would be a situation in which a patient suffered an episode of illness at a time when it was not expected or predicted by the prior course.

Intensity of symptoms

In patients who have a previous or pre-existing mental disorder, there may still be an element of PTI other than PTSD.

A marked deterioration in mental state soon after trauma is suggestive of a causative or aggravating effect.

Some patients have an episode of illness after trauma that is either more severe or longer lasting than previous episodes.

Patient perception

It is probable that less emphasis should be placed upon the patient's view of attribution than upon other factors. It is by no means suggested that the majority of patients would be intentionally misleading about the origin of illness. However, there is a normal human tendency to search for meaning and to look for causes or things to blame for problems.

In their search for an explanation for illness or difficulties, patients may even, in all honesty, blame traumatic events for problems which were clearly already present at the relevant time. Inappropriate diagnosis may be unhelpful or damaging and it is important that corroboration be sought where possible.

Diagnostic methods in PTSD

Symptom recognition instruments

By this is meant the various forms of instruments which list either the specific diagnostic symptoms of PTSD or a list of similar concepts, and ask potential sufferers to recognise or acknowledge their presence or absence in response to a prompt. The actual diagnostic criteria for DSM-IV PTSD and the diagnostic guidelines for ICD-10 PTSD are detailed in Table 7.1.

The symptom recognition instruments have the advantage of being simple and unambiguous. They also act as an aide memoire or prompt for the patient, and validate or legitimise symptoms of which the subject may be ashamed or which they may see as normal or deserved.

The disadvantages are similar. They delineate or suggest symptoms to which a subject need only agree. This is probably not a major problem for the majority of patients in a purely clinical setting where the only concern is provision of appropriate clinical management for a help-seeker. It may be a major problem when the situation is different or is less clear.

There are quite a large number of examples of this type of instrument. Some of them have been developed for particular projects and some have been more widely intended and used. There is no guarantee that those validated in a particular setting will be universally useful. A small number of such tools are described below.

Table 7.1. *Diagnostic criteria for PTSD*

A. The person has been exposed to a traumatic event in which both of the following were present:
1. the person experienced, witnessed, or was confronted with an event or events that involved actual or threatened death or serious injury, or a threat to the physical integrity of self or others
2. the person's response involved intense fear, helplessness, or horror. *Note.* In children, this may be expressed instead by disorganised or agitated behaviour.

B. The traumatic event is persistently re-experienced in one (or more) of the following ways:
1. recurrent and intrusive distressing recollections of the event, including images, thoughts, or perceptions. *Note.* In young children, repetitive play may occur in which themes or aspects of the trauma are expressed
2. recurrent distressing dreams of the event. *Note.* In children, there may be frightening dreams without recognisable content
3. acting or feeling as if the traumatic event were recurring (includes a sense of reliving the experience, illusions, hallucinations, and dissociative flashback episodes, including those that occur on awakening or when intoxicated). *Note.* In young children, trauma-specific re-enactment may occur
4. intense psychological distress at exposure to internal or external cues that symbolise or resemble an aspect of the traumatic event
5. physiological reactivity on exposure to internal or external cues that symbolise or resemble an aspect of the traumatic event.

C. Persistent avoidance of stimuli associated with the trauma and numbing of general responsiveness (not present before the trauma), as indicated by three (or more) of the following:
1. efforts to avoid thoughts, feelings or conversations associated with the trauma
2. efforts to avoid activities, places or people that arouse recollections of the trauma
3. inability to recall an important aspect of the trauma
4. markedly diminished interest or participation in significant activities
5. feeling of detachment or estrangement from others
6. restricted range of affect (e.g. unable to have loving feelings)
7. sense of a foreshortened future (e.g., does not expect to have a career, marriage, children, or a normal life span).

D. Persistent symptoms of increased arousal (not present before the trauma), as indicated by two (or more) of the following:
1. difficulty falling or staying asleep
2. irritability or outbursts of anger
3. difficulty concentrating
4. hypervigilance
5. exaggerated startle response.

Table 7.1. *(cont.)*

E. Duration of the disturbance (symptoms in Criteria B, C and D) is more than one month.

F. The disturbance causes clinically significant distress or impairment in social, occupational, or other important areas of functioning.
    Specify if:
        acute: if duration of symptoms is less than three months
        chronic: if duration of symptoms is three months or more.
    Specify if:
        with delayed onset: if onset of symptoms is at least six months after the stressor.

ICD-10 diagnostic guidelines for post-traumatic stress disorder
This disorder should not generally be diagnosed unless there is evidence that it arose within six months of a traumatic event of exceptional severity. A 'probable' diagnosis might still be possible if the delay between the event and the onset was longer than six months, provided that the clinical manifestations are typical and no alternative identification of the disorder (e.g. as an anxiety or obsessive-compulsive disorder or depressive episode) is plausible.

In addition to evidence of trauma, there must be a repetitive, intrusive recollection or re-enactment of the event in memories, daytime imagery, or dreams.

Conspicuous emotional detachment, numbing of feeling, and avoidance of stimuli that might arouse recollection of the trauma are often present but are not essential for the diagnosis.

The autonomic disturbances, mood disorder, and behavioural abnormalities all contribute to the diagnosis but are not of prime importance.

The late chronic sequelae of devastating stress, i.e. those manifest decades after the stressful experience, should be classified under F62.0.

Impact of Events Scale
Probably the best known and most widely used transparent measure of symptoms is the Impact of Events Scale (IES). This was actually developed by Horowitz (Horowitz, Wilner and Alvarez, 1979) before the publication of the definition of PTSD. However, it lists a series of intrusive and avoidance phenomena and produces a score for these two elements of the post-traumatic response. There are 15 items and they are clearly symptoms associated with the effect of a particular traumatic event. The subject marks a frequency of occurrence for each phenomenon from a pick-list of four.

The validity of the IES as an indicator of diagnosis of PTSD in the clinical setting has been investigated on a number of occasions (Horowitz *et al.*, 1980; Zilberg, Weiss and Horowitz, 1982; Schwarzwald *et al.*, 1987; Weisenberg *et al.*,

1987), and it has always been found to correlate highly with a clinical diagnosis of PTSD. It has been used in many research studies into PTSD (Maida *et al.*, 1989; Solomon, 1989; Neal *et al.*, 1994a; Koopman, Classen and Spiegel, 1994).

While Horowitz did initially suggest that the IES could be used over time to reflect individual change in scores and progress with treatment, he did not claim that scores could be used to reflect the severity of illness between subjects.

The Mississippi Scale for Combat-Related PTSD

Keane, Caddell and Taylor (1988) published a report of three linked studies into the Mississippi Scale for Combat-Related PTSD. This is a 35-item, self-report scale derived from DSM-III criteria. The aim of the studies was to explore the psychometric properties of the scale.

The scale was devised to identify Vietnam-related PTSD, and the subject groups reflect this. In the first study, 362 help-seeking Vietnam veterans confirmed the internal consistency of the instrument. They then demonstrated the high test–retest reliability of the instrument, and the third phase showed that the test's sensitivity was 0.93, specificity was 0.89, and overall hit rate was 0.90 when comparing Vietnam PTSD patients with two non-PTSD comparison groups.

Importantly, Keane pointed out that the test's usefulness lay within the context of a multi-axial approach to assess military-related PTSD. He did not see it as a stand-alone diagnostic tool.

The Mississippi Scale has been used in many studies and has also been used as one of the standards in the process of testing or validating other instruments and measures (Hammarberg, 1992; Hovens *et al.*, 1994).

In one study, 30 help-seekers without PTSD were asked to fake PTSD on the Mississippi Scale (Dalton *et al.*, 1989). Although they generally scored less than patients, 77% managed to score positive, and this is a reminder of the transparency of the instrument and need for other measures in addition.

A shorter form of the scale has been validated with Vietnam veterans (Hyer *et al.*, 1991; Fontana and Rosenheck, 1994). In addition, a civilian form has been developed (Vreven *et al.*, 1995), but studies show that this is of less value than the original used with Vietnam veterans and is a reminder that investigative findings may not generalise across different populations and different stressors.

PTSD Symptom Scale

Foa *et al.* (1993) looked at two versions of a PTSD Symptom Scale, the PSS. The scale contains 17 items according to DSM-IIIR criteria. The two versions are interview and self-report. Subjects were 46 recent rape and 72 non-sexual assault female victims. Both versions of the PSS had satisfactory internal consistency, high test–retest reliability, and good concurrent validity. Perhaps surprisingly, the self-report version of the PSS was more conservative than the interview version, with a lower sensitivity and 100% specificity. The positive predictive rates were 88% and 100% respectively. The comparator diagnostic method was the Structured Clinical Interview for DSM-IIIR. It is not clear whether this tool is useful in other settings.

Clinical diagnostic interview

This refers to the normal diagnostic interview conducted by a psychiatrist or other postgraduate specially trained mental health professional. In day-to-day clinical practice, this is the way in which most mental health diagnoses are made. There may or may not be additional tests or assessments which are used to aid in the diagnostic process.

While such interviews generally conform to a pattern, they are not specifically structured and there is a danger that decision making early in the process may lead to relevant information not being sought or identified as the interviewer narrows down the area of enquiry.

It is recognised that patients do not generally volunteer information about previous traumatic events for a range of reasons. It is therefore important that systematic enquiry be made.

In research situations, one of the problems of the standard clinical interview is that it does require a high degree of expertise, experience and specialist knowledge. Varying approaches are used across, and even within, professional disciplines. Because of the lack of structure, it is comparatively difficult to control reliability. It is generally not suitable for use by lay interviewers or what have been described as 'sub-professionals'.

The clinical interview is therefore most appropriately used in the clinical situation rather than in a research or adversarial setting.

Structured interview

There are a number of structured interviews which are used in the diagnosis and assessment of PTSD. Some of them are general diagnostic interviews used for a wide range of conditions. These have either been designed with PTSD in mind as one of the diagnoses likely to be considered or, more commonly, have a PTSD supplement added in. The other sort is the structured interview specifically designed and constructed for the diagnosis of PTSD alone.

Structured Clinical Interview for DSM-IIIR

The SCID was the structured interview used as the standard in the National Vietnam Veterans Readjustment Study (NVVRS), a congressionally mandated, large-scale American study (Kulka *et al.*, 1990; Jordan *et al.*, 1991; Weiss *et al.*, 1992; Schlenger *et al.*, 1992a, 1992b). It was compared with a range of other measures used in this study, which is widely held to be the definitive study of the prevalence of PTSD in Vietnam veterans. A number of versions of the SCID are available for use with different populations, and the original versions, both patient and non-patient, do not actually include systematic investigation for PTSD. A specific SCID-NP-V (Structured Clinical Interview for DSM-III, Non-patient, Veterans) version was developed by Kulka and Schlenger for the Vietnam veterans work.

The SCID has the advantages of being a diagnostic interview for a wide range of Axis-I diagnoses, of being widely accepted, and of being frequently used in both clinical and research settings.

The SCID has been used as the standard for assessment of other diagnostic measures (Solomon *et al.*, 1993). It has also been used in studies of a range of at-risk groups (Hovens *et al.*, 1992; Triffleman *et al.*, 1995).

There exists a separate SCID-D, the Structured Clinical Interview for DSM-IV for Dissociative Disorders. In one study, this was used with Vietnam veterans with and without PTSD. It was found that the PTSD subjects had higher overall dissociation scores and higher scores on all five dissociative symptom areas (Bremner *et al.*, 1993). This was a comparatively small study of 40 cases and 15 controls but has been seen as fuel in the argument about the position of PTSD in relation to dissociative disorders rather than anxiety disorders.

Diagnostic Interview Schedule

The Diagnostic Interview Schedule (DIS) of the National Institute of Mental Health (Robins, Helzer and Croughan, 1981) is a structured interview designed to aid in the diagnosis of a wide range of mental disorders. It has been used extensively in community studies as well as other settings. A PTSD module has been added to the revised version.

The DIS was the principal diagnostic interview used in the Vietnam Experience Study, one of the two big systematic studies of Vietnam veterans (Centers for Disease Control Vietnam Experience Study, 1988). The objection laid against its use by the supporters of the NVVRS study was that the DIS was then simply too insensitive to detect much of the PTSD recognised in that study. The VES found a lower prevalence of PTSD than the NVVRS. Perhaps surprisingly, much later Watson found that the DIS detected a higher rate of

PTSD than other measures, and was considered to be more sensitive and less specific (Watson *et al.*, 1994).

The Epidemiological Catchment Area Study used the DIS to diagnose a wide range of mental illnesses including PTSD in a large community study (Helzer, Robins and McEvoy, 1987).

Because of its use in other areas of mental health research, the DIS has been widely used and reported. It has been used in treatment outcome studies (Boehnlein *et al.*, 1985; Boudewyns *et al.*, 1991), in comorbidity studies (Cottler *et al.*, 1992; Kessler *et al.*, 1995), and in various high risk-groups (Hodgins and Cote, 1990; Gleason, 1993).

Clinician-Administered PTSD Scale

The Clinician-Administered PTSD Scale (CAPS) is a comparatively new structured interview which has become increasingly popular (Blake, 1990). The authors suggest that the CAPS (Blake *et al.*, 1995) is the most useful, in psychometric and reliability terms of the structured interviews available for diagnosing PTSD. It assesses the frequency and intensity of each PTSD symptom using standard prompt questions and explicit, behaviorally anchored rating scales, yielding both continuous and dichotomous scores for current and lifetime PTSD. It is a reliable and valid PTSD interview. It does not enquire about any other diagnoses and must be used in conjunction with some other form of enquiry for comorbidity or alternative diagnosis.

Neal has looked at the use of a computerized version of the CAPS (Neal *et al.*, 1994a) in a heterogeneous group of PTSD sufferers, finding 95% sensitivity and specificity rates.

The Dutch experience is a little less positive, with the CAPS correlating less well with the IES than did other measures. However, it was a slightly curious three-centre study with large numbers of subjects being excluded from it for a variety of reasons. The sensitivity was said to be 74%, and the specificity 84%.

When considering the value of all of the structured interviews, it is necessary to remember that they do not have some inherent mechanism for detecting pathognomonic signs of PTSD. They are not an independent test for the disorder. Rather, they seek to operationalise and standardise clinical assessment. They contain a systematic way of assessing the presence or absence of agreed clinical symptoms in such a way as to make reliably appropriate enquiry without missing things out or failing to follow up possibly significant symptom areas. This was brought into focus by a study (Blanchard *et al.*, 1995) of 100 road traffic accident victims with whom the CAPS was used. When the way in which the scoring rules for the interview were applied to the whole sample was changed, this led to variations in the rates of diagnosis of PTSD from 29% to 44%.

The PTSD Interview

Watson's Post-traumatic Stress Disorder Interview (PTSD-I) (Watson *et al.*, 1991) has been designed to correspond closely to DSM-III diagnostic criteria, give dichotomous and continuous scoring on each symptom as well as the entire syndrome, be easily administered, and be reliable and valid. Initial study was favourable in work on Vietnam veterans.

Watson has subsequently used the PTSD-I in a number of studies (Watson *et al.*, 1993; Watson, Anderson and Gearhart, 1995) and, in reviews of the psychometric properties of various diagnostic instruments, he has supported its use as a reliable and valid instrument (Watson, Juba and Anderson, 1989). He has suggested that when it comes to assessing severity of PTSD, the PTSD-I and the Mississippi Scale have better convergence than other measures, while for simple categorical diagnosis there is less difference between these measures than between the DIS and MMPI scale (Watson *et al.*, 1994). However, the PTSD-I scale does not appear to have been widely used by other groups of investigators.

The Structured Interview for PTSD

The SI-PTSD is a 13-item structured interview with anchor points for scores of 0 to 4 on each item from the clinical symptom criteria for PTSD. It was developed by Davidson *et al.* (Davidson, Smith and Kudler, 1989) during their work in pharmacological treatments of PTSD. The SCID was used as a standard comparator and in a sample of 41 cases the SI-PTSD was 96% sensitive and 80% specific when compared with the SCID.

The SI-PTSD was used in a French study of 58 consecutive female psychiatric inpatients with other presenting diagnoses (Darves *et al.*, 1995). The investigators, perhaps surprisingly, suggested that there was a 21% current and more than 60% lifetime prevalence of PTSD in these general psychiatric inpatients.

The SI-PTSD has also been used in drug treatment studies of PTSD (Duffy and Malloy, 1994).

Jackson Structured Interview for PTSD

This interview, developed by Keane (1985), is not only specific for PTSD, but it is also for combat-related PTSD and Vietnam combat-related PTSD. It is not generalisable to other situations.

Vietnam Era Stress Inventory
This instrument was also developed specifically for Vietnam veterans. It examines general psychosocial adjustment rather than simply (Wilson and Krauss, 1985). One part of it, the Stress Assessment Questionnaire, has been modified for use with other populations (Wilson, Smith and Johnson, 1985). It is not widely used now.

Other psychological tests

This group is intended to include a range of tests of varying psychometric properties which do not refer directly to the symptoms of PTSD as defined in DSM. They may have been specifically empirically constructed like the MMPI scales, or may represent the pragmatic use of pre-existing instruments, backed by empirical research.

Minnesota Multiphasic Personality Inventory scales
The MMPI is probably the most widely used psychological assessment instrument in history. It has been revised recently in the MMPI-2 (Hathaway and McKinley, 1989). Its usefulness is generally seen in that it produces a lot of data, has a wide normative base, and contains a number of internal validity scales to assess the subject's approach. This last was described by one patient by saying that the inventory was 'a lie detector', although this is an overestimate of the strength of the internal validity scales. It is named a 'personality' inventory, but was constructed around what could be called Axis 1 symptom areas and some personality traits. It has been exceedingly widely used in the USA, not only in clinical settings but in selection, and in assessments in high school. It has been much less popular in the UK for a range of reasons.

It is not surprising that attempts have been made to apply the MMPI to the diagnosis of PTSD. There are at least 50 publications which either specifically address the utility of the MMPI in diagnosis, or use it as part of the diagnostic process.

A number of different MMPI profiles have been associated with PTSD and there have been specific attempts to construct PTSD scales. The most popular of these is the PK scale of Keane (Keane, Malloy and Fairbank, 1984). This was based on a group of 200 Vietnam veterans with PTSD or another Axis 1 diagnosis, and was found to have an 82% diagnostic hit rate. There have been a number of attempts to confirm this finding, with varying results. Some have found the PK scale to be equally useful (Blanchard *et al.*, 1988), even in different groups such as World War II veterans (Query, Megran and McDonald, 1986) and in civilians (Koretzky and Peck, 1990). Others have been less successful (Gayton, Burchstead and Matthews, 1986). One study suggested that the PK scale had good sensitivity but a high false-positive rate (Tick, 1986) in a sample of 595 Vietnam veteran psychiatric inpatients, and suggested that the scale was useful for ruling out, but not for diagnosing, PTSD.

While Keane's scale was constructed by comparing PTSD with other diagnoses, that of Schlenger (Schlenger *et al.*, 1992b) compared PTSD Vietnam veterans with healthy veterans. It has been less widely reported, and needs completion of the full 567 questions of the MMPI, whereas the basic scales and PK can be derived from the first 370. As an aside, it has been noted that some studies have extracted the items for PK or PS scales from the MMPI and administered them rather than the MMPI. The validity of this procedure has not been established and there is no provision for assessing validity scales.

There have been a comparatively large number of studies into two related questions:

1. Can the MMPI detect those who fake PTSD?
2. Can people fake the MMPI?

One of the strengths of the MMPI is that it has internal validity scales. However, some investigators have suggested that high scores on the F validity scale suggesting over-reporting of symptoms, may, in themselves, be a symptom of PTSD, or a feature of those who have been exposed to combat (Hyer *et al.*, 1987). It has even been suggested that dissimulation may be an associated symptom of PTSD (Hyer *et al.*, 1989b). This last is, of course, a somewhat disturbing suggestion. At its simplest it suggests that faking illness is an indicator of PTSD rather than of faking! This would make any attempt to verify claimed symptoms meaningless. What seems more likely is that there is a perceived tendency for PTSD sufferers, and perhaps combat veterans in particular, to endorse a wide range of symptoms.

In one study, the traditional MMPI validity scales were used to discriminate between students and forensic inpatients who were instructed to fake bad, fake good, or report honestly (Bagby, Rogers and Buis, 1994) as regards PTSD symptoms and the MMPI generally. The scales were moderately good at detecting those who fake bad. There have been conflicting results, however, with some suggesting that it is possible to fake PTSD on the MMPI (Lees-Haley, 1989) despite the specific scales (Perconte and Goreczny, 1990), while others suggest that the MMPI is useful in detecting faking (Moller, 1988), even in the litigation situation (Lees-Haley, 1992), and even when the fakers have been given instruction in how they should fake symptoms (Wetter *et al.*, 1993). It seems clear that while the MMPI may be of value in the diagnosis of PTSD and the detection of dissimulation, it is not a definitive diagnostic tool in itself.

One interesting study (Schnurr, Friedman and Rosenberg, 1993) used the pre-existing fortuitous widespread application of the MMPI to large samples of normals to look at its predictive value in PTSD. Many American students have completed the MMPI. Schnurr looked at 131 such students and compared Vietnam veterans with those who were not there. She found that, overall, the adolescent MMPI scores pre-Vietnam were within the normal range both for veterans and for non-veterans. No scales predicted those who would or would not be exposed to greater or lesser degrees of violence. However, as a group, the hypochondriasis, psychopathic deviancy, masculinity–femininity, and paranoia scales were to some extent predictive of PTSD symptoms in those who were so exposed. This work was not without its critics (Shulman, 1994), but is a pointer to future interesting areas of research into the questions of vulnerability and prediction.

General Health Questionnaire

The GHQ is a self-report questionnaire devised by Goldberg. It was initially intended, and used, as a screening instrument in general practice to help identify psychiatric caseness in those using primary health care services. The original method of use of GHQ scores was to produce a dichotomous score of 'probable caseness' versus 'probable non-case'. However, the instrument, which is easy and quick to administer and complete, has been used in many other settings and validation has been extended. It is reasonable to point out that the GHQ is less effective at identifying chronic, fixed, and severe mental illness as originally used, because it focuses on recent symptoms and change of symptoms. It has been shown to underestimate chronic illness in the setting for which it was first devised.

Many studies have used the score on GHQ as a continuous or quantitative variable to denote severity of illness and this may not be wholly appropriate.

McFarlane is the investigator who has probably most influenced the use of the GHQ in PTSD. He used the GHQ as the definition of caseness in his famous studies of those involved in the Australian bush fires (McFarlane, 1987, 1988, 1989). This led to the widespread use of the GHQ to diagnose PTSD in those exposed to trauma, although the symptom content is quite clearly not specific to PTSD. It has been used in studies of rescuers (Feinstein and Dolan, 1991), survivors of a shipping disaster (Joseph *et al.*, 1993), and survivors of a terrorist bomb (Curran *et al.*, 1990).

It is still widely used in studies in which GHQ scores are employed as an indicator of severity of illness rather than of caseness. It is also frequently used in medicolegal settings, where its transparency and the quantitative interpretation of scores may be a problem. In an adversarial setting it is entirely obvious to the subject that marking all the responses in the right-hand column indicates illness or disability, as with the IES and others.

Millon Clinical Multiaxial Inventory

The original MCMI (Millon, 1983)was a 175-item true-false questionnaire yielding scores on 11 personality disorder categories and 9 clinical syndromes related to diagnoses in DSM-III. The later, 1987, MCMI-II (Millon, 1987) is a modification with two new categories and some modification, including an item weighting system. One of the principal arguments against the MCMI has been the large item overlap on the scales.

The MCMI has been used quite extensively with Vietnam veterans, both to search for particular personality profiles, and as a diagnostic tool (Robert, 1985; Piekarski, Sherwood and Funari, 1993; Munley *et al.*, 1995). In a pair of large-scale studies, the MCMI was used in a cluster analysis in Vietnam veterans with the result that it produced three clusters labelled as traumatic personality, schizoid influence, and antisocial influence. The last of these was seen to be the 'most healthy' cluster. Much of this work has been done by Hyer *et al.*

It has also been used in the study of adult survivors of sexual abuse (Alexander, 1993) and of perpetrators (Dutton, 1995).

The MCMI, like the MMPI, has been used in an attempt to detect malingering in the litigation situation.

When used as a measure of response to treatment (Funari, Piekarski and Sherwood, 1991), the MCMI has been shown to change over time, but has also demonstrated a deterioration across 17 of the 20 scales following a five-week intensive 'revivifying' treatment programme in 50 Vietnam veterans (Hyer *et al.*, 1989a).

It is not widely used in the UK.

Symptom Check List 90 – Revised

The SCL-90R is a widely used self-report measure of psychiatric symptomatology across a range of clinical areas. It was devised by Derogatis and gives severity scores across the range of included symptom groups as well as global severity measures. It is intended as a severity measure and to be used to measure change in symptomatology. Like the GHQ it is not specific to PTSD.

The measure has been used widely in mental health research and practice. It has been less frequently used in PTSD work but there are some studies. For example, it has been used in the investigation of Korean American riot victims (Kim-Goh *et al.*, 1995), abused children and their parents (Kelley, 1990), and office workers from a building in which there was a shooting incident (Creamer, Burgess and Pattison, 1992).

In addition, a subscale has been developed to screen for crime-related PTSD in female crime victims. The first study of 355 women (Saunders, Arata and Kilpatrick, 1990) found the 28-item scale to be of value. A concurrent validity study with the IES looked at 266 female crime victims and found both tests to be useful, with the IES having more false positives.

Penn Inventory

The Penn Inventory was devised by Hammarberg (1992). It consists of a series of 26 sets of scored sentence items. While it is obvious which responses are more likely to indicate pathology, and all sets are scored in the same direction, the items are not simply statements of the DSM criteria. It was initially standardised on Vietnam veterans, with veterans with PTSD scoring more than other veterans, who scored higher than non-veterans. A cut-off score of 35 has been used.

In phase one of the study, 52 PTSD cases, 15 veterans and 16 non-veterans were studied, with a resultant sensitivity of 90%, specificity of 100%, and positive predictive rate of 100%. There is a suggestion that the Penn may have value as a long-term indicator in that approximately half of the PTSD subjects in this study were assessed after completion of treatment and the predictive value was the same.

In phase two there was a total of 98 subjects, with results of 98% sensitivity, 94% specificity, and a positive predictive rate of 77%.

The final phase used complicated groups, with 22 veterans in treatment for PTSD, 17 consecutive admissions with PTSD, 18 other admissions, and 19 survivors of the Piper Alpha oil rig fire, 16 of whom had PTSD. The results for Vietnam veterans were sensitivity of 97%, specificity of 61%, and positive predictive rate of 84%. The results for the Piper Alpha group were sensitivity 94%, specificity 100%, positive predictive rate 100%.

The Penn Inventory has not yet been widely investigated.

Pathological diagnostic tests

At present there are no definitive pathological or physiological tests for PTSD despite a significant amount of research. Much of the work into the aetiology of PTSD has involved study of biochemical, neuro-endocrinological, or physiological research. It is the opinion of the author that one of the difficulties is that PTSD is not yet, despite DSM-IV, very clearly defined on a phenomenological basis. It is something of a catch-22 situation. It is not possible to find a simple definitive test for PTSD until we are quite certain what PTSD is and which subjects do and do not have PTSD. However, we cannot be certain which subjects do and do not have PTSD until we have a definitive test for it. That the boundaries between PTSD and other illnesses, or between PTSD and normal reaction, are unclear is demonstrated by the way that the diagnostic criteria have changed in successive revisions of DSM, and in the remarkably high level of comorbidity. While the empirical approach of DSM without a hierarchical structure is accepted, it is hard to think of any other condition in which 80% of sufferers also fulfil diagnostic criteria for a range of other conditions. It must raise doubts about the purity of the PTSD diagnosis.

Despite the absence of a single useful and widely applicable biological test for PTSD, books have been written on the subject (Giller, 1990). Friedman (1991) has provided a useful review.

Dexamethasone suppression test

It is not surprising that the dexamethasone suppression test (DST) has been used, given the comorbidity of depression and PTSD, as well as the overlap of symptoms. Theoretically, PTSD patients should be suppressors while those with depression should be non-suppressors (Friedman, 1988). In brief, DST is of little use in distinguishing PTSD from depression as the results may well differentiate in the directions indicated between groups but are not necessarily useful in individual patients. In addition, patients with both PTSD and depression have at times given conflicting results in studies (Kudler *et al.*, 1987; Halbreich *et al.*, 1988).

Yohimbine challenge

Yohimbine is an α-2 receptor antagonist which can induce flashbacks, panic and startle reflex, particularly in patients with panic disorder. Intravenous infusion has been used to demonstrate induction of panic and intrusive symptoms in a subgroup of PTSD patients (Krystal, 1993; Southwick *et al.*, 1993), and to show enhanced acoustic startle reflex in some (Morgan *et al.*, 1995). However, it has been suggested that these responses may be associated with comorbidity or other factors rather than being diagnostic of PTSD. There is no suggestion that this would be a universal diagnostic tool for PTSD.

Lactate infusion

Infusion of lactate has been used in a similar way to Yohimbine. It has been suggested that it can precipitate panic attacks (Rainey *et al.*, 1990). However, it has also been suggested that this response only occurs in patients with PTSD and panic disorder concurrently, so that this is unlikely to be a diagnostic tool of general use.

Cortisol and noradrenaline levels

It has been found generally (Mason *et al.*, 1986; Yehuda *et al.*, 1990), but not universally (Pitman and Orr, 1990), that urinary cortisol levels are lower in PTSD than in affective disorders. In addition, urinary noradrenaline levels are relatively high. In an extension of this work, Mason *et al.* (1988) have indicated that while neither of these measures can be used confidently to discriminate PTSD subjects from those with other major psychiatric disorders, the ratio of the two can do so, with 78% sensitivity and 89% specificity. This work is interesting but needs larger-scale replication. It requires careful collection of 24-hour specimens of urine and it has been suggested that there are difficulties with specimen preparation and methodology which might make generalised use as a simple clinical diagnostic tool difficult, even if the work were widely replicated.

Other pathological tests

The corticotrophin-releasing hormone test failed to distinguish PTSD (Smith *et al.*, 1989).

Thyrotrophin-releasing hormone tests are not diagnostic of PTSD (Reist *et al.*, 1995), although there are certainly abnormalities.

An MRI scan study of 26 cases and 22 controls showed a significant 8% reduction in volume in the right hippocampal region of the brain in a specific group of PTSD patients. This needs replication and extension (Bremner *et al.*, 1995).

Physiological tests

There has been, and continues to be, great interest in psychophysiological tests as a means of confirming the diagnosis in PTSD. It is obvious that self-report measures are very sensitive, but there is a hope that physiological measures will be more specific (Gerardi, Keane and Penk, 1989). Interest in such measures can probably be dated from Kardiner's description of problems similar to those in PTSD as a 'physioneurosis'.

A number of different physiological measures have been studied. Tests usually involve repeated measures in the three situations of neutrality, non-specific stress, and specific trauma-related stress conditions. The responses which have been studied with some success have included event related potentials in the brain (Paige *et al.*, 1990), heart rate, blood pressure, electromyography, skin reactivity (Blanchard *et al.*, 1982), and temperature. Much of this work has involved Blanchard, who has pointed out the problems and costs of adding in more and more measures, comparing the costs with the value (Blanchard, Kolb and Prins, 1991).

Overall it seems clear that the single most useful measure is the heart rate, or rather the change therein on exposure to relevant stressor stimuli either in vivo or in vitro. In the study quoted above, Blanchard *et al.* were able successfully to identify 83% of a group of 96 Vietnam veterans with and without PTSD.

The same tests have been used in other populations including World War II veterans (Orr *et al.*, 1993), road traffic accident victims (Blanchard, Hickling and Taylor, 1991), and other non-combat PTSD cases (Drescher, 1992).

There has been one experiment in attempts to dissimulate the physiological response (Gerardi, Blanchard and Kolb, 1989). In this, PTSD subjects were not able to fake well, but healthy volunteers were able to increase their physiological response to the relevant stimuli with advice or training. However, even in such circumstances, the test was able to differentiate the PTSD from the dissimulating group. There has also been interest in the potential use of such physiological evidence in forensic situations (Pitman and Orr, 1993).

It seems likely that physiological testing currently holds out the best hope for a diagnostic tool in PTSD which is free from reliance on patient report.

Multimodal assessments

The data presented above show clearly that there continues to be an absence of the 'gold standard' for the diagnosis of PTSD. The very search for it is hampered by its lack! How can you identify a gold standard when you have no gold standard to compare it with?

Most reviews over recent years have concentrated on the importance of multimodal assessment of potential PTSD cases. In particular two major reviews (Gerardi, Keane and Penk, 1989; Kulka *et al.*, 1991) have pointed out the need for this, and the dangers of over-reliance on a single diagnostic measure or index in the absence of a gold standard.

A number of the papers on multimodal assessment have involved Wolfe (Wolfe *et al.*, 1987; Keane, Wolfe and Taylor, 1987; Lyons *et al.*, 1988). While nobody has prescribed exactly which tests from the various groups should be used in which situations or in all situations, various lists of the type of measures which might be required have been produced. Suggested components have included:

- demographic information
- structured interviews
- psychometric tests
- interviewer rating scales
- psychophysiological testing
- behavioural observation
- review of previous records and contemporaneous information
- collateral confirmation of information.

There may well be a need or desire to use more than one test or measure in some categories. This may help improve validity, but it is important to remember that there is no increase in validity if different tests based on the same data are used as if they were independent. For example, there are a number of self-report questionnaires which ask about PTSD symptoms or about depressive symptoms. To use more than one of each of these will not increase diagnostic accuracy as it may be simple repetition.

Comparison of utility of diagnostic tools

The validation data for different tools used in the diagnosis or assessment of PTSD are very variable, both in quality and quantity.

Another problem is that many have been devised and standardised for specific groups of subjects, usually Vietnam veterans, but also rape victims and others. The assumption that such tools can be used in other groups may not be well founded. While a major justification for the development of the concept of PTSD was that the responses to various forms of trauma were similar rather than disparate, this does not necessarily mean that there is no variation or that investigation of all groups can use the same measures.

Not only may the diagnostic tools not necessarily be generalisable to different groups, but they may not be useful in all situations. The high sensitivity of self-report symptom questionnaires may be a major advantage in a population survey or general practice study, but may be of much less value in an adversarial situation such as litigation.

There has been some work done on the convergent validity of different measures.

Watson *et al.* (1994) compared the DIS PTSD module, the Mississippi Scale, the PK Scale of the MMPI, and the PTSD Interview of Watson in a group of 80 help-seeking Vietnam veterans. Perfect agreement in diagnosis of presence or absence of PTSD was found in 68% of subjects, with a further 16% having agreement on three of the four measures. All measures were highly inter-correlated. However, when used to measure severity in a continuous measure, the Mississippi and PTSD-I were more closely correlated than the others.

McFall *et al.* (1990) looked at the SCID, Mississippi, IES, PK of MMPI, and Vietnam Era Stress Inventory in 130 help-seeking Vietnam veterans. Using the SCID as the index, all measures were significantly correlated with it, the Mississippi Scale alone being able to account for 42% of the variance in PTSD symptoms measured by the SCID. Correlations between the different psycho-metric measures varied widely, with a strong correlation between the Mississippi and both the IES and PK, but no significant correlation between IES and PK.

In the UK, Neal *et al.* (1994a) looked at the SCL-90, IES and PK Scale in a mixed group of 70 patients referred to a PTSD unit. The paper seems to suggest that the PK Scale from the MMPI was used in isolation rather than as part of the MMPI, which would be surprising as this was not what was intended and some of the assumptions may not apply. The index measure was the CAPS. All three study measures produced high correlations with the CAPS intensity score. The IES gave the lowest apparent total misclassification rate at 11.4% when used dichotomously, while those for PK and SCL-90 were 18.6% and 21.4% respectively.

Summary

To summarise the situation as regards diagnosis and diagnostic methods is quite simple:

there is no gold standard.

This should colour diagnostic and assessment methods used by clinicians and researchers and has a number of implications.

- It is inappropriate to rely too heavily on a single index diagnostic or comparator measure.
- Diagnostic needs vary according to the situation, both as regards the subject group, and the reason for the diagnosis. In general, the more adversarial or contentious the situation, the more specific and robust methods need to be.

- The same diagnostic tools may not be suitable for all subjects in all situations.
- Transparent self-report symptom questionnaires are very sensitive, and are therefore useful as a screening tool.
- Physiological measures are possibly the most specific but the most difficult and expensive to apply.
- That psychometric measures produce apparently continuous scores does not necessarily imply that the score is a measure of severity. Rather, severity should be assessed in clinical terms and with particular reference to observed and reported disability. Similarly, it has not been adequately demonstrated that small changes in scores on any of the psychometric tests used specifically for PTSD represent significant clinical change.
- There is overwhelming agreement that a multimodal approach using the various areas outlined above is the most appropriate.
- Use of multiple measures with the same theoretical basis does not improve diagnostic accuracy but may lead to false complacency. It is necessary to use multiple measures from multiple modalities.
- Individual clinicians working with PTSD will probably naturally adopt a standard and consistent diagnostic approach while remaining alert to the development of new methods, for example in psychophysiology.
- Departments will necessarily have a common approach with appropriate training in application and interpretation of results as well as inter-rater testing.

References

Alexander, P.C. (1993). The differential effects of abuse characteristics and attachment in the prediction of long-term effects of sexual abuse. Special issue: Research on treatment of adults sexually abused in childhood. *Journal of Interpersonal Violence*, **8**, 3: 346–62.

Bagby, R.M., Rogers, R., and Buis, T. (1994). Detecting malingered and defensive responding on the MMPI 2 in a forensic inpatient sample. *Journal of Personality Assessment*, **62**: 2.

Blake D. (1990). A clinician rating scale for assessing current and lifetime PTSD: the CAPS-1. *Behaviour Therapist*, **18**: 187–8.

Blake, D.D., Weathers, F.W., Nagy, L.M., Kaloupek, D.G., Gusman, F.D., Charney, D.S. and Keane, T.M. (1995). The development of a clinician-administered PTSD scale. *Journal of Traumatic Stress*, **8**, 1: 75–90.

Blanchard, E.B., Hickling, E.J. and Taylor, A.E. (1991). The psychophysiology of motor vehicle accident related posttraumatic stress disorder. *Biofeedback and Self Regulation*, **16**, 4: 449–58.

Blanchard, E.B., Hickling, E.J., Taylor, A.E., Forneris, C.A., Loos, W. and Jaccard, J. (1995). Effects of varying scoring rules of the clinician-administered PTSD scale (CAPS) for the diagnosis of post-traumatic stress disorder in motor vehicle accident victims. *Behaviour Research and Therapy*, **33**, 4: 471–5.

Blanchard, E.B., Kolb, L.C., Pallmeyer, T.P. and Gerardi, R.J. (1982). A psychophysiological study of post traumatic stress disorder in Vietnam veterans. *Psychiatric Quarterly*, **54**, 4: 220–9.

Blanchard, E.B., Kolb, L.C. and Prins, A. (1991). Psychophysiological responses in the diagnosis of posttraumatic stress disorder in Vietnam veterans. *Journal of Nervous and Mental Disease*, **179**, 2: 97–101.

Blanchard, E.B., Wittrock, D., Kolb, L.C. and Gerardi, R. (1988). Cross-validation of a Minnesota Multiphasic Personality Inventory (MMPI) subscale for the assessment of combat-related post-traumatic stress disorder. *Journal of Psychopathology and Behavioral Assessment*, **10**, 1: 33–8.

Blank, A.S. (1994). Clinical detection, diagnosis, and differential diagnosis of posttraumatic stress disorder. *Psychiatric Clinics of North America*, **17**, 2: 351–83.

Boehnlein, J.K., Kinzie, J.D., Ben, R. and Fleck, J. (1985). One-year follow-up study of posttraumatic stress disorder among survivors of Cambodian concentration camps. *American Journal of Psychiatry*, **142**, 8: 956–9.

Boudewyns, P.A., Albrecht, J.W., Talbert, F.S. and Hyer, L.A. (1991). Comorbidity and treatment outcome of inpatients with chronic combat-related PTSD. *Hospital and Community Psychiatry*, **42**, 8: 847–9.

Bremner, J.D., Randall, P., Scott, T.M., Bronen, R.A., Seibyl, J.P., Southwick, S.M., Delaney, R.C., McCarthy, G., Charney, D.S. and Innis, R.B. (1995). MRI-based measurement of hippocampal volume in patients with combat-related posttraumatic stress disorder. *American Journal of Psychiatry*, **152**, 7: 973–81.

Bremner, J.D., Steinberg, M., Southwick, S.M., Johnson, D.R. and Charney, D.S. (1993). Use of the Structured Clinical Interview for DSM-IV dissociative disorders for systematic assessment of dissociative symptoms in posttraumatic stress disorder. *American Journal of Psychiatry*, **150**, 7: 1011–14.

Centers for Disease Control Vietnam Experience Study. (1988). Health status of Vietnam veterans; I. psychosocial characteristics. *Journal of the American Medical Association*, **259**, 18: 2701–8.

Cottler, L.B., Compton, W.M., Mager, D., Spitznagel, E.L. and Jancer, A. (1992). Posttraumatic stress disorder among substance users from the general population. *American Journal of Psychiatry*, **149**, 5: 664–70.

Creamer, M., Burgess, P. and Pattison, P. (1992). Reaction to trauma: a cognitive processing model. *Journal of Abnormal Psychology*, **101**, 3: 452–9.

Curran, P.S., Bell, P., Murray, A., Loughrey, G., Roddy, R. and Rocke, L.G. (1990). Psychological consequences of the Enniskillen bombing. *British Journal of Psychiatry*, **156**, 479–82.

Dalton, J.E., Tom, A., Rosenblum, M.L. and Garte, S.H. (1989). Faking on the Mississippi Scale for combat-related posttraumatic stress disorder. *Psychological Assessment*, **1**, 1: 56–7.

Darves, B.J.M., Benhamou, A.P., Degiovanni, A. and Lepine, J.P.G.P. (1995). Psychological trauma and mental disorders. *Annales Medico-Psychologiques*, **153**, 1: 77–81.

Davidson, J., Smith, R. and Kudler, H. (1989). Validity and reliability of the DSM-III criteria for posttraumatic stress disorder: Experience with a structured interview. *Journal of Nervous and Mental Disease*, **177**, 6: 336–41.

Drescher, K.D. (1992). Psychophysiological assessment of PTSD with survivors of non-combat traumatic experiences. *Dissertation Abstracts International*, **53**, 6–B: 31–52.

Duffy, J.D. and Malloy, P.F. (1994). Efficacy of buspirone in the treatment of posttraumatic stress disorder: An open trial. *Annals of Clinical Psychiatry*, **6**, 1: 33–7.

Dutton, D.G. (1995). Trauma symptoms and PTSD-like profiles in perpetrators of intimate abuse. *Journal of Traumatic Stress*, **8**, 2: 299–316.

Feinstein, A. and Dolan, R. (1991). Predictors of post-traumatic stress disorder following physical trauma: An examination of the stressor criterion. *Psychological Medicine*, **21**, 1: 85–91.

Foa, E.B., Riggs, D.S., Dancu, C.V. and Rothbaum, B.O. (1993). Reliability and validity of a brief instrument for assessing post-traumatic stress disorder. *Journal of Traumatic Stress*, **6**, 4: 459–73.

Fontana, A. and Rosenheck, R. (1994). A short form of the Mississippi Scale for measuring change in combat related PTSD. *Journal of Traumatic Stress*, **7**: 3.

Friedman, M.J. (1988). Toward rational pharmacotherapy for posttraumatic stress disorder: An interim report. *American Journal of Psychiatry*. **145**, 3: 281–5.

Friedman, M.J. (1991). Biological approaches to the diagnosis and treatment of posttraumatic disorder. *Journal of Traumatic Stress*, **4**, 1: 67–91.

Funari, D.J., Piekarski, A.M. and Sherwood, R.J. (1991). Treatment outcomes of Vietnam veterans with posttraumatic stress disorder. *Psychological Reports*, **68**, 2: 571–8.

Gayton, W.F., Burchstead, G.N. and Matthews, G.R. (1986). An investigation of the utility of an MMPI posttraumatic stress disorder subscale. *Journal of Clinical Psychology*, **42**, 6: 916–17.

Gerardi, R.J., Blanchard, E.B. and Kolb, L.C. (1989). Ability of Vietnam veterans to dissimulate a psychophysiological assessment or PTSD. *Behavior Therapy*, **20**, 1: 229–44.

Gerardi, R., Keane, T.M. and Penk, W.E. (1989). Utility: sensitivity and specificity in developing diagnostic tests of combat-related post-traumatic stress disorder (PTSD). Special issue: Post-traumatic stress disorder. *Journal of Clinical Psychology*, **45**, 5 (Suppl.) 691–703.

Giller, E.L. Jr (Ed.) (1990). *Biological Assessment and Treatment of Posttraumatic Stress Disorder*. Washington: American Psychiatric Press.

Gleason, W.J. (1993). Mental disorders in battered women: An empirical study. *Violence and Victims*, **8**, 1: 53–68.

Halbreich, U., Olympia, J., Glogowski, J., Carson, S., Axelrod, S. and Yeh, C.M. (1988). The importance of past psychological trauma and pathophysiological process as determinants of current biologic abnormalities. *Archives of General Psychiatry*, **45**, 3: 293–4.

Hammarberg, M. (1992). Penn Inventory for posttraumatic stress disorder: psychometric properties. *Psychological Assessment*, **4**, 1: 67–76.

Hathaway, S. and McKinley, J. (1989). MMPI-2. *MMPI-2 Manual for Administration and Scoring*. Minneapolis: National Computer Systems.

Helzer, J.E., Robins, L.N. and McEvoy, L. (1987). Post-traumatic stress disorder in the general population: Findings of the Epidemiologic Catchment Area survey. *New England Journal of Medicine*, **317**, 26: 1630–34.

Hodgins, S. and Cote, G. (1990). Prevalence of mental disorders among penitentiary inmates in Quebec. *Canada's Mental Health*, **38**, 1: 1–4.

Horowitz, M., Wilner, N. and Alvarez, W. (1979). Impact of Event Scale: A measure of subjective stress. *Psychosomatic Medicine*, **41**, 3: 209–18.

Horowitz, M.J., Wilner, N., Kaltreider, N., and Alvarez, W. (1980). Signs and symptoms of post traumatic stress disorder. *Archives of General Psychiatry*, **37**, 1: 85–92.

Hovens, J.E., Falger, P.R., Op, d.V.W., Schouten, E.G. and Van Duijn, H. (1992). Occurrence of current post traumatic stress disorder among Dutch World War II resistance veterans according to the SCID. *Journal of Anxiety Disorders*, **6**, 2: 147–57.

Hovens, J.E., Van der Ploeg, H.M., Klaarenbeek, M.T.A., Bramsen, I., Schreuder, J.N. and Rivero, W. (1994). The assessment of posttraumatic stress disorder: with the clinician administered PTSD scale: Dutch results. *Journal of Clinical Psychology*, **50**, 3: 325–40.

Hyer, L., Davis, H., Boudewyns, P.A. and Woods, M.G. (1991). A short form of the Mississippi Scale for combat-related PTSD. *Journal of Clinical Psychology*, **47**, 4: 510–18.

Hyer, L., Fallon, J.H., Harrison, W.R. and Boudewyns, P.A. (1987). MMPI overreporting by Vietnam combat veterans. *Journal of Clinical Psychology*. **43**, 1: 79–83.

Hyer, L., Woods, M.G., Bruno, R. and Boudewyns, P. (1989a). Treatment outcomes of Vietnam veterans with PTSD and the consistency of the MCMI. *Journal of Clinical Psychology*, **45**, 4: 547–52.

Hyer, L.A., Woods, M., Harrison, W.R., Boudewyns, P.A. and O'Leary, W.C. (1989b). MMPI F-K index among hospitalized Vietnam veterans. *Journal of Clinical Psychology*, **45**, 2: 250–54.

Jordan, B.K., Schlenger, W.E., Hough, R.L., Kulka, R.A., Weiss, D., Fairbank, J.A. and Marmar, C.R. (1991). Lifetime and current prevalence of specific psychiatric disorders among Vietnam veterans and controls. *Archives of General Psychiatry*, **48**, 3: 207–15.

Joseph, S., Yule, W., Williams, R. and Hodgkinson, P. (1993). Increased substance use in survivors of the Herald of Free Enterprise disaster. *British Journal of Medical Psychology*, **66**, 2: 185–91.

Keane, T.M. (1985). A behavioral approach to assessing and treating PTSD in Vietnam veterans. In *Trauma and Its Wake*. pp. 257–94. Ed. C.R. Figley. New York: Brunner/Maze.

Keane, T.M., Caddell, J.M. and Taylor, K.L. (1988). Mississippi Scale for combat-related posttraumatic stress disorder: Three studies in reliability and validity. *Journal of Consulting and Clinical Psychology*, **56**, 1: 85–90.

Keane, T.M., Malloy, P.F. and Fairbank, J.A. (1984). Empirical development of an MMPI subscale for the assessment of combat-related posttraumatic stress disorder. *Journal of Consulting and Clinical Psychology*, **52**, 5: 888–91.

Keane, T.M., Wolfe, J. and Taylor, K.L. (1987). Post-traumatic stress disorder: Evidence for diagnostic validity and methods of psychological assessment. *Journal of Clinical Psychology*, **43**, 1: 32–43.

Kelley, S.J. (1990). Parental stress response to sexual abuse and ritualistic abuse of children in day care centers. *Nursing Research*, **39**, 1: 25–9.

Kessler, R.C., Sonnega, A., Bromet, E., Hughes, M. and Nelson, C.B. (1995). Posttraumatic stress disorder in the National Comorbidity Survey. *Archives of General Psychiatry*, **52**, 12: 1048–60.

Kim-Goh, M., Suh, C., Blake, D.D. and Hiley-Young, B. (1995). Psychological impact of the Los Angeles riots on Korean–American victims: Implications for treatment. *American Journal of Orthopsychiatry*, **65**, 1: 138–46.

Koopman, C., Classen, C. and Spiegel, D.A. (1994). Predictors of posttraumatic stress symptoms among survivors of the Oakland/Berkeley, California, firestorm. *American Journal of Psychiatry*, **151**, 6: 888–94.

Koretzky, M.B. and Peck, A.H. (1990). Validation and cross-validation of the PTSD subscale of the MMPI with civilian trauma victims. *Journal of Clinical Psychology*, **46**, 3: 296–300.

Krystal, J.H. (1993). *Assessment of Noradrenergic Contributions to PTSD Pathophysiology. FEDRIP Database*. Washington: National Technical Information Service (NTIS).

Kudler, H., Davidson, J., Meador, K., Lipper, S. and Ely, T. (1987). The DST and posttraumatic stress disorder. *American Journal of Psychiatry*, **144**, 8: 1068–71.

Kulka, R.A., Schlenger, W.E., Fairbank, J.A., Hough, R.L., Jordan, B.K., Marmar, C. and Weiss, D.S. (1990). *Trauma and the Vietnam War Generation: Report of Findings from the National Vietnam Veterans Readjustment Study*. Brunner Mazel Psychosocial Stress Series No. 18. New York: Brunner Mazel.

Kulka, R.A., Schlenger, W.E., Fairbank, J.A. and Jordan, B.K. (1991). Assessment of posttraumatic stress disorder in the community: Prospects and pitfalls from recent studies of Vietnam veterans. Special section: Issues and methods in assessment of posttraumatic stress disorder. *Psychological Assessment*, **3**, 4: 547–60.

LaGuardia, R.L., Smith, G., Francois, R. and Bachman, L. (1983). Incidence of delayed stress disorder among Vietnam era veterans: the effect of priming on response set. *American Journal of Orthopsychiatry*, **53**, 1: 18–26.

Lees-Haley, P.R. (1986). Pseudo-posttraumatic stress disorder. *Trial Diplomacy Journal*, **9**, 4: 17–20.

Lees-Haley, P.R. (1989). Malingering post-traumatic stress disorder on the MMPI. *Forensic Reports*, **2**, 1: 89–91.

Lees-Haley, P.R. (1992). Efficacy of MMPI-2 validity scales and MCMI-II modifier scales for detecting spurious PTSD claims: F, F-K, Fake Bad scale, Ego Strength, Subtle–Obvious subscales, DIS, and DEB. *Journal of Clinical Psychology*, **48**, 5: 681–9.

Lillywhite, A.R. and Neal, L.A. (1993). The importance of severity as a factor in posttraumatic stress disorder. *British Journal of Psychiatry*, **163**: 837.

Lynn, E.J., and Belza, M. (1984). Factitious posttraumatic stress disorder: The veteran who never got to Vietnam. *Hospital and Community Psychiatry*, **35**, 7: 697–701.

Lyons, J.A. Gerardi, R.J., Wolfe, J. and Keane, T.M. (1988). Multidimensional assessment of combat-related PTSD: Phenomenological, psychometric, and psychophysiological considerations. *Journal of Traumatic Stress*, **1**, 3: 373–94.

Maida, C.A., Gordon, N.S., Steinberg, A. and Gordon, G. (1989). Psychosocial impact of disasters: Victims of the Baldwin Hills fire. *Journal of Traumatic Stress*, **2**, 1: 37–48.

Mason, J.W., Giller, E.L., Kosten, T.R. and Harkness, L. (1988). Elevation of urinary nor-epinephrine/cortisol ratio in posttraumatic stress disorder. *Journal of Nervous and Mental Disease*, **176**, 8: 498–502.

Mason, J.W., Giller, E.L., Kosten, T.R., Ostroff, R.B. and Podd, L. (1986). Urinary free-cortisol levels in posttraumatic stress disorder patients. *Journal of Nervous and Mental Disease*, **174**, 3: 145–9.

McFall, M.E., Smith, D.E., Roszell, D.K. Tarver, D.J., and Malas, K.L. (1990). Convergent validity of measures of PTSD in Vietnam combat veterans. *American Journal of Psychiatry*, **147**, 5: 645–8.

McFarlane, A.C. (1987). Life events and psychiatric disorder: The role of a natural disaster. *British Journal of Psychiatry*, **151**: 362–7.

McFarlane, A.C. (1988). The longitudinal course of posttraumatic morbidity: The range of outcomes and their predictors. *Journal of Nervous and Mental Disease*, **176**, 1: 30–39.

McFarlane, A.C. (1989). The aetiology of post-traumatic morbidity: Predisposing, precipitating and perpetuating factors. *British Journal of Psychiatry*, **154**: 221–28.

Millon, T. (1983). *Millon Clinical Multiaxial Inventory*, 3rd edition. Minneapolis: Interpretive Scoring Systems.

Millon, T. (1987). *Millon Clinical Multiaxial Inventory II. Manual for the MCMI-II.* Minneapolis: National Computer Systems.

Moller, C.U. (1988). Detection of faked post traumatic stress disorder on the MMPI. *Dissertation Abstracts International*, **48**, 11–B: 3421.

Morgan, C.A.I., Grillon, C., Southwick, S.M., Nagy, L.M., Davis, M., Krystal, J.H. and Charney, D.S. (1995). Yohimbine facilitated acoustic startle in combat veterans with post traumatic stress disorder. *Psychopharmacology*, **117**, 4: 466–71.

Munley, P.H., Bains, D.S., Bloem, W.D., Busby, R.M. and Pendziszewski, S. (1995). Posttraumatic stress disorder and the MCMI-II. *Psychological Reports*, **76**, 3: 939–44.

Neal, L.A., Busuttil, W., Herapath, R. and Strike, P.W. (1994a). Development and validation of the computerized clinician administered post-traumatic stress disorder scale-1-Revised. *Psychological Medicine*, **24**, 3: 701–6.

Neal, L.A., Busuttil, W., Rollins, J., Herepath, R., Strike, P. and Turnbull, G. (1994b). Convergent validity of measures of post-traumatic stress disorder in a mixed military and civilian population. *Journal of Traumatic Stress*, **7**, 3: 447–55.

Neal, L.A. and Rose, M.C. (1995). Factitious post traumatic stress disorder: a case report. *Medicine, Science and Law*, **35**, 4: 352–4.

Orr, S.P., Pitman, R.K., Lasko, N.B. and Herz, L.R. (1993). Psychophysiological assessment of posttraumatic stress disorder imagery in World War II and Korean combat veterans. *Journal of Abnormal Psychology*, **102**, 1: 152–9.

Paige, S.R., Reid, G.M., Allen, M.G. and Newton, J.E. (1990). Psychophysiological correlates of posttraumatic stress disorder in Vietnam veterans. *Biological Psychiatry*, **27**, 4: 419–30.

Perconte, S.T. and Goreczny, A.J. (1990). Failure to detect fabricated posttraumatic stress disorder with the use of the MMPI in a clinical population. *American Journal of Psychiatry*, **147**, 8: 1057–60.

Piekarski, A.M., Sherwood, R. and Funari, D.J. (1993). Personality subgroups in an inpatient Vietnam veteran treatment program. *Psychological Reports*, **72**, 2: 667–74.

Pitman, R.K. and Orr, S.P. (1990). Twenty-four hour urinary cortisol and catecholamine excretion in combat-related posttraumatic stress disorder. *Biological Psychiatry*, **27**, 2: 245–7.

Pitman, R.K. and Orr, S.P. (1993). Psychophysiologic testing for post-traumatic stress disorder: Forensic psychiatric application. *Bulletin of the American Academy of Psychiatry and the Law*, **21**, 1: 37–52.

Query, W.T., Megran, J. and McDonald, G. (1986). Applying posttraumatic stress disorder MMPI subscale to World War II POW veterans. *Journal of Clinical Psychology*, **42**, 2: 315–17.

Rainey, J.M.J., Manov, G., Aleem, A. and Toth, A. (1990). Relationships between PTSD and panic disorder concurrent psychiatric illness: effects of lactate infusions and erythrocyte lactate production. *Frontiers of Clinical Neuroscience*, Vol. 9. *Clinical Aspects of Panic Disorder*, pp. 47–54. Ed. J.C. Balleneger. New York: Wiley-Liss.

Reist, C., Kauffmann, C.D., Chicz Demet, A., Chen, C.C. and Demet, E.M. (1995). REM latency, dexamethasone suppression test, and thyroid releasing hormone stimulation test in posttraumatic stress disorder. *Progress in Neuropsychopharmacology and the Biology of Psychiatry*, **19**, 3: 433–43.

Robert, J.A. (1985). MCMI characteristics of DSM-III: Posttraumatic stress disorder in Vietnam veterans. *Journal of Personality Assessment*, **49**, 3: 226–30.

Robins, L., Helzer, J. and Croughan, J. (1981). National Institute of Mental Health Diagnostic Interview Schedule: its history, characteristics, and validity. *Archives of General Psychiatry*, **38**: 382–9.

Rosen, G.M. (1995). The Aleutian Enterprise sinking and posttraumatic stress disorder: Misdiagnosis in clinical and forensic settings. *Professional Psychology: Research and Practice*, **26**, 1: 82–7.

Salloway, S., Southwick, S.M. and Sadowsky, M. (1990). Opiate withdrawal presenting as posttraumatic stress disorder. *Hospital and Community Psychiatry*, **41**, 6: 666–7.

Saunders, B.E., Arata, C.M. and Kilpatrick, D.G. (1990). Development of a crime-related post-traumatic stress disorder scale for women within the Symptom Checklist-90–Revised. *Journal of Traumatic Stress*, **3**, 3: 439–48.

Schlenger, W.E., Kulka, R.A., Fairbank, J.A., Hough, R.L., Jordan, B.K.M.C.R. and Weiss, D.S. (1992a). Post traumatic stress disorder among Vietnam veterans findings from the National Vietnam Veterans: Readjustment Study. *American Journal of Epidemiology*, **136**, 8: 1034.

Schlenger, W.E., Kulka, R.A., Fairbank, J.A. and Hough, R.L. (1992b). The prevalence of post-traumatic stress disorder in the Vietnam generation: A multimethod, multisource assessment of psychiatric disorder. *Journal of Traumatic Stress*, **5**, 3: 333–63.

Schnurr, P., Friedman, M. and Rosenberg, S. (1993). Premilitary MMPI scores as predictors of combat-related PTSD symptoms. *American Journal of Psychiatry*, **150**, 3: 479–83.

Schwarzwald, J., Solomon, Z., Weisenberg, M. and Mikulincer, M. (1987). Validation of the Impact of Event Scale for psychological sequelae of combat. *Journal of Consulting and Clinical Psychology*, **55**, 2: 251–6.

Shulman, E. (1994). Predicting postcombat PTSD by using premilitary MMPI scores. *American Journal of Psychiatry*, **151**, 1: 156.

Smith, M.A., Davidson, J., Ritchie, J.C., Kudler, H., Lipper, S., Chappell, P. and Nemeroff, C.B. (1989). The corticotropin-releasing hormone test in patients with posttraumatic stress disorder. *Biological Psychiatry*, **26**, 4: 349–55.

Solomon, Z. (1989). Psychological sequelae of war: A 3-year prospective study of Israeli combat stress reaction casualties. *Journal of Nervous and Mental Disease*, **177**, 6: 342–6.

Solomon, Z., Benbenishty, R., Neria, Y., Abramowitz, M., Ginzburg, K. and Ohry, A. (1993). Assessment of PTSD: Validation of the revised PTSD Inventory. *Israel Journal of Psychiatry and Related Sciences*, **30**, 2: 110–15.

Southwick, S.M., Krystal, J.H., Morgan, C.A., Johnson, D., Nagy, L.M.N.A., Heninger, G.R. and Charney, D.S. (1993). Abnormal noradrenergic function in posttraumatic stress disorder. *Archives of General Psychiatry*, **50**, 4: 266–74.

Sparr, L.F. (1995). Post-traumatic stress disorder. Does it exist? *Neurology Clinics*, **13**, 2: 413–29.

Sparr, L.F. and Atkinson, R.M. (1986). Posttraumatic stress disorder as an insanity defense: Medicolegal quicksand. 138th Annual Meeting of the American Psychiatric Association, 1985, Dallas, Texas. *American Journal of Psychiatry*, **143**, 5: 608–13.

Sparr, L. and Pankratz, L.D. (1983). Factitious posttraumatic stress disorder. *American Journal of Psychiatry*, **140**, 8: 1016–19.

Spector, J. and Huthwaite, M. (1993). Eye-movement desensitisation to overcome post-traumatic stress disorder. *British Journal of Psychiatry*, **163**: 106–8.

Tick, E. (1986). The face of horror. *Psychotherapy Patient*, **3**, 2: 101–20.

Triffleman, E.G., Marmar, C.R., Delucchi, K.L. and Ronfeldt, H. (1995). Childhood trauma and posttraumatic stress disorder in substance abuse inpatients. *Journal of Nervous and Mental Disease*, **183**, 3: 172–6.

Vreven, D.L., Gudanowski, D.M., King, L.A. and King, D.W. (1995). The civilian version of the Mississippi PTSD Scale: a psychometric evaluation. *Journal of Traumatic Stress*, **8**, 1: 91–109.

Watson, C.G., Anderson, P.E. and Gearhart, L.P. (1995). Posttraumatic stress disorder (PTSD) symptoms in PTSD patients' families of origin. *Journal of Nervous and Mental Disease*, **183**, 10: 633–8.

Watson, C.G., Brown, K., Kucala, T., Juba, M., Davenport, E.C. and Anderson, D. (1993). Two studies of reported pretraumatic stressors' effect on posttraumatic stress disorder severity. *Journal of Clinical Psychology*, **49**, 3: 311–18.

Watson, C.G., Juba, M.P. and Anderson, P.E. (1989). Validities of five combat scales. *Psychological Assessment*, **1**, 2: 98–102.

Watson, C.G., Juba, M.P., Manifold, V., Kucala, T. and Anderson, P.E. (1991). The PTSD interview: Rationale, description, reliability, and concurrent validity of a DSM-III-based technique. *Journal of Clinical Psychology*, **47**, 2: 179–88.

Watson, C.G., Plemel, D., DeMotts, J., Howard, M.T., Tuorida, J., Moog, R., Thomas, D. and Anderson, D. (1994). A comparison of four PTSD measures' convergent validities in Vietnam veterans. *Journal of Traumatic Stress*, **7**, 1: 75–82.

Weisaeth, L. (1989a). Importance of high response rates in traumatic stress research. Special issue: Traumatic stress: empirical studies from Norway. *Acta Psychiatrica Scandinavica*, **80**, 355 (Suppl.): 131–7.

Weisaeth, L. (1989b). The stressors and the post-traumatic stress syndrome after an industrial disaster. Special issue: Traumatic stress: empirical studies from Norway. *Acta Psychiatrica Scandinavica*, **80**, 355 (Suppl.): 25–37.

Weisaeth, L. (1989c). A study of behavioural responses to an industrial disaster. Special issue: Traumatic stress: empirical studies from Norway. *Acta Psychiatrica Scandinavica*, **80**, 355 (Suppl.): 13–24.

Weisenberg, M., Solomon, Z., Schwarzwald, J. and Mikulincer, M. (1987). Assessing the severity of posttraumatic stress disorder: Relation between dichotomous and continuous measures. *Journal of Consulting and Clinical Psychology*, **55**, 3: 432–34.

Weiss, D.S., Marmar, C.R., Schlenger, W.E. and Fairbank, J.A. (1992). The prevalence of lifetime and partial post-traumatic stress disorder in Vietnam theater veterans. *Journal of Traumatic Stress*, **5**, 3: 365–76.

Wetter, M.W., Baer, R.A., Berry, D.T. and Robison, L.H. (1993). MMPI-2 profiles of motivated fakers given specific symptom information: A comparison to matched patients. *Psychological Assessment*, **5**, 3: 317–23.

Wilson, J.P. and.Krauss, G. (1985). Predicting post-traumatic stress disorders among Vietnam veterans. In *Post-Traumatic Stress Disorder and the War Veteran Patient*, pp. 102–47. Ed. W.E. Kelly. New York: Brunner Mazel.

Wilson, J.P., Smith, W.K. and Johnson, S.K. (1985). A comparative analysis of PTSD among various survivor groups. In *Trauma and Its Wake: The Study and Treatment of Post Traumatic Stress Disorders*, pp. 142–12. Ed. C.R. Figley. Brunner Mazel. Psychosocial Stress Series, No. 4. New York: Brunner Mazel.

Wolfe, J., Keane, T.M., Lyons, J.A. and Gerardi, R.J. (1987). Current trends and issues in the assessment of combat-related posttraumatic stress disorder. *Behavior Therapist*, **10**, 2: 27–32.

Yehuda, R., Southwick, S.M., Nussbaum, G., Wahby, V.S., Giller, E.L. and Mason, J.W. (1990). Low urinary cortisol excretion in patients with posttraumatic stress disorder. *Journal of Nervous and Mental Disease*, **178**, 6: 366–9.

Zilberg, N.J., Weiss, D.S. and Horowitz, M.J. (1982). Impact of Event Scale: a cross-validation study and some empirical evidence supporting a conceptual model of stress response syndromes. *Journal of Consulting and Clinical Psychology*, **50**, 3: 407–14.

CHAPTER 8

MANAGEMENT AND OUTCOME OF POST-TRAUMATIC ILLNESS

There is a definite paucity of empirical data about the treatment and the outcome of PTI other than PTSD and acute stress disorder. In acute stress disorder the data are sparse and mostly based upon either intervention in combat stress disorder, or on uncontrolled trials or case data.

Even in the most closely studied area, that of PTSD, there is insufficient evidence to say that there is a single specific treatment strategy which is the most appropriate to be used in every case or in the typical case of PTSD. In the same way, there is considerable controversy about the prognosis in PTSD.

ICD-10 suggests that PTSD is essentially of good prognosis (World Health Organisation, 1992) when it says 'the course is fluctuating but recovery can be expected in the majority of cases'.

However, it also points out that 'in a small proportion of patients the condition may show a chronic course over many years and a transition to an enduring personality change'. It is suggested, therefore, that PTSD may precede a type of personality change which is 'a chronic, irreversible sequel of stress disorder'. The notes to the specific diagnosis in ICD-10 indicate that such a change should only be diagnosed following extreme and prolonged traumatic events and not following brief life-threatening experiences such as road traffic accidents. The diagnostic guidelines are somewhat vague. The prognosis for this condition, which is not present in DSM-IV but is akin to the concept of DESNOS (Worzel, 1992), is effectively of inevitable poor prognosis as it is necessary for the changes in personality to have been present for two years before the diagnosis can be made, and because it is described as 'enduring'.

In essence, it seems to be that ICD-10 says that the prognosis is generally good but if it is not good and problems are chronic, then in certain circumstances the diagnosis should be changed. Recovery can be anticipated except following extreme trauma when there may be permanent and irreversible personality change. It does not explain why some of those who are not exposed to catastrophic trauma develop chronic illness, except to hint at the role of personal vulnerability factors. This does not really accord with most of the research, which shows a less than clear link between severity of trauma and outcome, and which, unlike ICD-10, does not indicate that vulnerability factors are irrelevant in extreme situations.

Most of the studies of PTSD do not clearly demonstrate a good prognosis, and this will be discussed further. However, it seems clear that many of the larger and more robust studies have involved later, more entrenched, and perhaps more resistant cases, so that there may have been inherent bias towards a poor prognosis.

It is the intention in this chapter to consider briefly any relevant changes to the management of mental disorders when they follow trauma, to consider prognosis and management of acute stress disorder, and then to focus on the prognosis of PTSD and the various strategies used in management. There is very little written about the first, and almost all of the work around acute stress disorder concerns the specific situation of battle shock or combat stress reaction. The PTSD work still has an emphasis on Vietnam, but there is an increasing body of data on other traumata.

Other mental illnesses following trauma

There really is a shortage of work on this subject except that associated with bereavement, and perhaps work looking at comorbidity, particularly with substance abuse. While Neal and also Sparr (Sparr and Boehnlein, 1990; Neal, 1994) have warned us of the dangers of forcing people into a diagnosis of PTSD when it really does not fit, nevertheless there has been an increasing focus in recent years on PTSD as if it were the only possible problem after trauma. This is clearly inappropriate and inaccurate. There is very good evidence that a wide range of mental disorders may be associated with trauma. Each should be treated on its own merits, taking into account the effects of trauma. There should be a careful assessment of the presence or absence of PTSD, but if it is not present then the treatment should be aimed at the presenting condition. If there is 'dual diagnosis', then both disorders will need attention.

This chapter will make no attempt to detail the treatment of a whole range of possible post-traumatic illnesses or of individual comorbid illnesses as the treatments should essentially be those recognised for the various conditions.

Treatment of PTI

The most useful principle concerning treatment of other mental illnesses following trauma is that it should be tailored to the presenting condition. In other words, depression should be treated as depression, phobic disorder as phobia etc. It is not appropriate to treat all illness which follows trauma as PTSD. The process of engaging in treatment will need recognition of the influence of the trauma, and the principle of normalisation of responses in an abnormal situation is of importance. A difficulty which may be practically met with patients is the belief that the symptoms, of whatever type, are a direct consequence of the trauma. The symptoms are therefore seen as understandable and neither worthy of, nor susceptible to, treatment. Rather, they are something that must be endured. It is in this area that engagement and establishment of treatment in PTI may differ from the same condition in other circumstances. Once a therapeutic alliance has been established, treatment should probably be that of the presenting condition, although the therapist must be aware of specific post-traumatic issues which may emerge and must be prepared to treat them pragmatically.

Treatment of comorbid disorders

There is debate about methodology of management of disorders comorbid with PTSD. There is plenty of evidence of the frequency with which comorbidity is seen. There is some suggestion that comorbid disorders may interfere with completion of treatment or adversely affect prognosis (Boudewyns *et al.*, 1991a). Should PTSD be treated first, second, or concurrently?

The answer must, at present, be a pragmatic one. If comorbid disorders prevent engagement in treatment for PTSD, then they may well need to be treated first, or at least brought under control. If PTSD is aggravating pre-existing illness, then it may need to be addressed first. If the interrelationship is unknown or so complicated that it cannot be disentangled, then it may be most appropriate to treat the symptoms which are causing most distress and are most accessible or amenable to treatment first.

An obvious example is substance abuse. There may seem to be a need to establish abstinence before the subject is in a position to engage in treatment. However, if the substance abuse is a conscious attempt to control distressing symptoms, usually intrusive, then the increase in symptom distress following withdrawal may be too much to cope with in addition to preventing engagement. Jelinek has pointed out that such situations need careful assessment (Jelinek and Williams, 1984) as the relationship between PTSD and, for example, alcohol abuse, may be very complicated. It should be remembered that substance misuse may be a common reason for patients dropping out of treatment (Boudewyns *et al.*, 1991b).

When considering treatment of comorbidity with affective disorders such as depression, the situation is clearer. Antidepressant therapy for sufferers is likely to be helpful. It may also have a significant positive effect on the intrusive symptoms of PTSD. Severe depression may, of course, impair engagement in treatment. The doses of antidepressants needed to affect PTSD symptomatology may be relatively high.

Acute stress disorder

Acute stress disorder is a new diagnosis, introduced in ICD-10 and DSM-IV. There is a temptation to extrapolate from experience in related areas such as combat psychiatry, battle shock, and the previous concept of gross stress disorder. However, there is, and can be, no evidence that these situations are all equivalent. There should be caution in extrapolating from one to the other.

There is little empirical research on acute stress reactions, and an absence of randomised controlled trials. While there have been papers written on acute stress reactions at least since the First World War, even the more recent ones have been descriptive rather than trial designs (Cardena and Spiegel, 1993; Koopman, Classen and Spiegel, 1994).

The major importance of acute stress disorder seems to be in its predictive value for PTSD. It is suggested that most of those who will develop PTSD will have had an acute stress reaction, although most of those with acute stress reactions will not go on to have PTSD. This opinion is certainly supported by the Israeli combat stress reaction work, which has consistently shown that soldiers who suffer such reactions, even if they respond to treatment, have higher rates of PTSD than controls (Solomon, 1989). This finding has been consistent, and the occurrence of a combat stress reaction in Israeli soldiers is still predictive of PTSD-related problems 18 years later (Solomon and Kleinhauz, 1996).

Combat psychiatry principles

For some time, basic principles of combat psychiatry have been influential in military medical planning. They stem to a great extent from observations in the

First World War that the large numbers of British First World War shell shock cases evacuated to hospitals such as Netley and Moss Side had low rates of recovery and, particularly, low rates of return to active service. As the new pro-grammes of in-theatre forward treatment in special units was established, recovery rates increased dramatically. The principles of combat psychiatry were established as:

proximity
immediacy
expectancy.

A fourth, simplicity, has crept in to the planning.

It should be understood that the purpose of these principles of treatment of acute psychiatric problems in the trauma of combat was to return soldiers quickly to duty and to avoid overwhelming the evacuation and treatment chain. Solomon and others have studied the application of these principles in Israel, where the geography of the country both assists and enforces them. Israel's wars have not been fought overseas. Soldiers who are not treated in field hos-pitals are necessarily treated in civilian 'home' hospitals. The results from the Israeli studies (Solomon and Benbenishty, 1986) have shown that all three of the original principles are associated with improved outcome after combat stress reaction. The outcome measures were return to active military duty and presence or absence of PTSD a year later. Other authors have also shown the advantages of treating soldiers with combat-related acute stress reactions in a military setting and with expectancy (Margalit *et al.*, 1994).

It is important to note that the Israeli experience suggests that the progno-sis for soldiers exposed to combat who develop acute reactions is not good, even when they are treated apparently effectively. Although those who are treated in accordance with the principles of proximity, immediacy and expectancy appear to do better, combat stress reaction cases still have higher rates of PTSD than controls at one, two and three years (Solomon, 1989). The rate of PTSD at one year in such treated patients was 59%, compared with 16% for control combat soldiers (Solomon *et al.*, 1987).

Proximity

By proximity is meant the idea that sufferers should be treated as near to the site of the trauma as possible. The logic is obvious, at least with soldiers who are expected to stay in the theatre of war and return to fighting. However, it may be applicable to the civilian who is involved in a trauma at work or the person whose home is in the zone of damage of some disaster.

In military terms, the sufferer is treated as near to the front line as possible, without being entirely removed from the zone of danger. As the sufferer does not leave the area of potential further danger or trauma, the symptoms are not reinforced or perpetuated by the reduction of anxiety associated with escape from the feared situation. For the civilian, the dangerous link between removal from work or home and reduction of anxiety is hopefully not made.

Immediacy

In the combat situation, immediacy also reinforces the importance of maintaining the soldier role. For civilian and military victims, immediacy is congruent with general crisis intervention theory, which suggests that early intervention is likely to be more powerful than the same intervention later.

Following road traffic accidents there is evidence that early intervention has more effect than delayed contact (Bordow and Porritt, 1979), although there is also more recent evidence from a well-constructed trial that immediate intervention has no effect in the long term (Brom, Kleber and Hofman, 1993), even though it is generally appreciated by victims.

While it seems entirely logical that immediate intervention will be appropriate for individuals exposed to trauma, the actual evidence for improved efficacy is really confined to combat situations.

Where there is a clear advantage to both proximity and immediacy is, of course, in the situation in which an ad hoc group of people is involved in a traumatic event. There are ideological and economical reasons for intervening with them as a group. This may only be possible if done in the immediate aftermath.

Those who were involved in providing psychotherapy for the survivors of the Beverly Hills club fire have suggested that one of the reasons why such a high proportion of the survivors seen did not complete therapy, and in particular why a significant number 'fled' from therapy was that a number of the therapists had not been present in the make-shift mortuaries in the immediate aftermath, while others had (Lindy *et al.*, 1983). It was hinted that only those who had been exposed to the carnage and had been involved so early were acceptable or were able to act as therapists for this particular group. However, when we consider that the study involved 22 therapists and 30 patients, of whom 17% did not enter therapy and only 50% completed therapy, it seems dangerous to make generalisations.

Expectancy

Expectancy has come to be seen as an important principle because of the observed high invaliding rates of soldiers with shell shock early in the First

World War. It has become accepted that in order to avoid this loss of man-power, as well as the chronic disability that goes with it, there should be a con-scious expectation from all that the combat stress reaction victim is still a soldier and will inevitably return to his functional role.

This may be a significant dilemma for the mental health professional if the concept of expectancy means the expectation that the patient will return to the front line in a new tank after the last one burned out beneath him but he escaped with his life. The counter-argument is, of course, that expectancy inevitably involves expectation of 'exposure' while removal from danger involves 'avoidance' which is likely to be reinforcing. Nevertheless, this will inevitably be a dilemma for the therapist and is one of the many arguments for supervision and support for therapists involved in this difficult area of work.

The expectancy argument may be just as important for civilian trauma victims but is not usually, except in the case of some of the emergency services, a question of whether or not to send the victim back to a situation in which they can anticipate somebody trying to kill them.

The idea that an early return to duties in the case of work-related trauma is of importance seems to have been accepted by employers in a range of potentially dangerous occupations. The author has been involved with planning and provi-sion of services in a range of employment sectors, and has observed others.

- Some financial institutions are aware that following the all too frequent robberies or attempted robberies, there is a potential problem of pro-longed staff absence. They insist on staff being seen at the place of work within 48 hours, and of involved staff's absence being traced. They provide 'counselling'. Clinical psychologists employed by banking institu-tions in the USA have described their experiences and given recommenda-tions for those involved in dealing with this particular group (Manton and Talbot, 1990).
- Some, at least, of British Rail's regions (now the new franchisee compa-nies) have programmes for the re-introduction to driving of train drivers who have been involved in deaths or injuries on the track. Perhaps surpris-ingly, this is not an uncommon occurrence. In Denmark it occurs about once a week (Tang, 1994), and on London Underground about twice a week (Farmer et al., 1992). Treatment strategies have been evolved (Williams et al., 1994), some of which include graded exposure in vivo by riding the foot-plate and gradually resuming driving responsibilities.
- Some bus companies have similar programmes with the inevitable 'coun-selling' plus re-assessments before resuming full duties.

- The principles of combat psychiatry have been used to help miners involved in mine disasters to return to the pits (Badenhorst and Van Schalkwyk, 1992).
- Both fire services (McCloy, 1992) and police forces (Duckworth, 1991) have also set up immediate, proximate, and expectant treatment or intervention programmes to keep staff at work.
- Armed Forces medical services have, not surprisingly, established standard operating procedures which include responses to acute stress reactions.

Simplicity

Simplicity has been added as part of the military model of early intervention in acute stress disorder. The reasons are pragmatic, as most major military planning for much of the second half of the twentieth century has focused on a possible major confrontation on the land-mass of Northern Europe. The numbers involved mean that simplicity is essential if it is to work. There have been a small number of reviews of the process in the generally available press (Kentsmith, 1986; Belenky, 1987; Margalit *et al.*, 1994), and obviously detailed plans have been made for specific situations.

While the concept of simplicity has not been empirically tested, it is attractive, and is likely to be of value to employers who wish to ensure that there is an agreed response to acute stress disorders which is likely to be actioned even in the comparative chaos of the aftermath of trauma.

Treatment of acute stress disorders

Much of the specific advice about treatment of acute stress disorders is based upon theoretical approaches or upon personal experience rather than empirical research. Even when based on personal series of many cases, there is an absence of control groups. It seems a consistent feature of the literature that most victims find the intervention helpful and positive, but there is thus far no firm evidence that any of the interventions used prevent PTSD or other PTI in the long term. This is an important point to reinforce. Apart from some degree of success in the particular case of combat stress reactions, there has not yet been any demonstration that interventions in acute stress disorders affect long-term outcome. There is a real need for a controlled trial, not only of intervention for non-complaining trauma survivors, but also of treatments for those with identified difficulties.

A number of treatment methods have been used thus far.

Psychological debriefing

This process, which is described in more detail in Chapter 10 when considering prevention of PTI, was originally developed for use with rescue and emergency personnel (Mitchell, 1983; Dyregrov, 1989; Armstrong *et al.*, 1995).

It was clearly initially intended to be preventive and to be used with all those involved in the traumatic situation, initially emergency services personnel, and later victims. However, it has now come to be used as a therapeutic tool for those showing signs of psychological disturbance in the immediate aftermath of trauma. The theory is that it helps people to recognise and validate feelings and reactions, to confront inappropriate assumption of personal responsibility, to recognise the universality of the reaction, and to normalise reactions. Thus it leads the way to integration of the event.

Individual dynamic psychotherapies

The common factor in an individual psychotherapeutic approach to acute stress disorder is remembering followed by 'working through' of the trauma, with the intention that memories be restructured such that they are manageable.

Various techniques may be used to access and explore memories, including hypnosis (Spiegel and Cardena, 1990) and abreaction.

The process can be closely likened to brief grief work and the same processes logically used. In the process it is necessary to face rather than repress painful memories, with the aim being not that those painful memories are not there any longer, but that they have become bearable and controllable. The hoped-for end-product is that the trauma still happened and the individual was affected by it but has not been permanently robbed of autonomy by the event and has been able to move on.

Group therapies

The use of group therapies for soldiers affected by trauma has a long history which has been reviewed by Terr (1992). Indeed the work with soldiers has had a major influence on the development of group therapies in general.

It is hardly surprising that after Vietnam, group therapies were widely used with what were later to become known as PTSD sufferers. Both conventional group therapies and what came to be known as 'rap groups' developed (Galloucis and Kaufman, 1988).

A particular form of early intervention group treatment which has been developed for use following group experience of trauma is that of the 'mini-marathon group' (Rahe *et al.*, 1990; Terr, 1992). This has been used with heterogeneous groups who have experienced a common trauma, not only with homogeneous groups such as a fire-fighting crew. It is not specifically aimed at those identified as 'ill' rather than survivors in general. Empirical evidence of outcome is not yet available. There are three stages:

1. sharing of information
2. sharing of symptoms
3. sharing of coping strategies and suggestions of self-help.

Terr also suggests that at the end of the session there should be a brief period devoted to sharing of stories of survival and heroism as an acknowledgement of the ability of the human spirit to overcome adversity.

Cognitive–behavioural therapies

There is considerable work surrounding cognitive–behavioural work and PTSD. The logic in application to acute stress disorder is the same, although there is no empirical evidence for or against efficacy. Major components include exposure, cognitive restructuring, and skills training.

Exposure is an important part of many treatment programmes and one with which sufferers can easily identify. Everybody has heard of the old adage about getting back onto a horse after falling off. While the practice may be difficult, the theory is acceptable to most. Graded exposure *in vitro* or *in vivo*, flooding, and implosion may be used.

Cognitive restructuring aims to re-attribute meaning to memories, attempting to 'correct' the common problems of inappropriate guilt and self-recrimination.

Skills training may be particularly valuable in helping victims interact with family members who were not involved in the trauma (Carroll *et al.*, 1991) and with work-mates or others with whom there is a need for regular contact in the immediate aftermath of events.

Drug treatment

It seems to be generally accepted by researchers and practitioners that drug treatment has a limited role to play in acute stress disorder. However, there is little definite evidence either way. Davidson has suggested that for acute stress disorder any drug intervention should be much more brief than is accepted for PTSD (Davidson, 1992). This would be in accord with all of the other advice for management of acute responses.

Benzodiazepines may be seen as an effective way of reducing anxiety in the immediate aftermath of any trauma or loss event and it certainly seems true that they are effective at reducing intrusive if not avoidance and dissociative symptoms (Forster, 1992). It should be remembered that anxiety and anxiety symptoms are part of the normal response to traumatic events. It may be inappropriate, and actually hinder integration, to damp down anxiety completely. It is also possible that use of benzodiazepines in this way, attempting completely to ablate symptoms, may increase the likelihood of inappropriate use and of dependence and tolerance problems. It seems logical that those with a history of benzodiazepine dependence should not be prescribed these drugs. In addition, of course, benzodiazepines do tend to have a mood-lowering effect.

Despite this, benzodiazepines may have a part to play in helping induce sleep in the early post-traumatic period and in helping reduce anxiety and intrusive symptoms to a level at which the sufferer is able to take part in his treatment.

Almost by definition, the usefulness of all *antidepressants* in acute stress disorder must be limited. There is about a two-week lag period before antidepressants have a significant effect on mood, and they will therefore inevitably take too long to work. Some people use sedating antidepressants for what is essentially the side-effect of promoting sleep through sedation.

Propranolol has been suggested to have an acute effect in reducing intrusive symptoms. However, the evidence of efficacy in acute use is sparse and seems to be based on a small pilot study of 11 children that was off–on–off in nature. The subject group were children acutely distressed after abuse (Famularo, Kinscheriff and Fenton, 1988). Their intrusive symptoms were reported to be reduced when taking propranolol compared with either before or after the drug treatment period. A follow-up of the pilot does not seem to have been published.

Neuroleptic or antipsychotic medication has not generally been promoted as being of major value in acute stress disorder.

Post-traumatic stress disorder

It is perhaps surprising that a condition which has been the subject of so much research and publication is not one for which a clear and simple treatment plan can be written. A wide range of treatment strategies has been used in the relatively few years since PTSD was defined, but there have been few randomised controlled trials of treatment. In 1992 a retrospective review of published articles was only able to find 11 randomised controlled trials using DSM criteria (Solomon, Gerrity and Muff, 1992). It suggested that there was evidence for effect of drug therapy, some better evidence for efficacy of behavioural treatments, and the possibility of efficacy of psychodynamic therapies.

At the time of writing it is not possible to define a best practice treatment for PTSD. The major areas of treatment interest appear to be:

psychotherapeutic
pharmacological
cognitive–behavioural
psychosocial
integrated.

To some extent the separation is artificial as most centres seem to tend nowadays to have an empirical problem-centred approach to management rather than a dogmatic one.

A problem with studying psychotherapies and other treatments for PTSD has always been assessment of outcome. McFarlane has reviewed the question of psychotherapy efficacy, pointing out that most types of psychotherapy have been used, but few validated (McFarlane, 1994). There are, of course, many concerns about 'proof' of efficacy of psychological treatments, and particularly of psychotherapies. Randomised controlled trials are difficult to perform or assess and this well-studied problem will not be explored here. However, McFarlane has specifically pointed out that one of the problems in assessing efficacy of treatments for PTSD is that it is very difficult actually to decide what constitutes improvement. This argument has been nicely seen in assessment of the Koach project in Israel.

The Koach project (Solomon *et al.*, 1992a) is not simply a psychotherapeutic project based on a single psychotherapeutic ideology. It is a partially residential, partly outpatient treatment programme for Israeli combat veterans with chronic PTSD in which therapists are also veterans and the treatment is multimodality, and focused significantly around the concept of returning to the status of 'warrior'. It uses psychodynamic, behavioural and psychosocial elements. There has been debate about the outcome measures and suggestions that the patients, the therapists, and objective assessors assess outcome differently (Bleich *et al.*, 1992). The therapists endorse efficacy of the project (Shalev *et al.*, 1992), subjects are positive towards it (Solomon *et al.*, 1992a) and would recommend it to others, although objective testing shows little improvement in actual symptomatology. Some comparative study has suggested that, in symptom terms, Koach subjects do worse than chronic PTSD controls without treatment (Solomon *et al.*, 1992a).

It is probably important to examine carefully claims of efficacy of treatments in PTSD. There may be differences in assessment depending upon whether patient satisfaction, objective test results, or observed function is used as the outcome measure. Another difficulty is that of duration of response. For example, Perconte has shown that more than 50% of patients responding successfully to a partial hospitalisation treatment programme relapse to such an extent that they require further hospital admission within two years (Perconte, Griger and Bellucci, 1989). Another prospective study of 39 veterans completing a 90-day treatment programme showed 48% improved and 13% deteriorated at the end of treatment, with a return to baseline levels of objective measures of symptomatology for all groups one year later (Hammarberg and Silver, 1994). These are obviously not very encouraging results, and fuel concern about the positive attitude to prognosis expressed in ICD-10.

A further problem with assessment of outcome is that there is no definite evidence that it is safe to assume that outcome in different groups of sufferers is the same. Simple observation of the various studies certainly seems to suggest that outcome in Vietnam veterans is worse over time than that in many civilian groups exposed to trauma, especially single episodes.

Psychotherapies

It is clear that in the years just before the definition of PTSD the focus of treatment for Vietnam veterans was in the psychotherapies. This is not surprising. It was the way in which treatment was orientated in America at the time. There was an acceptance that the 'post-Vietnam syndrome' or PTSD was not due to the commotio cerebri postulated as being caused by expanding gases from exploding shells in World War I, but due to psychological assault on the person. Perhaps there was also a recognition that about half of cases had been previously diagnosed as schizophrenia (Zarcone, *et al.* 1977) and treated with neuroleptics.

When PTSD was defined there continued to be a focus upon the psychotherapies, both individual and group, and both inpatient and outpatient. A wide range of different therapies has been used. There is, however, a lack of empirical evidence of efficacy. Hendin (1983) has reviewed the use of psychotherapy in PTSD.

Group psychotherapy has considerable support and is still proposed by some as the principal line of treatment (Makler *et al.*, 1990; Koller, Marmar and Kanas, 1992), suggesting weekly groups over at least a year or more, and using those groups particularly to address issues of isolation, guilt and helplessness. The success or efficacy of group therapy is not clear. One study of 40 cases receiving group therapy plus medication as required showed no improvement in symptomatology following treatment, and no relationship between symptom level and the duration of treatment (Frueh *et al.*, 1994).

The treatment efficacy of brief individual psychodynamic psychotherapy has been compared with that of hypnosis, desensitisation, and a waiting-list control in a group of 112 subjects who had developed PTSD following varied events such as road traffic accidents, bereavement etc. (Brom, Kleber and Defares, 1989). All active treatments had some superiority over the waiting-list condition.

While Marmar would suggest that brief psychotherapy is most suitable for those who have suffered from PTSD for several years (Marmar, 1991), others have suggested that earlier treatment and brief and focused treatment are most appropriate (Prout and Schwarz, 1991). Prout and Schwarz suggest five stages of treatment:

1. supporting adaptive coping skills and strategies
2. normalising experiences and sensations
3. decreasing avoidance
4. producing an alternative attribution of meaning
5. facilitating the integration or re-integration of self.

There are a number of other reports or descriptions of the suggested phases or process of dynamic therapies. Lindy has produced an outline of the methodology of psychoanalytic therapy with PTSD patients (Lindy, 1986).

Horowitz has been influential in the use of individual brief psychotherapy in post-traumatic situations, producing guidelines for treatment some years before the definition of PTSD (Horowitz, 1973, 1979), which continue to be of value in understanding the process of changing symptoms in PTSD and the methods used in psychotherapeutic treatment (Horowitz, 1986; Horowitz *et al.*, 1994). His work has often focused upon the phasic nature of PTSD symptoms, with intrusive symptoms often emerging episodically against a background of avoidance symptoms.

Brende has written on a number of treatment modalities including hypnotherapy (Brende and Benedict, 1980) and combined individual and group therapy (Brende, 1981). He has also described a phasic treatment for combat-related PTSD (Brende and Parson, 1987).

1. The stabilisation of target symptoms.
2. Confronting emotional detachment, smouldering rage, and self-destructive symptoms.
3. Simultaneously controlling intrusive memories and uncovering traumatic experiences.
4. Resolving guilt and facing grief.

5.   Re-integration of self.

6.   Finding atonement with God, self and others.

It has been suggested that in Holocaust survivors there should be three phases of therapy (Erdreich, 1984):

1.   building a relationship

2.   the processing of neuroses

3.   integration of the restructured memories.

Most of the different types of psychotherapy have been used in PTSD at some time. Ego-state therapy (Phillips, 1993) has been used and case histories presented.

Transcendental meditation has been compared with brief psychotherapy for three months in the treatment of post-Vietnam 'adjustment difficulties' in a small study with group sizes of eight (Brooks and Scarano, 1985). A positive effect was found for transcendental meditation but not for brief psychotherapy.

Gestalt therapy, including re-enactment and verbal repetition, has been used in Vietnam veterans with PTSD (Crump, 1984).

It has been suggested that spiritual ideas and spiritual healing in group therapy may sometimes be important (Jimenez, 1993; Decker, 1993).

Frankl was a Holocaust survivor who invented logotherapy and worked with other Holocaust survivors. It is suggested that his 'will to meaning' principle means that his form of psychotherapy is of value to those with PTSD in helping them to identify and assimilate traumatic memories and then use them (Lantz, 1992; Chung, 1995).

The Royal Air Force 12-day group treatment programme which has treated groups of mixed trauma survivors with PTSD, although eclectic, used psychological debriefing (Busuttil et al., 1995) as its main treatment modality, reporting good outcome at one year.

Sociodrama (Baumgartner, 1986) has been used in PTSD.

Pharmacological treatment

The physiological and neuro-endocrinological investigation of PTSD provides support for the theoretical value of a number of different medications in PTSD. There is clear evidence of some dysfunction or alteration in noradrenergic centres, in locus coeruleus function, in serotonin activity and of problems of impulse control. There is also interest in the kindling and sensitisation process.

This, therefore, provides support for the investigation of the value of drugs such as the various types of antidepressants, membrane-stabilising drugs, and noradrenergic-blocking drugs.

A practical point about drug treatment in PTSD is that there is a perception amongst therapists that compliance with treatment may often be poor. There is at least as much need as usual to explain clearly to patients about lag-times before response can be expected, and about side-effects of medication. There is a need for close monitoring of compliance and to beware of early discontinuation or alteration in treatment.

Antidepressants

All of the types of antidepressants in current use have been tried in PTSD. A psychotropic drug directory (Bazire, 1996) notes that no drugs are specifically licensed for the treatment of PTSD in the UK. The drugs listed in this directory as having some recognised potency are all antidepressants, while each of the other drugs reported as being used is considered to be of less definite efficacy.

There has been prolonged debate about whether antidepressants have any actual effect upon PTSD or whether their effect is only upon the associated depressive symptoms. The former seems the case. The biochemical findings in PTSD go some way to explaining why there should be some effect and why it is difficult to separate it from an antidepressant effect. There is a general consensus that antidepressants are of some value but not totally efficacious. It has been suggested, with some experimental evidence (Sutherland and Davidson, 1994), that tricyclics and other antidepressants have an effect upon intrusive but not upon other symptoms of PTSD. It is held that maximum response to the antidepressants may take several months.

A pilot project involving 158 patients with PTSD has shown that the combination of fluoxetine, amitriptyline, and the anticonvulsant benzodiazepine clonazepam seems to be effective when used with a multimodality treatment programme (Burdon et al., 1991). There seems to be significant symptom response within 72 hours and further symptom amelioration over a longer period. This is a good indication of the fact that it is generally accepted that treatment of PTSD requires more than a single therapeutic element.

The *tricyclic antidepressants* used in trials have been imipramine, desipramine, and amitriptyline. They have mostly been used in open trials or series of cases, but there have been a few controlled trials.

Amitriptyline has been used in double-blind controlled comparisons with placebo (Davidson *et al.*, 1993). In the original study of 40 people with an eight-week treatment period, Davidson found amitriptyline to be superior to placebo (Davidson *et al.*, 1990).

Imipramine was said to be effective in an open trial of ten patients (Burstein, 1984). Controlled trials have often compared imipramine with phenelzine and placebo, and have tended to be confusing. In a study of 34 cases (Frank *et al.*, 1988), imipramine was better than phenelzine which was better than placebo. However, in another trial of 60 cases (Kosten *et al.*, 1991) phenelzine was superior to imipramine and people continued to take this drug longer than they did the imipramine.

Desipramine was compared with placebo in a double-blind crossover trial involving 18 cases by Reist (Reist *et al.*, 1989). Little effect was seen and what effect there was could be seen only on the depressive symptoms. However, critics suggest that the duration of the trial was too short and the PTSD measures used were insensitive so that a type two error was inevitable. Other studies have found some effect of desipramine (Reist *et al.*, 1995).

The older *monoamine oxidase inhibitor (MAOI) antidepressants* have also been tried in PTSD. In an open trial of ten cases described as a pilot, Davidson (Davidson, Walker and Kilts, 1987) found a positive effect, while another open trial involving 25 Israeli veterans (Lerer *et al.*, 1987) found little benefit. It has been suggested from studies of Indochinese trauma survivors that MAOIs have a positive effect (DeMartino, Mollica and Wilk, 1995). A small double blind crossover trial found no significant benefit from phenelzine (Shestatzky, Greenberg and Lerer, 1988). Given the problems of side-effects and drug–drug interactions of this group of drugs, they are unlikely to be of primary importance in management of PTSD. There has, however, been suggestion that the new reversible MAOIs should be investigated for possible value in the management of PTSD (Priest *et al.*, 1995).

It seems inevitable that the *serotonin re-uptake inhibitor antidepressants* should have been tried in PTSD. The connection between impulse control and serotonin, and that with intrusive thoughts or ruminations seems obvious. The drugs investigated have been fluoxetine, fluvoxamine, and sertraline. There has also been considerable pre-clinical work on sertraline.

Fluoxetine has been noted to have a positive effect in open trials (Davidson, Roth and Newman, 1991; McDougle *et al.*, 1991; Nagy *et al.*, 1993). In one such trial it was particularly noted to reduce the frequency of explosive outbursts in 13 of 18 subjects (Shay, 1992). In a randomised double-blind five-week controlled trial with placebo it was significantly more effective than the placebo (Van Der Kolk *et al.*, 1994). Of the 64 subjects, about half were Vietnam veterans and half not. The latter group did better than veterans with fluoxetine. The drug also had an antidepressant effect in addition to its effect on PTSD. It should be noted that most reports of fluoxetine in PTSD have used relatively high doses of about 80 mg daily over prolonged periods.

Fluvoxamine had a modest but significant effect in the 17 of 24 patients who completed four weeks of treatment (de Boer *et al.*, 1992).

Sertraline was used in a series of 80 patients and was of significant benefit (Kline *et al.*, 1994). In a trial of nine patients with comorbidity of PTSD and alcohol related problems, it was effective in reducing symptom scores and drinking behaviour (Brady, Sonne and Roberts, 1995).

Mood-stabilising drugs

There is some considerable interest in whether there is a place for the drugs which are prescribed for mood stabilisation in the treatment of bipolar disorder in the management of patients with PTSD. The presence of explosive outbursts, of impulsivity, and of irritability and mood swings suggests that these drugs may be of some value. It has been pointed out that there are, as of yet, no controlled trials of these drugs in PTSD (Keck, McElroy and Friedman, 1992), but there is still considerable interest in their possible efficacy.

Sodium valproate has been the subject of single case reports (Berigan and Holzgang, 1995) and of an open trial of 15 cases (Fesler, 1991) in which it has been said to have been of value.

Lithium has been said, in open treatment reports of two (Forster *et al.*, 1995) and four (Kitchner and Greenstein, 1985) cases, to be effective in reducing irritability and explosive behaviour.

Carbamezapine has also been used and is said to be of some value.

Other drugs

Quite a range of drugs has been used in PTSD at various times. However, there are no significant controlled trials. It seems clear that drug treatment is not the whole answer in PTSD. Even the antidepressants which have been shown to have some effect have not been found to be 'curative'.

Propranolol has been used to control some of the physical symptoms of anxiety for many years. It has been reported to have been used in PTSD (Wolf, Alavi and Mosnaim, 1987) but the only trial of such treatment was in children, as has been noted above (Famularo, Kinscheriff and Fenton, 1988). There is no good evidence of its general value in PTSD.

Clonidine has been said to be of benefit in Vietnam veterans with PTSD. Specifically, it has been used in Cambodian refugees, particularly in combination with imipramine (Kinzie and Leung, 1989), with one paper suggesting a beneficial effect in a group of 68 severely traumatised refugees. Case reports in other patients have supported the beneficial effect (Iruela *et al.*, 1991) and the effect of the drug on the locus coeruleus gives some theoretical back-up to its use.

Benzodiazepines have been discussed in the section on acute stress disorder. While they may have brief value in reducing arousal and anxiety symptomatology to a level at which a sufferer may be able to enter treatment, there are significant potential problems of tolerance, dependency and abuse. In conversation with a group of Argentinean psychiatrists, they reported a significant problem of benzodiazepine dependence in veterans following the Falklands War, but no published reports have been seen.

Alprazolam, specifically has been used. However, a double-blind crossover trial of ten subjects showed a modest effect upon anxiety but no significant effect upon PTSD symptoms (Braun *et al.*, 1990). In addition, a series of eight cases of severe withdrawal symptoms in Vietnam veterans with PTSD who had been taking alprazolam regularly has been reported (Risse *et al.*, 1990).

Buspirone has been reported as of value in PTSD on a number of occasions. There has been a report of three cases who responded to buspirone (Wells *et al.*, 1991), an open trial of eight cases (Duffy and Malloy, 1994), and 7 of 12 Vietnam veterans with PTSD are said to have responded (Fichtner and Crayton, 1994). There is need for a controlled trial.

Neuroleptics are generally considered to be of little value in PTSD per se. There has been a single case report of response to thioridazine (Dillard, Bendfeldt and Jernigan, 1993) but there is no evidence that this is an observation which can be generalised.

Cognitive and behavioural treatments

It is in this area that the best evidence for efficacy exists. A relatively wide range of interventions has been tried with varying degrees of success, but it is generally the case that exposure-based therapies seem to be beneficial. In addition to exposure treatment, anxiety management treatments appear to be effective (Foa and Rothbaum, 1989).

Cognitive–behavioural therapy was found to be effective in treatment of a group of 19 sexually abused girls (Deblinger, McLeer and Henry, 1990).

The principle of restructuring cognitions and challenging maladaptive thought processes and assumptions is a significant part of many treatment schemes.

Exposure therapies have been presented in various ways, both *in vitro* and *in vivo*. Because of the nature of the traumatic events, the former is by far the more common. Different forms of in-vitro exposure are used. One important practical point is that therapists must make their patients aware that they can expect significant increases in anxiety with direct exposure treatment. This is something which must be recognised and contained in treatment and the patient must be prepared and must realise that it is essential to recovery. Otherwise a flight from treatment can be anticipated.

Systematic desensitisation has been shown to be effective. In this method the subject trains in relaxation before being exposed to fear-provoking imagery. The method has been found to be effective, but to involve prolonged treatment. In a study of eight Vietnam veterans with PTSD and eight controls (Peniston, 1986), using electromyography feedback to aid relaxation, a period of two years of treatment resulted in improvement in the treated group. A further study of 15 cases and controls showed significant changes in MMPI scores after 30 sessions of treatment using brainwave feedback (Coolican, Grogan and Vassar, 1989). Improvement was maintained at 30 months.

However, it became recognised that relaxation was not a necessary component of the therapy, and it was perceived that it might prolong treatment. Direct imaginal exposure or flooding was seen to be at least as effective (Boudewyns *et al.*, 1990).

Flooding and implosive therapies have been used widely (Lyons and Keane, 1989). In a randomised controlled trial of treatment in Vietnam veterans, implosive or flooding therapy showed an improvement in anxiety and intrusive symptoms but not avoidance symptoms at the end of treatment and again six months later (Keane *et al.*, 1989). Others have published case reports of flooding therapy for victims from other trauma in addition to the reports on Vietnam veterans. However, it cannot be assumed that implosive treatment is free of risk. A series of six cases in which there was significant deterioration in associated symptoms other than anxiety during implosive treatment has been described (Pitman *et al.*, 1991) and the dangers pointed out.

Other methods of exposure have included techniques such as taped imaginal exposure (Bisson and Jones, 1995). This method involves production of a first person, current tense, account of the traumatic event which is refined, audio-taped, and used regularly as a means of exposure. Sixteen of 18 consecutive patients were able to use this therapy and improved. Similar techniques have been previously used in Australia (Vaughan and Tarrier, 1992) and called image habituation training.

Muss has developed a system called rewind (Muss, 1991). He says that this was initially developed for a single person and is a method which involves an imaginative exposure technique in which the outcome of the traumatic event is wound backwards in time on a visualised cinema screen and then changed so that there is a different outcome and therefore cognitive restructuring is facilitated.

One of the most keenly investigated variations of exposure in recent years is eye movement desensitisation and reprocessing (EMDR). This process, first discussed in the author's unit as an amusing 'oddity' in new treatments, is the subject of nearly 30 papers indexed in Medline, and more elsewhere. It has been taken very seriously and has been the subject of much research and not a little controversy.

It was described by Shapiro as involving the client being induced to make large rhythmic saccadic eye movements while visualising or holding in mind a traumatic memory (Shapiro, 1989). It is said that often as little as one session can result in sustained anxiety reduction, changed meaning of the memory, and reduction of intrusive symptoms. It is a method which has been hotly disputed and questioned (Herbert and Mueser, 1992; Lohr *et al.*, 1992). Even the alleged origin of the method, which is said to have been a serendipitous discovery of a response, has been challenged (Rosen, 1995). However, Silver and others found EMDR to be superior to relaxation and to biofeedback (Silver, Brooks and Obenchain, 1995) and a pilot study (Forbes, Creamer and Rycroft, 1994) showed significant response after few treatments.

Not all investigators have agreed however. Vaughan and others did not find EMDR to be superior to image habituation training or muscle relaxation (Vaughan *et al.*, 1994), and a study of 23 subjects which intentionally used variations of the system suggested that the eye movements were not an essential part of the treatment effect (Renfrey and Spates, 1994).

The consensus view seems to be that whether or not the eye movements or the specific sort of eye movements are the secret of the treatment, this treatment does have some significant effect upon intrusive symptoms.

Psychosocial interventions

Psychosocial interventions have generally been seen as a part of a multimodal or eclectic treatment package. Figley has produced a detailed review of the importance of family and social support (Figley, 1986).

It is necessary to take into account the position of the victim in the world and in society. For example, healed burns victims are recognised to be likely to need significant psychosocial interventions to enable them to reintegrate into society (Blumenfield and Schoeps, 1992) in addition to their needs concerning possible PTSD symptomatology.

Often victims will need help in readjustment in the family situation and in other relationships (Allen and Bloom, 1994). There is clearly a place for marital therapy (Bagarozzi, 1994), and for therapeutic recreation (Lawney, 1982) particularly in groups.

There has been some interest in the role of work and vocational adjustment (Pendorf, 1990) in rehabilitation in PTSD in Vietnam veterans. This is an area of considerable interest. Not only is there a suggestion, although disputed, that combat veterans with PTSD have significant difficulty settling into work, but it is not uncommon for events at work to be the source of the PTSD. As noted above, a number of employers recognise this and it is important that employers become involved in programmes like graded exposure or return to work.

Other specific interventions which may be of value include anger management and practical problem issues such as debt counselling.

Integrated approaches to treatment of PTSD

Over the years, most units specialising in the treatment of PTSD have developed specific treatment packages. While these initially tended to focus only on psychodynamic therapies, it is inevitable that with time they have developed to meet perceived and measured needs. Either there is an 'adding on' of treatment modalities as they become available or a pragmatic addition of treatments for specific problem areas. There are two methods of development. There may either be a fixed treatment programme for cohorts of patients or there may be a problem-orientated approach in which there is an arsenal of therapeutic interventions available which are selected and fitted together in order to respond to the particular needs and problems of each individual patient so that treatment is individually packaged but in a 'menu' system. A range of programmes have published their methodology and sometimes their results, although they seldom produce controlled trials of the whole package rather than individual elements.

One package for Vietnam veterans, which is based primarily on group treatment using psychotherapeutic, cognitive–behavioural, and Gestalt strategies, is deemed to be unsuitable for those who are unwilling or unable to verbalise their difficulties (Besyner, 1985). The author accepts that verbal therapies will not eliminate all intrusive symptoms so relaxation therapy and visual imagery are included, as are specific symptom-focused tactics. A very similar theoretical model with the addition of EMDR and focus on timing has been used with Desert Storm cases (Viola and McCarthy, 1994). Another inpatient programme adding psychoeducational processes and art therapy has been described in male survivors of sexual abuse (Zaidi, 1994).

Perconte has championed the concept of partial hospitalisation for group treatment of PTSD (Perconte, 1986; 1987). The approach is eclectic and its aims include:

- verbalisation of problems
- abreaction of emotions
- communication of feelings to patients' families
- modification of stereotyped maladaptive behaviours
- social desensitisation and reintegration.

It has already been noted that relapse rates following this intensive form of treatment for people with long-standing, severe PTSD are high, and that not all benefit or even complete treatment, although some improvement is maintained at two years despite the relapse rate.

Forman and Havas (1990) have drawn attention to the observation that a number of Vietnam veterans have not received treatment for PTSD. They focus on the public health aspects of the condition, the effects upon relationships, family life and employment, and describe an inpatient-based eclectic treatment and rehabilitation programme.

This emphasis on the importance of social reintegration is overtly discussed in the description of the second generation programme for treatment of Vietnam veterans (Johnson *et al.*, 1994). This concept indicates that first generation treatment involves attempts to access and work through unresolved war trauma and to reduce core symptoms of PTSD. The second generation treatment then focuses on attempts to reintegrate the sufferer in the social context of family, work and society.

As can be seen, much of the work around integrated treatment programmes, specifically those involving hospitalisation or partial hospitalisation, has been aimed at particular groups of PTSD sufferers, and essentially at service personnel. Most of it has involved Vietnam veterans, but also Falklands and Gulf War veterans and others. It is understandable that specific treatment programmes would be set up for these groups. Not only is it recognised that there may be significant numbers requiring treatment, but they may be considered an essentially homogeneous group for whom a prepared package and group approach may be particularly appropriate. All three armed services in the UK have used such courses and the Royal Air Force and Royal Navy have published results (Busuttil *et al.*, 1995; Nevison, Flower and Naish, 1996). Each of them has included PTSD sufferers from other forms of trauma in their groups. There is a debate as to whether inclusion of such outsiders is intrusive or is helpful in normalising and emphasising universality. At times, the opening up of groups may be a pragmatic decision if accumulating a homogeneous group will involve indeterminate waiting and there are patients presenting from various sources.

The idea of setting up treatment programmes for all PTSD sufferers in most cities is attractive but currently probably impractical, at least in the UK where the National Health Service funds most health care. There is a conscious and centrally directed move towards almost total concentration of resources of mental health services to what is described as severe and enduring mental illness, a concept which may well be considered not to include PTSD. In addition, although Epidemiological Catchment Area (ECA) studies and other epidemiological work may suggest a lifetime prevalence of PTSD of 1% or more, the perception is that far fewer present seeking help. In an unpublished work the author surveyed local consultant psychiatrists about their experience of PTSD. Few had many cases in treatment. About half said that they saw clients for medicolegal assessment more commonly than they had patients referred for treatment. In the UK there are a number of small groups of experts offering tertiary referrals for PTSD treatment and most cities have clinical psychologists or consultant psychiatrists who have a particular interest. They are not always easy to find. The absence of specialist inpatient units may or may not be a problem. There is, as of yet, little evidence of the superior efficacy of inpatient programmes over best practice outpatient care.

Summary

- The evidence for efficacy of treatments in post-traumatic illnesses is not very extensive.
- Although it is generally accepted, and clearly stated by ICD-10, that the prognosis of PTI is good, the studies do not really reflect this, perhaps as most studies have been carried out on chronic and severe cases.
- Assessment of outcome of treatment of PTI and of PTSD in particular is made more difficult by the fact that therapist, patient and external assessor using objective tests may perceive response to treatment as being quite different.

- Assessment should also be long term as in PTSD the relapse rate is high.
- In PTI other than the specific stress disorders, treatment should be appropriate to the diagnosis. It is necessary to take into account the trauma in the process of engagement and in assessing for comorbid PTSD. However, it is wrong to apply a 'standard' treatment regime for PTSD when a different post-traumatic diagnosis applies.
- When there is comorbid illness the order of treatment of conditions should be pragmatic and dictated by the clinical situation rather than dogma.
- In acute stress disorder there may well be a role for the combat psychiatry principles of proximity, immediacy, expectancy, and simplicity in applying treatment. Drugs are of limited value. Recovery can be expected, but some will go on to have PTSD. There is some evidence that in combat-related problems the combat psychiatry interventions may reduce the very high rate of PTSD following combat shock, but residual rates remain high. There is not yet evidence of reduction of PTSD following civilian trauma.
- Problems in treatment of established PTSD include probable high rates of difficulties in engaging, dropping out of treatment, and non-compliance with medications.
- Treatments are not without adverse effects. Exposure will increase intrusive symptoms at first. Complete abolition of anxiety with anxiolytics may interfere with further treatment.
- Treatment strategies in PTSD have been traditionally based upon psychotherapy but the best evidence of efficacy is for exposure-based therapy and for medication.
- Most interest in PTSD treatment at present is in:
     integrated or co-ordinated eclectic treatment approaches
     cognitive behavioural work based on exposure and including techniques such as flooding, EMDR and taped imaginal exposure
     drug treatment, specifically antidepressants, especially specific serotonin reuptake inhibitors, and perhaps mood stabilisers
     psychosocial and psychoeducational problem-based interventions
     psychotherapies of a range of types, both individual and group.
- It is probable that the best general approach is an eclectic one. Psychotherapeutic skills will be needed to engage the patient and to prepare them for exposure techniques which will temporarily increase symptomatology. Medication such as SSRIs may be a useful adjunct. There is a need to normalise responses and to help the patient to re-

integrate and restructure maladaptive cognitions. Specific problems in family, work and other relationships or anger management will need to be addressed.

References

Allen, S.N. and Bloom, S.L. (1994). Group and family treatment of post-traumatic stress disorder. *Psychiatric Clinics of North America*, **17**, 2: 425–37.

Armstrong, K., Lund, P., McWright, L. and Tichenor, V. (1995). Multiple stressor debriefing and the American Red Cross: the East Bay Hills fire experience. *Social Work*, **40**, 1: 83–90.

Badenhorst, J.C. and Van Schalkwyk, S.J. (1992). Minimizing post traumatic stress in critical mining incidents. *Employee Assistance Quarterly*, **7**, 3: 79–90.

Bagarozzi, D.A. (1994). Identification, assessment and treatment of women suffering from post traumatic stress after abortion. *Journal of Family Psychotherapy*, **5**, 3: 25–54.

Baumgartner, D.D. (1986). Sociodrama and the Vietnam combat veteran: A therapeutic release for a wartime experience. *Journal of Group Psychotherapy, Psychodrama and Sociometry*, **39**, 1: 31–9.

Bazire, S. 1996. *Psychotropic Drug Directory 1991. The Professionals' Pocket Handbook and Aide Memoire*. London: Lundbeck Ltd.

Belenky, G.L. (1987). Varieties of reaction and adaptation to combat experience. *Bulletin of the Menninger Clinic*, **51**, 1: 64–79.

Berigan, T.R. and Holzgang, A. (1995). Valproate as an alternative in post-traumatic stress disorder: a case report. *Military Medicine*, **160**, 6: 318.

Besyner, J.K. (1985). Multimodal inpatient treatment of Vietnam combat veterans with post-traumatic stress disorder. 92nd Annual Convention of the American Psychological Association. *Psychotherapy in Private Practice*, **3**, 4: 43–7.

Bisson, J.I. and Jones, N. (1995). Taped imaginal exposure as a treatment for post-traumatic stress reactions. *Journal of the Royal Army Medical Corps*, **141**, 1: 20–24.

Bleich, A., Shalev, A., Shoham, S. and Solomon, Z. (1992). PTSD: Theoretical and practical considerations as reflected through Koach: An innovative treatment project. *Journal of Traumatic Stress*, **5**, 2: 265–71.

Blumenfield, M. and Schoeps, M. (1992). Reintegrating the healed burned adult into society: psychological problems and solutions. *Clinical Plastic Surgery*, **19**, 3: 599–605.

de Boer, M., Op den Velde, W., Falger, P.J., Hovens, J.E., De Groen, J.H. and Van Duijn, M. (1992). Fluvoxamine treatment for chronic PTSD: A pilot study. 2nd European Conference on Traumatic Stress, 1990, Noordwijk, Netherlands. *Psychotherapy and Psychosomatics*, **57**, 4: 158–63.

Bordow, S. and Porritt, D. (1979). An experimental evaluation of crisis intervention. *Psychology Bulletin*, **84**: 1189–217.

Boudewyns, P.A., Albrecht, J.W., Talbert, F.S. and Hyer, L.A. (1991a). Comorbidity and treatment outcome of inpatients with chronic combat-related PTSD. *Hospital and Community Psychiatry*, **42**, 8: 847–9.

Boudewyns, P.A., Hyer, L., Woods, M.G. and Harrison, W.R. (1990). PTSD among

Vietnam veterans: An early look at treatment outcome using direct therapeutic exposure. *Journal of Traumatic Stress*, **3**, 3: 359–68.

Boudewyns, P.A., Woods, M.G., Hyer, L. and Albrecht, J.W. (1991b). Chronic combat-related PTSD and concurrent substance abuse: Implications for treatment of this frequent 'dual diagnosis'. *Journal of Traumatic Stress*, **4**, 4: 549–60.

Brady, K.T., Sonne, S.C. and Roberts, J.M. (1995). Sertraline treatment of comorbid posttraumatic stress disorder and alcohol dependence. *Journal of Clinical Psychiatry*, **56**, 11: 502–5.

Braun, P., Greenberg, D., Dasberg, H. and Lerer, B. (1990). Core symptoms of posttraumatic stress disorder unimproved by alprazolam treatment. *Journal of Clinical Psychiatry*, **51**, 6: 236–8.

Brende, J.O. (1981). Combined individual and group therapy for Vietnam veterans. *International Journal of Group Psychotherapy*, **31**, 3: 367–78.

Brende, J.O. and Benedict, B.D. (1980). The Vietnam combat delayed stress response syndrome: hypnotherapy of 'dissociative symptoms'. *American Journal of Clinical Hypnosis*, **23**, 1: 34–40.

Brende, J.O. and Parson, E.R. (1987). Multiphasic treatment of the Vietnam veterans. *Psychotherapy in Private Practice*, **5**, 2: 51–62.

Brom, D., Kleber, R.J. and Defares, P.B. (1989). Brief psychotherapy for posttraumatic stress disorders. *Journal of Consulting and Clinical Psychology*, **57**, 5: 607–12.

Brom, D., Kleber, R.J. and Hofman, M.C. (1993). Victims of traffic accidents: Incidence and prevention of post-traumatic stress disorder. *Journal of Clinical Psychology*, **49**, 2: 131–40.

Brooks, J.S. and Scarano, T. (1985). Transcendental meditation in the treatment of post-Vietnam adjustment. Special issue: Paradigm shifts: Considerations for practice. *Journal of Counseling and Development*, **64**, 3: 212–15.

Burdon, A.P., Sutker, P.B., Foulks, E.F., Crane, M. and Thompson, K.E. (1991). Pilot program of treatment for PTSD. *American Journal of Psychiatry*, **148**, 9: 1269–70.

Burstein, A. (1984). Treatment of post-traumatic stress disorder with imipramine. *Psychosomatics*, **25**, 9: 681–7.

Busuttil, W., Turnbull, G., Neal, L.A., Rollins, J., West, A.G., Blanch, N. and Herepath, R. (1995). Incorporating psychological debriefing within a brief group psychotherapy programme for the treatment of PTSD. *British Journal of Psychiatry*, **167**, 4: 495–502.

Cardena, E. and Spiegel, D. (1993). Dissociative reactions to the San Francisco Bay area earthquake of 1989. *American Journal of Psychiatry*, **150**, 3: 474–8.

Carroll, E.M., Foy, D.W., Cannon, B.J. and Zwier, G. (1991). Assessment issues involving the families of trauma victims. *Journal of Traumatic Stress*, **4**, 1: 25–40.

Chung, M. (1995). Reviewing Frankl's Will to meaning and its implications for psychotherapy dealing with post-traumatic stress disorder. *Medicine in War*, **11**, 1: 45–55.

Coolican, M., Grogan, J. and Vassar, E. (1989). Helping survivors survive. *Nursing*, **19**, 8: 52–7.

Crump, L.D. (1984). Gestalt therapy in the treatment of Vietnam veterans experiencing PTSD symptomatology. *Journal of Contemporary Psychotherapy*, **14**, 1: 90–98.

Davidson, J.R. (1992). Drug therapy of post-traumatic stress disorder. *British Journal of Psychiatry*, **160**: 309–14.

Davidson, J.R., Kudler, H.S., Saunders, W.B., Erickson, L., Smith, R.D., Stein, R.M., Lipper, S. and Hammett, E.B. (1993). Predicting response to amitriptyline in post-traumatic stress disorder. *American Journal of Psychiatry*, **150**, 7: 1024–9.

Davidson, J., Kudler, H., Smith, R., Mahorney, S.L., Lipper, S., Hammett, E.B., Saunders, W.B. and Cavener, J.O. (1990). Treatment of posttraumatic stress disorder with amitriptyline and placebo. *Archives of General Psychiatry*, **47**, 3: 259–66.

Davidson, J.R., Roth, S. and Newman, E. (1991). Fluoxetine in post-traumatic stress disorder. *Journal of Traumatic Stress*, **4**, 3: 419–23.

Davidson, J., Walker, J.I. and Kilts, C. (1987). A pilot study of phenelzine in the treatment of post-traumatic stress disorder. *British Journal of Psychiatry*, **150**: 252–5.

Deblinger, E., McLeer, S.V. and Henry, D. (1990). Cognitive behavioral treatment for sexually abused children suffering post-traumatic stress: Preliminary findings. *Journal of the American Academy of Child and Adolescent Psychiatry*, **29**, 5: 747–52.

Decker, L.R. (1993). Beliefs, post-traumatic stress disorder, and mysticism. Special issue: Trauma and transcendence. *Journal of Humanistic Psychology*, **33**, 4: 15–32.

DeMartino, R., Mollica, R.F. and Wilk, V. (1995). Monoamine oxidase inhibitors in post-traumatic stress disorder. Promise and problems in Indochinese survivors of trauma. *Journal of Nervous and Mental Disease*, **183**, 8: 510–15.

Dillard, M., Bendfeldt, F. and Jernigan, P. (1993). Use of thioridazine in post-traumatic stress disorder. *Southern Medical Journal*, **86**, 12: 1276–8.

Duckworth, D.H. (1991). Managing psychological trauma in the police service: from the Bradford fire to the Hillsborough crush disaster. *Journal of the Society of Occupational Medicine*, **41**, 4: 171–3.

Duffy, J.D. and Malloy, P.F. (1994). Efficacy of buspirone in the treatment of post-traumatic stress disorder: An open trial. *Annals of Clinical Psychiatry*, **6**, 1: 33–7.

Dyregrov, A. (1989). Caring for helpers in disaster situations: Psychological debriefing. *Disaster Management*, **2**, 1: 25–9.

Erdreich, M. (1984). A traumata-oriented psychotherapy. *Dynamische Psychiatrie*, **17**, 5: 419–31.

Famularo, R., Kinscheriff, R. and Fenton, T. (1988). Propranolol treatment for childhood PTSD, acute type. A pilot study. *American Journal of Diseases of Children*, **142**, 11: 1244–7.

Farmer, R., Tranah, T., O. Donnell I. and Catalan, J. (1992). Railway suicide: the psychological effects on drivers. *Psychological Medicine*, **22**, 2: 407–14.

Fesler, F.A. (1991). Valproate in combat-related posttraumatic stress disorder. *Journal of Clinical Psychiatry*, **52**, 9: 361–4.

Fichtner, C.G. and Crayton, J.W. (1994). Buspirone in combat-related posttraumatic stress disorder. *Journal of Clinical Psychopharmacology*, **14**, 1: 79–81.

Figley, C.R. (1986). Traumatic stress: the role of the family and social support system. In *Traumatic Stress Theory, Research and Intervention*. pp. 39–54. Ed. C.R. Figley, *Brunner/Mazel Psychosocial Stress Series, No. 8. Trauma and Its Wake, Vol. II*. New York: Brunner Mazel.

Foa, E.B. and Rothbaum, B.O. (1989). Behavioural psychotherapy for post-traumatic stress disorder. Special issue: Behavioural psychotherapy into the 1990s. *International Review of Psychiatry*, **1**, 3: 219–26.

Forbes, D., Creamer, M. and Rycroft, P. (1994). Eye movement desensitization and reprocessing in posttraumatic stress disorder: A pilot study using assessment measures. *Journal of Behavior Therapy and Experimental Psychiatry*, **25**, 2: 113–20.

Forman, S.I. and Havas, S. (1990). Massachusetts' Post Traumatic Stress Disorder Program: a public health treatment model for Vietnam veterans. *Public Health Reports*, **105**, 2: 172–80.

Forster, P. (1992). Nature and treatment of acute stress reactions. In *Responding to Disaster: A Guide for Mental Health Professionals*, pp. 25–52. Ed. L. Austin. Washington: American Psychiatric Press.

Forster, P.L., Schoenfeld, F.B., Marmar, C.R. and Lang, A.J. (1995). Lithium for irritability in post-traumatic stress disorder. *Journal of Traumatic Stress*, **8**, 1: 143–9.

Frank, J.B., Kosten, T.R., Giller, E.L. and Dan, E. (1988). A randomized clinical trial of phenelzine and imipramine for posttraumatic stress disorder. *American Journal of Psychiatry*, **145**, 10: 1289–91.

Frueh, B.C., Mirabella, R.F., Chobot, K. and Fossey, M. (1994). Chronicity symptoms in combat veterans with PTSD treated by the VA Mental Health System. *Psychological Reports*, **75**, 2: 843–8.

Galloucis, M. and Kaufman, M.E. (1988). Group therapy with Vietnam veterans: A brief review. *Group*, **12**, 2: 85–102.

Hammarberg, M. and Silver, S.M. (1994). Outcome of treatment for post-traumatic stress disorder in a primary care unit serving Vietnam veterans. *Journal of Traumatic Stress*, **72**: 195–216.

Hendin, H. (1983). Psychotherapy for Vietnam veterans with posttraumatic stress disorders. *American Journal of Psychotherapy*, **37**, 1: 86–99.

Herbert, J. and Mueser, K. (1992). Eye movement desensitization: a critique of the evidence. *Journal of Behavior Therapy and Experimental Psychiatry*, **23**, 3: 169–74.

Horowitz, M.J. (1973). Phase oriented treatment of stress response syndromes. *American Journal of Psychotherapy*, **27**, 4: 506–15.

Horowitz, M.J. (1986). Stress-response syndromes: A review of posttraumatic and adjustment disorders. *Hospital and Community Psychiatry*, **37**, 3: 241–9.

Horowitz, M.J. and Kaltreider, N.B. (1979). Brief therapy of the stress response syndrome. *Psychiatric Clinics of North America*, **2**, 2: 365–77.

Horowitz, M.J., Milbrath, C., Ewert, M., Sonneborn, D. and Stinson, C. (1994). Cyclical patterns of states of mind in psychotherapy. *American Journal of Psychiatry*, **151**, 12: 1767–70.

Iruela, L.M., Gilaberte, I., Oliveros, S.C. and Rojo, V. (1991). Clonidine-imipramine therapy. *Journal of Nervous and Mental Disease*, **179**, 5: 304.

Jelinek, J.M. and Williams, T. (1984). Post-traumatic stress disorder and substance abuse in Vietnam combat veterans: Treatment problems, strategies and recommendations. *Journal of Substance Abuse Treatment*, **1**, 2: 87–97.

Jimenez, M.J.J. (1993). The spiritual healing of post traumatic stress disorder at the Menlo Park Veteran's Hospital. *Studies in Formative Spirituality*, **14**, 2: 175–88.

Johnson, D.R., Feldman, S.C., Southwick, S.M. and Charney, D.S. (1994). The concept of the second generation program in the treatment of post-traumatic stress disorder among Vietnam veterans. *Journal of Traumatic Stress*, **7**, 2: 217–35.

Keane, T.M., Fairbank, J.A., Caddell, J.M. and Zimering, R. (1989). Implosive (flooding) therapy reduces symptoms of PTSD in Vietnam combat veterans. *Behavior Therapy*, **20**, 2: 245–60.

Keck, P.E., McElroy, S.L. and Friedman, L.M. (1992). Valproate and carbamazepine in the treatment of panic and posttraumatic stress disorders, withdrawal states, and behavioral dyscontrol syndromes. *Journal of Clinical Psychopharmacology*, **12**, 1(Suppl.): 36–41.

Kentsmith, D.K. (1986). Principles of battlefield psychiatry. *Military Medicine*, **151**, 2: 89–96.

Kinzie, J.D. and Leung, P. (1989). Clonidine in Cambodian patients with posttraumatic stress disorder. *Journal of Nervous and Mental Disease*, **177**, 9: 546–50.

Kitchner, I. and Greenstein, R. (1985). Low dose lithium carbonate in the treatment of post traumatic stress disorder: Brief communication. *Military Medicine*, **150**, 7: 378–81.

Kline, N.A., Dow, B.M., Brown, S.A. and Matloff, J.L. (1994). Sertraline efficacy in depressed combat veterans with posttraumatic stress disorder. *American Journal of Psychiatry*, **151**, 4: 621.

Koller, P., Marmar, C.R. and Kanas, N. (1992). Psychodynamic group treatment of post-traumatic stress disorder in Vietnam veterans. *International Journal of Group Psychotherapy*, **42**, 2: 225–46.

Koopman, C., Classen, C. and Spiegel, D.A. (1994). Predictors of posttraumatic stress symptoms among survivors of the Oakland/Berkeley, California, firestorm. *American Journal of Psychiatry*, **151**, 6: 888–94.

Kosten, T.R., Frank, J.B., Dan, E., McDougle, C.J. and Giller, E.L. (1991). Pharmacotherapy for posttraumatic stress disorder using phenelzine or imipramine. *Journal of Nervous and Mental Disease*, **179**, 6: 366–70.

Lantz, J. (1992). Using Frankl concepts with PTSD clients. *Journal of Traumatic Stress*, **5**: 3.

Lawney, D.J. (1982). Role of therapeutic recreation in the treatment of post traumatic stress disorder. *Leisure Information Newsletter*, **8**, 4: 9–11.

Lerer, B., Bleich, A., Kotler, M., Garb, R., Hertzberg, M. and Levin, B. (1987). Posttraumatic stress disorder in Israeli combat veterans: Effect of phenelzine treatment. *Archives of General Psychiatry*, **44**, 11: 976–81.

Lindy, J.D. (1986). An outline for the psychoanalytic psychotherapy of PTSD. In *Traumatic Stress Theory, Research and Intervention*. pp. 195–212. Ed. C.R. Figley. *Brunner/Mazel Psychosocial Stress Series, No. 8. Trauma and It's Wake, Vol. II.* New York: Brunner Mazel.

Lindy, J.D., Green, B.L., Grace, M. and Titchener, J. (1983). Psychotherapy with survivors of the Beverly Hills Supper Club fire. *American Journal of Psychotherapy*, **37**, 4: 593–610.

Lohr, J., Kleinknecht, R., Conley, A., Dal, C.S., Schmidt, J. and Sonntag, M. (1992). A methodological critique of the current status of eye movement desensitization (EMD). *Journal of Behavior Therapy and Experimental Psychiatry*, **23**, 3: 159–67.

Lyons, J.A. and Keane, T.M. (1989). Implosive therapy for the treatment of combat-related PTSD. *Journal of Traumatic Stress*, **2**, 2: 137–52.

Makler, S., Sigal, M., Gelkopf, M., Bar, K.B. and Horeb, E. (1990). Combat-related, chronic posttraumatic stress disorder: Implications for group-therapy intervention. *American Journal of Psychotherapy*, **44**, 3: 381–95.

Manton, M. and Talbot, A. (1990). Crisis intervention after an armed hold-up: guidelines for counsellors. *Journal of Traumatic Stress*, **3**: 4507–26.

Margalit, C., Rabinowitz, S., Ezion, T. and Solomon, Z. (1994). Treatment of post-traumatic stress disorders: An applied rear-echelon approach. *Military Medicine*, **159**, 5: 415–18.

Marmar, C.R. (1991). Brief dynamic psychotherapy of post-traumatic stress disorder. *Psychiatric Annals*, **21**, 7: 405–14.

McCloy, E. (1992). Management of post-incident trauma: a fire service perspective. *Occupational Medicine*, **42**, 3: 163–6.

McDougle, C.J., Southwick, S.M., Charney, D.S. and StJames, R.L. (1991). An open trial of fluoxetine in the treatment of posttraumatic stress disorder. *Journal of Clinical Psychopharmacology*, **11**, 5: 325–7.

McFarlane, A.C. (1994). Individual psychotherapy for post-traumatic stress disorder. *Psychiatric Clinics of North America*, **17**, 2: 393–408.

Mitchell, J.T. (1983). When disaster strikes. The critical incident stress debriefing process. *Journal of Emergency Medical Services*, **8**: 36–9.

Muss, D.C. (1991). A new technique for treating post-traumatic stress disorder. *British Journal of Clinical Psychology*, **30**, 1: 91–2.

Nagy, L.M., Morgan, C.A., Southwick, S.M. and Charney, D. (1993). Open prospective trial of fluoxetine for posttraumatic stress disorder. *Journal of Clinical Psychopharmacology*, **13**, 2: 107–13.

Neal, L. (1994). The pitfalls of making a categorical diagnosis of post traumatic stress disorder in personal injury litigation. Medicine Science Law, **34**, 2: 117–22.

Nevison, C., Flower, J. and Naish, P. (1996). The post-traumatic stress management course at RN Hospital, Haslar. *Journal of the Royal Navy Medical Service*, **82**, 1: 9–14.

Pendorf, J.E. (1990). Vocational rehabilitation for psychiatric inpatient Vietnam combat veterans. *Military Medicine*, **155**, 8: 369–71.

Peniston, E.G. (1986). EMG biofeedback-assisted desensitization treatment for Vietnam combat veterans post-traumatic stress disorder. *Clinical Biofeedback and Health: An International Journal*, **9**, 1: 35–41.

Perconte, S.T. (1986). Partial-hospitalization treatment of posttraumatic stress disorder (PTSD). *International Journal of Partial Hospitalization*, **3**, 4: 219–29.

Perconte, S.T. (1987). Efficacy of partial-hospitalization treatment of post-traumatic stress disorder (PTSD): Preliminary results and follow-up. *International Journal of Partial Hospitalization*, **4**, 1: 29–35.

Perconte, S.T., Griger, M.L. and Bellucci, G. (1989). Relapse and rehospitalization of veterans two years after treatment for PTSD. *Hospital and Community Psychiatry*, **40**, 10: 1072–3.

Phillips, M. (1993). The use of ego-state therapy in the treatment of posttraumatic stress disorder. *American Journal of Clinical Hypnosis*, **35**, 4: 241–9.

Pitman, R.K., Altman, B., Greenwald, E., Longpre, R.E., Macklin, M.L., Poire, R.E. and Steketee, G.S. (1991). Psychiatric complications during flooding therapy for post-traumatic stress disorder. *Journal of Clinical Psychiatry*, **52**, 1: 17–20.

Priest, R.G., Gimbrett, R., Roberts, W. and Steinert, J. (1995). Reversible and selective inhibitors of monoamine oxidase A in mental and other disorders. *Acta Psychiatrica Scandinavica*, **91**, S386: 40–43.

Prout, M.F. and Schwarz, R.A. (1991). Post traumatic stress disorder, a brief integrated approach. *International Journal of Short-Term Psychotherapy*, **6**, 2: 113–24.

Rahe, R.H., Karson, S., Howard, N.S.Jr, Rubin, R.T. and Poland, R.E. (1990). Psychological and physiological assessment on American hostages freed from captivity in Iran. *Psychosomatic Medicine*, **52**, 1: 1–16.

Reist, C., Kauffmann, C.D., Chicz Demet, A., Chen, C.C. and Demet, E.M. (1995). REM latency, dexamethasone suppression test, and thyroid releasing hormone stimulation test in posttraumatic stress disorder. *Progress in Neuropsychopharmacology and the Biology of Psychiatry*, **19**, 3: 433–43.

Reist, C., Kauffmann, C.D., Haier, R.J., Sangdahl, C., De Met, E.M., Chicz DeMet, A. and Nelson, J.N. (1989). A controlled trial of desipramine in 18 men with post-traumatic stress disorder. *American Journal of Psychiatry*, **146**, 4: 513–16.

Renfrey, G. and Spates, C.R. (1994). Eye movement desensitization: A partial dismantling study. *Journal of Behavior Therapy and Experimental Psychiatry*, **25**, 3: 231–9.

Risse, S.C., Whitters, A., Burke, J., Chen, S., Scurfield, R.M. and Raskind, M.A. (1990). Severe withdrawal symptoms after discontinuation of alprazolam in eight patients with combat-induced posttraumatic stress disorder. *Journal of Clinical Psychiatry*, **51**, 5: 206–9.

Rosen, G.M. (1995). On the origin of eye movement desensitization. *Journal of Behavior Therapy and Experimental Psychiatry*, **26**, 2: 121–2.

Shalev, A., Spiro, S.E., Solomon, Z. and Bleich, A. (1992). Positive clinical impressions: I. Therapists' evaluations. *Journal of Traumatic Stress*, **5**, 2: 207–16.

Shapiro, F. (1989). Eye movement desensitization: A new treatment for post-traumatic stress disorder. *Journal of Behavior Therapy and Experimental Psychiatry*, **20**, 3: 211–17.

Shay, J. (1992). Fluoxetine reduces explosiveness and elevates mood of Vietnam combat vets with PTSD. *Journal of Traumatic Stress*, **5**, 1: 97–101.

Shestatzky, M., Greenberg, D. and Lerer, B. (1988). A controlled trial of phenelzine in posttraumatic stress disorder. *Psychiatry Research*, **24**, 2: 149–55.

Silver, S.M., Brooks, A. and Obenchain, J. (1995). Treatment of Vietnam War veterans with PTSD: a comparison of eye movement desensitization and reprocessing, biofeedback, and relaxation training. *Journal of Traumatic Stress*, **8**, 2: 337–42.

Solomon, S., Gerrity, E. and Muff, A. (1992). Efficacy of treatments for posttraumatic stress disorder. An empirical review. *Journal of the American Medical Association*, **268**, 5: 633–8.

Solomon, Z. (1989). A 3-year prospective study of post-traumatic stress disorder in Israeli combat veterans. *Journal of Traumatic Stress*, **2**, 1: 59–73.

Solomon, Z. and Benbenishty, R. (1986). The role of proximity, immediacy, and expectancy in frontline treatment of combat stress reaction among Israelis in the Lebanon War. *American Journal of Psychiatry*, **143**, 5: 613–17.

Solomon, Z., Bleich, A., Shoham, S. and Nardi, C. (1992a). The 'Koach' project for treatment of combat-related PTSD: Rationale, aims, and methodology. *Journal of Traumatic Stress*, **5**, 2: 175–93.

Solomon, Z. and Kleinhauz, M. (1996). War-induced psychic trauma: an 18-year follow-up of Israeli veterans. *American Journal of Orthopsychiatry*, **66**, 1: 152–60.

Solomon, Z., Shalev, A., Spiro, S.E. and Dolev, A. (1992b). Negative psychometric outcomes: Self-report measures and a follow-up telephone survey. *Journal of Traumatic Stress*, **5**, 2: 225–46.

Solomon, Z., Spiro, S.E., Shalev, A. and Bleich, A. (1992). Positive clinical impressions: II. Participants' evaluations. *Journal of Traumatic Stress*, **5**, 2: 217–23.

Solomon, Z., Weisenberg, M., Schwarzwald, J. and Mikulincer, M. (1987). Posttraumatic stress disorder among frontline soldiers with combat stress reaction: The 1982 Israeli experience. *American Journal of Psychiatry*, **144**, 4: 448–54.

Sparr, L.F. and Boehnlein, J.K. (1990). Posttraumatic stress disorder in tort actions: Forensic minefield. *Bulletin of the American Academy of Psychiatry and the Law*, **18**, 3: 283–302.

Spiegel, D. and Cardena, E. (1990). New uses of hypnosis in the treatment of posttraumatic stress disorder. 143rd Annual Meeting of the American Psychiatric Association, 1990, New York. *Journal of Clinical Psychiatry*, **51 (Suppl.)**: 39–43.

Sutherland, S.M. and Davidson, J.R. (1994). Pharmacotherapy for post traumatic stress disorder. *Psychiatric Clinics of North America*, **17**, 2: 409–23.

Tang, D. (1994). Psychotherapy for train drivers after railway suicide. *Social Sciences Medicine*, **38**, 3: 477–8.

Terr, L.C. (1992). Mini-Marathon groups: Psychological 'first-aid' following disasters. *Bulletin of the Menninger Clinic*, **56**, 1: 76–86.

Van Der Kolk, B.A., Dreyfuss, D., Michaels, M., Shera, D., Berkowitz, R., Fisler, R. and Saxe, G. (1994). Fluoxetine in posttraumatic stress disorder. *Journal of Clinical Psychiatry*, **55**, 12: 517–22.

Vaughan, K., Armstrong, M.S., Gold, R., O'Connor, N., Jenneke, W. and Tarrier, N. (1994). A trial of eye movement desensitization compared to image habituation training and applied muscle relaxation in post-traumatic stress disorder. *Journal of Behavior Therapy and Experimental Psychiatry*, **25**, 4: 283–91.

Vaughan, K. and Tarrier, N. (1992). The use of image habituation training with post-traumatic stress disorders. *British Journal of Psychiatry*, **161**: 658–64.

Viola, J.M. and McCarthy, D.A. (1994). An eclectic inpatient treatment model for Vietnam and Desert Storm veterans suffering from posttraumatic stress disorder. *Military Medicine*, **159**, 3: 217–20.

Wells, B., Chu, C., Johnson, R., Nasdahl, C., Ayubi, M., Sewell, E. and Statham, P. (1991). Buspirone in the treatment of posttraumatic stress disorder. *Pharmacotherapy*, **11**, 4: 340–43.

Williams, C., Miller, J., Watson, G. and Hunt, N. (1994). A strategy for trauma debriefing after railway suicides. *Social Sciences Medicine*, **38**, 3: 483–7.

Wolf, M.E., Alavi, A. and Mosnaim, A.D. (1987). Pharmacological interventions in Vietnam veterans with post traumatic stress disorder. *Research Communications in Psychology, Psychiatry and Behavior*, **12**, 3: 169–76.

World Health Organisation (1992). *International Classification of Diseases*, 10th edition, Geneva: WHO.

Worzel, M.A. (1992). Pilot study to validate criteria for proposed new DSM IV category: Disorders of extreme stress not otherwise specified (DESNOS). *Dissertation Abstracts International*, **52**, 9–B: 4991–2.

Zaidi, L.Y. (1994). Group treatment of adult male inpatients abused as children. *Journal of Traumatic Stress*, **7**, 4: 718–27.

Zarcone, V. *et al.* (1977). Psychiatric problems of Vietnam veterans. *Comprehensive Psychiatry*, **18**, 1: 1–53.

CHAPTER 9

MEDICOLEGAL ASPECTS OF POST-TRAUMATIC ILLNESS

In this chapter we will look at the medicolegal connotations of PTI. Where there is a need specifically to address legal practice, the focus will be quite clearly upon the interaction of PTI and law in England and Wales. Aspects of American law have been addressed widely elsewhere, for example by Sparr (Sparr and Boehnlein, 1990) and others. Indeed, almost all of the work concerning PTI and criminal law, as well as much of that concerning civil law, comes from America. There are a number of useful books and pamphlets which specifically address the legal side of the psychiatric injury issues (Napier and Wheat, 1995) (Law Commission 1995) in England and Wales, or in areas with similar basis of law (Mullany and Handford, 1993). An attempt will be made in this chapter to examine both criminal and civil legal issues from the point of view of the expert clinician.

Probably more than any other form of mental illness, PTI is associated with medicolegal issues. It seems that in almost every case of PTI, be it PTSD or another condition, there is at least the potential for some form of legal or quasi-legal consequence. There are a number of obvious areas of possible concern:

- PTI may be presented as a defence or mitigating factor in criminal cases
- PTI may be a consequence of criminal behaviour
- PTI may be a consequence of a civil wrong.

In the last two cases the sufferer with PTI can hope to gain some recompense for his suffering, which is the consequence of the action or negligence of another. In the first the sufferer will have some expectation of being exculpated or at least of having his punishment reduced because of his mental condition.

In general, wherever PTI is involved in the legal process there is a likelihood of some benefit accruing to the sufferer.

Where the diagnosis is one of PTSD, there is a clear statement of causation in the diagnostic process. PTSD cannot be diagnosed without identification of a particular event which is accepted as having caused the PTSD.

The situation is not so clear-cut with other PTI. There is a need both to identify the condition through the normal diagnostic procedure, and also to describe and justify the relationship with the causal event. This latter is often more difficult than the simple process of syndromal diagnosis. A simple temporal sequence of events does not, of itself, demonstrate a causal link. There is a need to demonstrate that the illness, or the particular episode of illness, has been caused or substantially contributed to, by the event.

PTI as a defence or as mitigation

Most of the literature concerning this subject comes from America and concerns PTSD and Vietnam. One of the factors leading to interest in what were originally called the 'readjustment problems' of Vietnam veterans was the reported dramatic involvement of Vietnam veterans in criminal behaviour. It began to be suggested that this criminal behaviour was a legacy of Vietnam and directly caused by the unpopular war and the way in which veterans had been ignored or disparaged by those at home.

Is PTI really associated with criminal behaviour?

For PTI other than PTSD there has never been any specific suggestion that there is a direct association with criminal behaviour in the sufferer. The same is certainly not true for PTSD. The research has been carried out amongst Vietnam veterans and, as has been suggested above, initial interest was raised mostly by reports in the lay press, initially of single cases, but then forming a body of opinion that Vietnam veterans had very high rates of criminal behaviour which was a consequence of their military training and of their service in Vietnam. Not surprisingly, such unscientific reports caused considerable debate, with one side saying that Vietnam was producing a legacy of a generation of criminals while others suggested that there was no increase in criminal behaviour.

Many figures were quoted, with variable basis in fact. For example, one paper in 1986 which reviewed the question of criminality and PTSD suggested that 25% of those who served in Vietnam had 'encountered serious legal difficulties'

(Marciniak, 1986). In fact, this paper quotes an earlier paper by Erlinder (1983) at length. Erlinder's paper, which in itself also quoted another source, suggested that 25% of those Vietnam veterans exposed to heavy combat had faced criminal charges, without detailing severity. If this were considered to be accurate, then the figure of 25% of those exposed to heavy combat would equate to 10% or less of Vietnam veterans.

Do Vietnam veterans have higher than expected rates of criminal behaviour?
Despite considerable research, this question has not been clearly answered. There are a number of reasons for this, including the fact that different states in America have separate penal systems, and that veteran status was not recorded electronically.

An important review addressed the question in 1989 (Beckerman and Fontana, 1989). Boman's disputed claim that in 1975 30% of all of the male prisoners in the USA were Vietnam veterans was noted in this study but not necessarily confirmed.

Where studies have been carried out on prison populations, the results seem to have varied depending upon who has done the research. For example, self-help project studies have generally disagreed with many of the findings of the US Department of Justice Study of 1979.

This study looked at 12 000 prisoners. It found that 25% of prisoners were military veterans who had taken part in a war at some time, and that 15% were Vietnam veterans. Black veterans were not found to be over-represented for their proportion of all Vietnam veterans. The Vietnam veteran prisoners identified in this study did not seem typical of Vietnam veterans in general as only 50% had been honourably discharged from service, 60% had been imprisoned before service, and 25% had been imprisoned during military service. In other words, this study seemed to find that the group of Vietnam veterans who were criminals was principally comprised of those criminals who had also been to Vietnam.

Other studies have tended to confirm that 11% to 15% of prison inmates have been Vietnam veterans.

Card (1983) looked at 1000 general Vietnam veterans. Obviously the sample was biased in one direction as all of the sample was at liberty and there were no current prisoners included. It was found that only 18% of Vietnam veterans had been arrested, and that only 20% of these had been arrested for any form of violent offence. It was also found that increased combat exposure was associated with arrest. Rather more surprisingly, Vietnam veterans were found generally to be no more likely to be arrested than other veterans or non-veterans, but if they were arrested they were more likely to be convicted.

It seems, in summary, that Vietnam veterans have a higher than average rate of arrest but that most arrests are for non-violent offences. The increase in rates is not very dramatic when compared with the relevant control population of young adult males who are generally responsible for most crime and make up much of the prison population.

Is criminal behaviour in Vietnam veterans associated with PTSD?
Even if there is a higher rate of criminal behaviour in the population of Vietnam veterans this does not, in itself, prove that PTSD is associated with criminal behaviour as not all veterans have PTSD.

In an important paper Sparr (Sparr, Reaves and Atkinson, 1987) refers to one reason why any increase in criminal behaviour might be found in Vietnam veterans, which is 'McNamara's 100 000'. Prior to Vietnam there were legally established minimum physical and mental entry standards for the armed forces. McNamara's 100 000 was ostensibly a rehabilitation programme for the poor. It lowered the legal entry standards and as a consequence 345 000 people entered the forces who would previously have been excluded because they would not have passed the entry criteria. Not surprisingly, there was an increased representation of disadvantaged black soldiers (41%). In addition, these particular soldiers had a higher rate of exposure to combat, at 40%. If a significant percentage of McNamara's men of all races did, as could be expected, come from poorer homes and disadvantaged backgrounds with lower academic achievement, it would not be surprising if they were seen to have a higher rate of criminal behaviour with or without PTSD. Their numbers were such as potentially to influence significantly the findings in the population of Vietnam veterans.

A moderately sized study in Iowa (Shaw *et al.*, 1987) compared incarcerated Vietnam veterans with a random sample of Vietnam veterans in the community. One problem with the study was that the response rate was higher in the community sample than in the prisoners. Both groups had high but essentially equal rates of PTSD, at 39% and 37%. The prisoner group, however, had higher rates of antisocial personality and of substance abuse.

Another study looked at the relationship between pre-adult antisocial behaviour, combat exposure, and adult antisocial behaviour in 118 help-seeking Vietnam veterans. It found that pre-adult behaviour and combat exposure each separately influenced adult antisocial behaviour. While PTSD was not correlated with pre-adult behaviour, it was correlated with both combat exposure and post-trauma adult antisocial behaviour.

PTI and criminal behaviour

The relationship between PTI and criminal behaviour is not very clear but is not a close one.

- There is no suggestion that PTI other than PTSD is associated with criminal behaviour.
- The association with PTSD is really only supported by the particular case of Vietnam. While there have been anecdotal case reports, studies of no other patient groups have even tentatively identified a relationship between PTSD and crime thus far. However, even with Vietnam veterans, although there is some evidence that they probably have an excess of primarily non-violent crime, the evidence that such behaviour is strongly related to PTSD rather than to previous personality or military training and experience is not strong.
- As Sparr has stated 'criminality and violence in veterans is not prima facie evidence of PTSD'. Although irritability and outbursts of anger are symptoms of PTSD, criminal behaviour is not.
- Even if a veteran offender has PTSD, this does not necessarily mean that the PTSD has caused the offence.
- There is no evidence of an association between PTSD caused by trauma other than combat, and criminal behaviour.

PTI and defendants

While it is recognised that most of the published work has come from America, the focus here will be on the law in England and Wales, pointing out differences as appropriate.

In general there are three main ways in which a diagnosis of PTI may be used to influence the judicial process.

1. Fitness to plead.
2. The insanity defence.
3. Mitigation.

Fitness to plead

If a defendant is unable to take part in the proceedings of a criminal trial due to mental illness, his fitness to plead may be decided by a jury specially empanelled for the purpose. This is, of course, an uncommon occurrence as it is difficult to see the advantages for anyone. It is more common for a defendant to be admitted as a result of an order under the Mental Health Act (1983) for assessment and treatment prior to the trial.

Given the English test of fitness to plead, it would be hard to envisage the question arising in connection with PTSD or the vast majority of PTIs. It is difficult to see how PTSD symptoms would disable the ability to challenge jurors, instruct counsel etc.

There is, however, a small amount of literature on the American equivalent of 'competence to stand trial'. There is a description (Daniels, 1984) of one case of alleged non-violent crime in which it was claimed that the irritability and impulsivity consequent upon PTSD interfered with the defendant's ability to co-operate with his counsel and with the judicial process. As a consequence, an adjournment was allowed for the defendant to undergo inpatient treatment. Following treatment the defendant was apparently able to take an active part in the trial and to co-operate with his legal advisers.

The author goes on to suggest that it is possible that many of the Vietnam veterans in prison may have ended up there because they had displayed their 'underlying rage and generalised distrust' in the court-room. This might explain the observation in a study quoted earlier that Vietnam veterans were no more likely to be arrested than non-veterans, but if arrested were more likely to be convicted. However, 'generalised distrust', while often cited as a feature of Vietnam veterans, is not a specific symptom diagnostic of PTSD.

Irritability is a symptom of PTSD. It must nevertheless be unreasonable, and for policy reasons unacceptable, to suggest that because they are likely to be irritable and volatile, PTSD sufferers are, as a group, unfit to stand trial. However, it is easy to see that the sort of verbally violent outburst which is not uncommon, at least in combat-induced PTSD, is unlikely to improve the light in which a defendant is seen by the court.

PTSD as an insanity defence

This section refers to PTSD rather than PTI because if other post-traumatic illnesses are raised as an insanity defence, then the questions raised are the same as those raised when the particular illness occurs in the absence of trauma.

Again, most of the literature comes from America and refers to Vietnam veterans. Indeed the question of the insanity defence for PTSD in Vietnam veterans has been a major source of interest in the USA, particularly following a small number of famous or infamous cases. That responses to an insanity defence for PTSD have varied markedly in America is probably related to the fact that different states have different penal codes. Indeed a few states have abolished the insanity defence completely, some replacing it with a 'guilty but mentally ill' verdict.

The most commonly used concept of insanity in America differs significantly from the McNaughten rules as used in England and Wales. The American Law Institute Model Penal Code states that a person is to be considered legally insane if 'at the time of such conduct as a result of mental disease or defect he lacks substantial capacity either to appreciate the criminality of his conduct or to conform his conduct to the requirements of the law'. This different definition helps explain some of the verdicts which, from the English point of view, seem surprising.

Packer (1983) reviewed PTSD and the insanity defence. Initially he questioned the concept of PTSD as a 'mental disease', pointing out that some DSM conditions such as schizophrenia were quite clearly mental diseases, but that others such as nicotine dependence and sexual dysfunctions probably were not. Thus inclusion in DSM does not, per se, mean that a disorder is a mental disease. Indeed, DSM contains a caveat that it is intended for clinical purposes and does not necessarily fulfil forensic functions. Packer suggests that only when PTSD results in impaired contact with reality as shown in the dissociative features of true flashbacks, can a sufferer be considered to have been 'insane' at the relevant time.

Packer goes on to make the very important point that 'simply because we understand the motivation for a particular behaviour does not mean that the individual is not legally responsible for that behaviour'. Criminal behaviour may be explicable in terms of a response to trauma but this does not, of itself, remove responsibility. Child sexual abuse may be explained in terms of the perpetrator having been a victim himself, or delinquent behaviour may be explained in terms of home conditions. Packer suggests that if crimes were negated because the behaviour was explicable, then it is likely that there would be a dramatic negative effect upon society.

Lipkin (Lipkin, Scurfield and Blank, 1983) agrees that the insanity defence is really only applicable when the defendant has carried out the act in a dissociative state such as a flashback. He also points out that such behaviours are not only rare, but are not predictive of recurrence. This last is particularly important because if the 'mad' behaviour cannot be predicted to be likely to happen again, what is the purpose of the special treatment or disposal of the perpetrator.

Many papers quote Sparr's list of nine criteria indicative of unconscious flashbacks as the explanation for a criminal act, and which can be used to help decide whether or not to give an opinion that the relevant behaviour was a consequence of the PTSD rather than a motivated act. These criteria are:

1.   the behaviour is unpremeditated and sudden
2.   it is uncharacteristic of the defendant

3. there is a history of the defendant having been involved in actual events which seem to be re-enacted in the incident
4. there is some degree of amnesia for the event
5. the behaviour lacks current motivation
6. the triggers for the event are relevant to the initial trauma
7. the defendant is mostly unaware of the specific ways in which he has re-enacted events
8. the choice of victim is fortuitous or accidental
9. the defendant has symptoms of PTSD.

There have been a number of cases in which PTSD sufferers have successfully pleaded 'not guilty by reason of insanity' (NGRI) because the alleged offences, usually violent ones, occurred during a flashback and showed the features described by Sparr and listed above. In England, Bisson (1993) has discussed the issues when describing the case of a soldier, who had previously been exposed to trauma in Northern Ireland, carrying out an armed abduction while in a dissociative state. He too focuses on the rarity of such events.

The most exciting and newsworthy NGRI cases have, of course, been the factitious or controversial ones, although these are by no means the only cases which have been heard, and some others seem much more straightforward and reasonable.

Packer describes the case of Mr A who held up a gun shop, stole a number of weapons, and was subsequently quietly arrested when he was found in an empty field shooting at a derelict building. The action was unpremeditated, uncharacteristic, apparently unmotivated, and the choice of target unexplained. It was found that much of his behaviour was reminiscent of a documented incident in Vietnam, and Mr A had only patchy memory of the incident and his actions. He had PTSD symptoms and in this non-controversial case was subsequently found NGRI.

The case of Arizona versus Jensen is rather different. This man was convicted of two murders in 1973 when he killed two teenagers. He managed to gain a retrial in 1985 on the grounds that he had been suffering from PTSD at the time but that as PTSD was not defined until 1980 it was not considered at his trial. At the retrial it was difficult to confirm Mr Jensen's military history. Although he gave a wide range of differing accounts of the relevant incident, his main claim was that the sound of a plane overhead made him think that he was back in Vietnam and he believed that the teenagers were North Vietnamese soldiers so he captured and executed them. Evidence was given that not only would it have been against orders and practice for him to act in this way, but that Mr Jensen had no military experience of having been in any such situation. It was not accepted that he had carried out the killings during a flashback and he was again found guilty.

One of the most notorious cases was that of Pard versus US, a civil matter in which Mr and Mrs Pard sued the US government and Veterans Administration for $9 500 000 for failure to diagnose and treat PTSD. Mr Pard had been found NGRI on three counts of attempted murder in a situation in which he was also wounded in firing which involved the police. He claimed that if he had been properly diagnosed and treated, his mental health would have been better, the offences would not have happened, he would not have been injured, and he would not have lost consortium with his wife. Not surprisingly, given the nature of the case and the possibility of a precedent being set, the authorities were not prepared to concede the facts as alleged, and Mr Pard's story was investigated further than it had been for the original criminal case. He claimed that he was in a helicopter gun ship in Vietnam that had 400 confirmed kills, that he had rescued a general who had been shot down, that he had shot unarmed children in self-defence on a mission, that he had been wounded in an attack, and that he had been awarded the Distinguished Flying Cross and the Bronze Star. However, evidence was given at trial that he had flown in an administrative helicopter, and that all the other claims were untrue. The court ruled that he had not had PTSD and that therefore the government and Veterans Administration were not negligent. Nevertheless, however, the finding of NGRI still stood even though his claims were said to be untrue, as the trial had already been completed.

While it seems at least possible that violent behaviour might be associated with PTSD given that irritability is one of the symptoms, it is less easy to see how PTSD could be used for a NGRI defence in non-violent cases including such matters as tax evasion.

US versus Tindall is one of the most famous of such cases. Tindall was one of 15 people involved in a major drug-smuggling ring. That he had been involved in smuggling a large amount of cannabis was not in doubt, but he entered a NGRI plea. In Vietnam, Tindall had, with other members of the ring, flown in a Cobra helicopter gun-ship. It was alleged that he had symptoms of PTSD on his return and that, when he was refused a civil pilot's licence, he was psychologically devastated. He joined the drug-smuggling ring, which ran the scheme like a paramilitary operation. It was put forward that he had an 'action addiction' which made him take part in the smuggling operation. The jury found that Mr Tindall was not legally responsible for his actions during the six months when he took part in the smuggling operation and flew in large amounts of drugs. He was found not guilty by reason of insanity.

It is hard to accept that this and similar cases would result in the same verdict in the UK. Indeed, they have not been universally welcomed in the USA and some authors have suggested that they are incorrect. This is, if anything, more concerning when one considers that the consequences of a finding of NGRI are different in England and the USA. In the former, detention in a special hospital at Her Majesty's pleasure can be expected, while in the latter a brief treatment package or non-custodial disposal is quite possible.

It is not surprising, given the dramatic nature of some of the cases, that there have been suggestions that PTSD has been grossly overused as an insanity defence in Vietnam veterans. One study has examined this issue (Appelbaum *et al.*, 1993). The investigators looked at all NGRI pleas entered in 49 counties in America over a single period. They found 8163 cases in which the question of NGRI was raised. In only 28 of these cases (0.3%) was PTSD mentioned. The defendants with PTSD were not demographically different from other NGRI cases. However, the outcome of cases was somewhat different in that defendants with PTSD were more likely to be found guilty than others who claimed insanity, but were nevertheless less likely to get a custodial sentence, with the equivalent of probation orders with conditions of treatment being common. The study, therefore, refuted the idea that PTSD was being used excessively in NGRI cases. Although some PTSD and NGRI cases tended to attract a lot of media attention, they were not a common occurrence.

PTSD as mitigation

In the UK it is much more common for mental illness to be raised as a mitigating factor rather than the entering of a NGRI plea. This is entirely logical as there are few occasions when it is in the defendant's interest to be detained indefinitely in a special hospital, as is the likely consequence of a finding of NGRI. The case is heard and, if the defendant is found guilty, then various mitigating factors may be raised after the verdict so that they can be taken into account when the sentence is decided.

As previously noted, in a number of American states this is not the case. They have abandoned the idea of insanity as a defence and have introduced a verdict of 'guilty but mentally ill'. The effect of this is the same as that when a mental illness is considered in mitigation.

In the UK, in the particular case of alleged murder, there is no reason why PTSD, which is a mental disorder as defined in both ICD-10 and DSM-IV should not, in theory, be used as grounds for 'diminished responsibility'. The effect is again the same, in that the sentence, instead of being the fixed sentence for murder, can be determined taking the relevance of the mental illness into account.

In fact, there have not yet been a very large number of cases in the UK in which PTSD has been put forward in mitigation before sentencing. There have been a number of unreported court martial cases in which the response of the court appears to have been variable, some being more lenient than others. The most infamous must surely be that of a Lance Sergeant in the Foot Guards who threatened himself and others with a loaded weapon when he had been drinking; consultant psychiatrists for both defence and the court diagnosed that he was suffering from PTSD due to his experiences in the Falklands. Despite this, he was sentenced to two years and dismissed. A civil case was settled out of court. At the European Court of Human Rights it was held that he had not received the impartial hearing that he had the right to expect, but this was a comment upon the process of court martial, not upon the verdict or sentence.

Bisson has reported two cases tried at crown court, but unfortunately does not record the sentences. It would be interesting to know the responses of courts in general to the presentation of PTSD in mitigation. Given the description of the main case reported by Bisson, it seems very likely that such a case in America would result in a verdict of NGRI.

Anecdotally reported cases have resulted in the defendant being sentenced to a probation order with condition of treatment when found guilty.

PTI following crime

Victims of crime

That PTSD or PTI can follow crime has been demonstrated elsewhere and will not be addressed in depth here. The association of PTSD with crime appears to be related to the severity of the crime and is a function of violence and intrusion. It is therefore hardly surprising that some of the highest rates of PTSD have been detected in victims of rape and of abusive violence to women. It seems likely that this accounts for the commonly observed excess of PTSD in women in community studies.

A major issue concerning the diagnosis of PTSD in victims of crime is the reluctance of victims to speak out and the consequent need actively to screen for PTI. Many victims of crime will not spontaneously report PTI, even at medical consultation.

It is probably important to remember that a criminal investigation and involvement in the adversarial and public situation of a criminal case may, in itself, aggravate symptoms and adversely affect a precarious psychological balance.

The management of PTI, including PTSD, in victims of crime is not generally different from that in victims of other trauma. By definition, patients will have been exposed to major traumatic events. There will always be a need for consideration of the patient's sensitivities.

Compensation for victims

In the UK, the Criminal Injuries Compensation Board (CICB) has provided compensation to victims of crime. There is no requirement for the perpetrator to be identified and successfully prosecuted. Mental health professionals may become involved either at the request of the CICB or of the defendant's advisors.

There is no requirement for a victim to have legal representation in order to make a CICB claim. Ordinarily the victim will complete a form in application. The board will then, where appropriate, contact those who have provided medical care to the victim and request that they provide a brief report, for which there is a predetermined fee scale. The CICB will consider the evidence, including medical reports, and will make an award where appropriate.

In some cases the victim will seek legal representation, either initially or on appeal against a board decision. The solicitor may then request a full medicolegal report, the fee for which will come out of the victim's final award. This is more likely where the claim is of high value, for example where the victim has been rendered unfit to work for a long period.

The government did introduce a scheme by which the CICB did not provide recompense for loss of earnings and a simple tariff scheme was used for all injuries. However, this was effectively retracted and victims can again gain recompense for financial loss consequent upon criminal injuries.

PTI and civil wrongs

In civil law, the mental health professional is most likely to be involved as an expert witness in personal injury litigation. The action usually follows an alleged tort, a 'civil wrong by act or omission other than breach of contract, in respect of which damages can be claimed by a victim from a wrongdoer for a loss or injury' (Weller, 1990).

The question of the nature of damages and of recompense is important. It is the author's experience that many plaintiffs with PTI harbour a belief that litigation will somehow bring 'justice'. Many think that the person who caused their problems will be 'in the dock', will be found 'guilty', and will be 'punished'. They do not realise that the case is about compensation at law, and that the successful outcome will be the receipt of damages, described in 1880 by Lord Blackburn as 'that sum of money which will put the party who has been injured, or who has suffered, in the same position as he would have been in if he had not sustained the wrong for which he is now getting compensation or reparation'.

Those who act as expert witnesses in such cases will have heard many plaintiffs say that they are not pursuing the case for money. For some this is true and these people, more than most, will inevitably feel disappointed or let down after the case is settled. Some will want 'their day in court' and their chance to speak out, and will therefore feel betrayed or cheated at the fact that the vast majority of cases settle out of court.

Others say not that they are not after money, but that 'no amount of money' will make up for their damages. They too are likely to be disappointed. The assessment of damages will almost never be correct. It is a single final payment to consider the long-term future as well as the past. When it comes to factors such as future loss of earnings, costs of future medical and social care, and future medical prognosis, there must be a massive element of guesswork. While it is possible to predict statistically a group of cases, it is not possible to predict accurately the course of a single case over many years.

Another factor likely to affect plaintiffs adversely is the finding that neither the person who hurt them in a road traffic accident, nor the employer who failed to provide a safe place of work, will personally pay for their wrongdoing. Indeed, if they actually get to court, neither will probably be present. Inevitably it will be an insurance company that foots the bill, an organisation with which the plaintiff has had no dealings.

The majority of plaintiffs have a pragmatic approach to the litigation, seeking reparation for their losses and allowing their legal advisers to run the case. A few are simply seeking as much money as they can get. Others, however, are on a search for 'justice', or for 'revenge'. From the comments above it is clear that they will inevitably be disappointed. In the process they will be hurt and annoyed by the adversarial process in which the defendants deny that the wrong ever happened and at the same time say that even if it did it was the plaintiff's fault. Clinicians will often see patients who are in the process of litigation and who hang their whole future on its outcome. Patients will even say that they will enter into possibly curative treatment if and when their lawyer says that it is all right to do so. There is a danger of the clinician also focusing on the outcome of the litigation and expecting matters to improve dramatically when it is over.

While the end of litigation may mean an end to going over events with various strangers, it is obvious that litigation is unlikely to leave the patient happy and satisfied. There is no evidence that PTI clears up when the litigation ends (Merskey and Woodforde, 1972; Cohen, 1987). Even though litigation obviously rewards disability rather than recovery, to delay treatment or rely upon the end of litigation for a miracle cure is inappropriate and is unlikely to be successful.

Psychiatric injury or nervous shock

'Nervous shock' is a term used for many years by the courts. It seems to refer to psychological injury which is more than a normal reaction to a traumatic event. In practice it appears to have been synonymous with a defined psychiatric illness. Normal reactions such as fear, sadness, grief are not nervous shock, and, in English law, they do not result in compensation but are to be borne as part of the normal course of life. The phrase nervous shock is being replaced by 'psychiatric injury'.

Until comparatively recently, there could be no relief in damages for mental shock at all. Indeed, it has been over a period of a 100 years, and particularly over the last 25 years or so, that the subject has been established and examined. The course has been similar, if recently somewhat accelerated and expanded, in the USA. As Slovenko (1994) reports, as late as 1896 a New York court said 'If the right of recovery (for mental distress in negligence cases without physical impact or injury) should once be established, it would naturally result in a flood of litigation in cases where the injury complained of may be easily feigned without detection and where the damages must rest upon mere conjecture or speculation'. It went on to elaborate the risks of fraudulent claims and also said that it would be against policy to allow such a right because of the widely increased burden on the defendant.

Courts seem to have been seriously preoccupied with this fear that plaintiffs will pull the wool over their eyes and succeed in spurious claims. UK courts have also pushed the 'flood-gates' argument hard, and, to a lesser extent the widened range of possible claims against the defendant. They have talked about the problem of objective confirmation of 'nervous shock', and the danger of spurious cases. Quite why they have been so afraid that there would be legions of people making false claims is not clear, although perhaps the recent news reports which claim 'staged' accidents and organised fraud in the US involving the medical and legal professions providing a 'production line' of cases may suggest that their fears were not totally unfounded. Nevertheless, the average psychiatric injury case is not worth a huge sum of money.

A brief history of nervous shock

Michael Napier, a leading solicitor who specialises in both personal injury and mental health litigation, has several times listed the important cases in the history of nervous shock and litigation in the courts of the UK and of areas with similar systems, such as Australia, New Zealand and Canada (Napier, 1991, 1993).

- Until 1890 there were no damages awarded for nervous shock unless there was also physical injury.
- Until 1925 it was possible to gain damages for nervous shock or psychiatric injury suffered through fear of injury or death for oneself. However, one could not receive damages for psychiatric injury caused by fear for someone else such as a child.
- By 1932 it had been established that relief could be gained for nervous shock induced by fear for a close relative but not for other people of lesser relationship.
- In 1942 it was established that there was no duty of care on a defendant when a third person developed nervous shock after witnessing the death or injury of a stranger and therefore no compensation was payable.
- In 1964, for the first time a father who did not actually witness the accident to his son but who heard the screams and ran there immediately afterwards, was awarded compensation.
- It was held in 1967 that a mother could not receive damages for nervous shock which was caused by being told of an incident which had happened to her children. It was held that there was no duty of care.
- In 1984 a woman who went to hospital and saw her family still covered in blood and being treated was awarded damages for nervous shock sustained.

Hillsborough

The consequence of this very abbreviated synopsis of the major events in the development of case-law regarding psychiatric injury is the position in English law which stood and was then examined in detail and solidified following the Hillsborough disaster cases (Teff, 1992; Pugh and Trimble, 1993). At

Hillsborough nearly 100 football supporters were killed and 400 injured in a crush in the ground before the start of a planned FA cup semi-final. Television cameras were present and the scenes were widely broadcast.

In order for the claims of victims to succeed there had to be:

1. a duty of care
2. negligent execution of that duty
3. damages as a consequence.

Clearly the police force had a duty of care to those present, and they admitted negligence. For the survivors who were injured either physically or psychiatrically in the Leppings Lane end of the ground, the case was straightforward. However, it was for the 'secondary' victims that this case was important.

Various friends and relatives claimed nervous shock as a consequence of watching the disaster unfold on television or hearing it on the radio. None of the claimants saw the bodies of loved ones for at least eight hours.

The courts eventually clarified that only the degree of relationship of spouse, child or parent would normally qualify for relief, although conceivably evidence could be given of another relationship which was unusually close and loving. Thus it would normally be expected that siblings, fiancees and grandparents would not qualify.

In addition, the claimants failed as they were not proximate enough to the incident. They did not arrive quickly enough to be considered to have seen the immediate aftermath of the incident. They did not see it with their unaided eyes and the television coverage did not identify individuals. Indeed, the defendants could rely upon the code of practice which insists that television companies may not show the suffering of recognisable individuals. (If they had, then presumably any potential claim would have had to have been made against the television company.)

All the 'secondary victims' failed in their claims.

Road traffic accidents

The specific association between road traffic accidents and PTI appears to have become of increasing interest, with a number of recent studies. Vehicle accidents vary enormously in severity and cannot be considered always to be equivalent to each other. They are a very common source of personal injury litigation.

Road traffic accidents are a good example of the danger of assuming that all PTI is PTSD. Rates for PTSD vary from less than 10% (Malt, 1988) to 46% (Blanchard et al., 1994). However, there is good evidence of a range of other post-traumatic illnesses which are common in road traffic accidents. These include major depression, anxiety states, and phobic symptoms (Ritter, 1993; Brom, Kleber and Hofman, 1993; Blanchard *et al.*, 1995a 1995b).

Blanchard has shown that PTI is more common following a road traffic accident when there is a previous history of depression and of another road traffic accident.

Nervous shock in personal injury cases

At times, it can seem difficult for the medical expert to understand who succeeds and who fails in personal injury cases. From the medical point of view, the PTI of the man sitting in a coach outside Hillsborough watching the television and hearing the screams come over the wall is as obviously a result of the disaster as that of the woman who is dragged alive from the crush. However, the one does not have a case at law and the other does.

In order for a case to succeed, the three factors detailed above must apply.

1. A duty of care to:
   (a) a primary victim
   (b) a secondary victim who is:
       (i) sufficiently proximate in relationship to a primary victim and
       (ii) sufficiently proximate to the event in space and time
   (c) a rescuer.
2. Negligence by the defendant.
3. Disability as a consequence of the incident. In psychiatric injury terms this means effectively that there must be an identifiable psychiatric illness which must have been caused or significantly contributed to or aggravated by the negligent act.

The role of the expert

There is no intention to attempt to produce instructions or suggestions as to how to prepare and present an expert opinion in court. However, there are nevertheless a number of points which need to be presented.

Whether in a criminal or civil case, the relationship between the mental health expert and the person being examined is very different from that in the clinical setting. While there is no suggestion that the legal fear of legions of dissimulating claimants is based in reality, the interviewee nevertheless has a lot resting on the outcome of the case. If he is a defendant, his freedom may be involved. More commonly he is a litigant who genuinely feels aggrieved and he is inevitably aware that his responses may determine to a great extent the size of any award.

In such circumstances even the most honest of subjects is likely to at least solidly describe, if not exaggerate, his symptoms. Some will be prepared to go further.

In this situation there is a real need for the expert to hold as close as possible to demonstrable facts. Neal (1994) has written to point out the dangers and pitfalls of pushing people into DSM diagnostic categories. There is increasing pressure from legal advisors and others to make diagnoses of PTSD as this is readily recognised by courts. There is a danger of producing the diagnosis when it is incorrect and perhaps of missing other genuine relevant diagnoses. Sparr and Boehnlein (1990) remind us of Tanay's point that the production and presentation of a psychiatric diagnosis are not processes with the precision of a Swiss watch mechanism. They point out also that the courts have no particular interest in the actual specific diagnosis, and there is no reason why they should do so. What the court wishes to know is whether they can be confident that a psychiatric illness is or was present, and what its relationship is to the relevant event. The court is interested in the expert's confidence in the presence or absence of a relevant illness, not its name. There is no presumption that only PTSD is relevant after trauma.

The dangers of this insistence on specific diagnoses is emphasised by the fact that there is no definitive diagnostic test for PTSD or many other illnesses. If we look at PTSD itself, there is real and legitimate concern about the educative or training effect of the diagnostic process, as well as the transparency of psychometric tests.

If a structured interview such as the CAPS is used, it prompts the patient with each symptom, asking leading questions as to both frequency and intensity. While this may be extremely useful in a clinical setting in which the patient can be expected to respond accurately, there can be no such comfortable assumption in a legal setting.

In the same vein, a whole series of questionnaires have been used to diagnose PTSD, as described in Chapter 7. While they may be useful at screening for PTSD in a clinical population, and may correlate well with measures such as the CAPS, none of them has been validated in a genuine adversarial position. The evidence is that specificity drops dramatically in the adversarial situation and that positive tests can be fabricated by motivated subjects.

The only tests which appear to have the likelihood of being robust against dissimulation are physiological tests. However, as Pitman and Orr point out (Pitman and Orr, 1993), this has not yet been argued out and accepted in court.

In general, it is essential that the expert relies upon documented evidence and independent corroboration, and maintains his independent, and healthily sceptic, stance.

References

Appelbaum, P.S., Jick, R.Z., Grisso, T. and Givelber, D. (1993). Use of posttraumatic stress disorder to support an insanity defense. *American Journal of Psychiatry*, **150**, 2: 229–34.

Beckerman, A. and Fontana, L. (1989). Vietnam veterans and the criminal justice system: A selected review. *Criminal Justice and Behavior*, **16**, 4: 412–28.

Bisson, J.I. (1993). Automatism and post-traumatic stress disorder. *British Journal of Psychiatry*, **163**: 830–32.

Blanchard, E.B., Hickling, E.J., Taylor, A.E. and Loos, W. (1995a). Psychiatric morbidity associated with motor vehicle accidents. *Journal of Nervous and Mental Disease*, **183**, 8: 495–504.

Blanchard, E.B., Hickling, E.J., Taylor, A.E., Loos, W.R. and Gerardi, R.J. (1994). Psychological morbidity associated with motor vehicle accidents. *Behaviour Research and Therapy*, **32**, 3: 283–90.

Blanchard, E.B., Hickling, E.J., Vollmer, A.J., Loos, W.R., Buckley, T.C. and Jaccard, J. (1995b). Short-term follow-up of post-traumatic stress symptoms in motor vehicle accident victims. *Behaviour Research and Therapy*, **33**, 4: 369–77.

Brom, D., Kleber, R.J. and Hofman, M.C. (1993). Victims of traffic accidents: Incidence and prevention of post-traumatic stress disorder. *Journal of Clinical Psychology*, **49**, 2: 131–40.

Card, J.J. (1983). *Lives After Vietnam*. Lexington, Mass.: DC Heath.

Cohen, R.I. (1987). Post traumatic stress disorder: does it clear up when the litigation is settled. *British Journal of Hospital Medicine*, **37**, 6: 485.

Daniels, N. (1984). Post-traumatic stress disorder and competence to stand trial. *Journal of Psychiatry and Law*, **12**, 1: 5–11.

Erlinder, C.P. (1983). Post-traumatic stress disorder, Vietnam veterans and the law: A challenge to effective representation. *Behavioral Sciences and the Law*, **1**, 3: 25–50.

Law Commission (1995). *Liability for Psychiatric Illness*. Law Commisson Consultation Paper No. 137. London: HMSO.

Lipkin, J.O., Scurfield, R.M. and Blank, A.S. (1983). Post-traumatic stress disorder in Vietnam veterans: Assessment in a forensic setting. *Behavioral Sciences and the Law*, **1**, 3: 51–67.

Malt, U. (1988). The long term psychiatric consequences of accidental injury: a longitudinal study of 107 adults. *British Journal of Psychiatry*, **153**: 810–18.

Marciniak, R.D. (1986). Implications to forensic psychiatry of post-traumatic stress disorder: A review. *Military Medicine*, **151**, 8: 434–7.

Merskey, H. and Woodforde, J.M. (1972). Psychiatric sequelae of minor head injury. *Brain*, **95**, 3: 521–8.

Mullany, N.J. and Handford, P.R. (1993). *Tort Liability for Psychiatric Damage*. Sydney: The Law Book Company Ltd.

Napier, M. (1991). The medical and legal trauma of disasters. *Medico Legal Journal*, **59**, 3: 157–79.

Napier, M. (1993). The medical and legal response to post traumatic stress disorder. *In Choices and Decisions in Health Care*, pp. 205–39. Ed. A. Grub. Chichester: John Wiley & Sons.

Napier, M. and Wheat, K. (1995). *Recovering Damages for Psychiatric Injury*. London: Blackstone Press Ltd.

Neal, L. (1994). The pitfalls of making a categorical diagnosis of post traumatic stress disorder in personal injury litigation. *Medicine Science and the Law*, **34**, 2: 117–22.

Packer, I.K. (1983). Post-traumatic stress disorder and the insanity defense: A critical analysis. *Journal of Psychiatry and Law*, **11**, 2: 125–36.

Pitman, R.K. and Orr, S.P. (1993). Psychophysiologic testing for post-traumatic stress disorder: Forensic psychiatric application. *Bulletin of the American Academy of Psychiatry and the Law*, **21**, 1: 37–52.

Pugh, C. and Trimble, M.R. (1993). Psychiatric injury after Hillsborough. *British Journal of Psychiatry*, **163**: 425–9.

Ritter, G. (1993). Psychic disturbances after whiplash injuries. *Nervenheilkunde*, **12**, 6: 247–9.

Shaw, D.M., Churchill, C.M., Noyes, R. and Loeffelholz, P. (1987). Criminal behavior and post-traumatic stress disorder in Vietnam veterans. *Comprehensive Psychiatry*, **28**, 5: 403–11.

Slovenko, R. (1994). Legal aspects of post-traumatic stress disorder. *Psychiatric Clinics of North America*, **17**, 2: 439–46.

Sparr, L.F. and Boehnlein, J.K. (1990). Posttraumatic stress disorder in tort actions: Forensic minefield. *Bulletin of the American Academy of Psychiatry and the Law*, **18**, 3: 283–302.

Sparr, L.F., Reaves, M.E. and Atkinson, R.M. (1987). Military combat, posttraumatic stress disorder, and criminal behavior in Vietnam veterans. *Bulletin of the American Academy of Psychiatry and the Law*, **15**, 2: 141–62.

Teff, H. (1992). The Hillsborough football disaster and claims for 'nervous shock'. *Medicine Science Law*, **32**, 3: 251–4.

Weller, M.P.I. (1990). Compensation for psychiatric disability. *In Principles and Practice of Forensic Psychiatry*, pp. 1101–16. Ed. R. Bluglas and P. Bowden. Essex: Longman.

CHAPTER 10

PREVENTION OF POST-
TRAUMATIC ILLNESS

There is considerable interest in the prevention of PTI. Popular opinion and the involvement of the media mean that it has now become entirely routine, if not somehow mandatory, for officially sanctioned efforts to be put in place to prevent PTI. At the time of writing, the most recent example has perhaps been the tragic killing of children in a school in Dunblane. As usual, there were the immediate reports of the arrival of 'trained counsellors' to help the survivors and the bereaved to cope. In conversation recently researchers have commented upon the difficulties in conducting a controlled trial of counselling or psychological debriefing after disasters because of the reluctance of survivors to become part of the control groups. Everybody in the general population knows that disaster is followed by some form of counselling or intervention and they are wary about being left out. There is a widespread assumption that such intervention is at least helpful, if not essential.

However, as recently as 1994, Lundin has said 'it is not quite clear that it is possible to prevent post traumatic stress disorder by means of early psychological support, counselling, or psychotherapeutic treatment' (Lundin, 1994). However, despite this, he nevertheless expresses the view, which is no doubt held by many who work in the management or provision of health services, that there is a 'basic human duty' to try to do so. Interestingly, he sees the introduction in DSM-IV of the new category of acute stress disorder as a step in the process of trying to prevent PTI.

In fact, if we look at the evidence, it is necessary to go further than Lundin and accept that it is far from clear that it is possible to prevent PTSD and PTI with the techniques which have been championed. Indeed, we need to examine the evidence that there is any way to prevent PTI.

What is prevention?

It is necessary to be clear about what is meant by prevention of PTI in general, and of PTSD in particular. There are various ways in which the issue can be addressed and various authors have looked at increasing 'orders' or layers, of victims, of increasing distance from the initial event. For example, Richards (1994) and others (Tarrier, 1995), have called for the recognition of, and have described, primary, secondary and tertiary preventive measures. Others have pointed out the importance of secondary victims such as children (Rosenheck and Nathan, 1985), wives (Pugh and Trimble, 1993), or bystanders and rescuers (Duckworth, 1991) (Pugh and Trimble, 1993), and even those involved in providing the preventive treatment (Talbot, 1990). Some authors talk of primary, secondary and tertiary victims.

In order to simplify matters and to allow consideration of the evidence, the question of prevention will be simplified to primary and secondary prevention, where primary means work before the trauma, and secondary means work after the event. We will also consider the place and the effect of early intervention, which is differentiated from secondary prevention in that early intervention is actually aimed at those already identified as having some sort of problems.

Primary prevention

Logic dictates that one sure way to prevent PTI is to prevent people being exposed to traumatic events. If traumatic events must occur, it is logical to minimise exposure to such events, to prepare those people who must be so exposed, and to select for necessary exposure only the people least likely to suffer PTI after such exposure.

Reducing exposure to traumatic events

In an ideal world, war, violent crime, natural disasters and human tragedies would not occur. Clearly there are ways in which governments could reduce the incidence of these events. For example enforcement in some countries of laws preventing additional storeys being surreptitiously added to existing buildings might prevent the subsequent collapse of such buildings and the death and trauma which ensue. However, mental health professionals have little or no influence in preventing such occurrences. They must look at ways to minimise the consequences.

Who needs to be exposed?

An aspect which is often forgotten in planning and rather more so in practice is controlling exposure. It seems very obvious that when there is any form of traumatic event the minimum number of people possible should be exposed to that trauma. This is obviously something which can be most easily applied to secondary potential victims such as rescuers, other workers, by-standers and relatives.

As an example, consider a major road traffic accident. Inevitably, a small number of police officers, fire-fighters, paramedics, and perhaps other health professionals will need to be on the scene and actually involved in the rescue at the time. They will necessarily be exposed to the full horror of the traumatic incident. However, it is likely that varying numbers of other people will arrive at the scene. By-standers who have not been immediately involved in rescue before the arrival of the professionals have no need actually to be exposed to the carnage. Is it not logical that back-up or standby emergency services personnel should be held outside the actual scene until it has been decided that they are definitely going to have to be used?

Rescuer-type patients have been seen who were traumatised by incidents in which they did not play a direct active role but in which they attended either in a management rather than operational role, or in case they were going to be needed. In such situations there is no need for the officer actually to enter, for example, a crashed aeroplane with bodies inside. In a standby or reinforcement role, he or she should be briefed but not involved unless their services are actually needed. In a staff role the officer can be briefed by operational staff. His or her credibility will have been established by previous experiences while in an operational role and by the respect they have earned from their staff.

Even emergency personnel may be tempted to 'rubber-neck'. This should be prevented. It seems at least possible that those rescuers who are fully occupied and busy may be less traumatised than those who enter the situation passively as by-standers, as reserve personnel, or as staff managers, and are helpless to make any change to the situation.

Controlling exposure

This may seem the opposite to the previous point, but where possible individual exposure to trauma should be controlled and restricted. There may be a need to bring in relief rescuers. Simple logic suggests that precautions should be taken to prevent carers and rescuers being allowed to work to the point of exhaustion and inevitable failure.

One stratagem with body-handlers has been to avoid any individual being involved in the whole process for an individual corpse of discovery, identification, removal, transport, storage, preparation, post-mortem, further preparation, and return to family. In order to avoid too close identification with individual victims, staff are expected to play a restricted part in any one case.

Primary victims should be made safe and removed from the immediate scene and from excess danger as soon as is possible. They should not be left helpless to watch their companions dead and dying while rescue efforts continue.

Is exposure important?

Although reducing exposure in the ways suggested seems entirely logical, it must be said that there is a paucity of evidence that exposure to trauma predicts PTI. While the Vietnam research has suggested that perhaps as much as 35% of the variance of post-traumatic morbidity is attributable to degree of exposure, McFarlane's work after the Ash Wednesday fires found significantly less than 10% of the variance accounted for by exposure in both fire-fighters and victims.

Selecting those most likely to cope

This is obviously something which can only be applicable to those who are, by reason of their employment, more than usually likely to be exposed to traumatic events. Much of the interest stems from the search by the armed forces to exclude from their ranks those who are most likely to 'break down'. While the British government was no doubt concerned that more than 30 000 people were still in receipt of psychiatric medical pensions at the start of the Second World War, the interest of the army has been in preventing the loss of manpower and the disruption caused by psychiatric casualties during the actual mission. Such personnel were seen as having an adverse effect upon their peers as well as reducing manpower.

In fact the detailed selection procedures used by armies have been relatively unsuccessful in excluding those who break down. It is, anyway, a potentially problematic tactic, particularly in a situation in which soldiers are not volunteers. Chapter 4 has considered predisposing factors to PTI. One of the few things which has been convincingly demonstrated to predict PTI is a history of previous emotional problems. Such problems are common, and in a conscription situation it might be anticipated that a policy of total exclusion of personnel with such a history from any actual combat situation would be open to abuse.

Other employers who expect their employees to have a higher than average risk of being exposed to traumatic events may consider selection based on previous history in a number of areas as well as upon a current assessment. However, the situation remains far from clear. There are obvious potential problems if large numbers of potential employees are excluded from employment because of a factor in their personal or family history which is known to be associated with an increased risk of PTSD. Quite apart from the practical point that most of those people would not develop PTSD, there will be potential issues of equity and of discrimination.

There is a wide range of employees who are likely to be exposed to traumatic incidents and situations in their work. The requirements for an infantry soldier, a policeman and a bank clerk are not the same. The last of these is far more likely to be the victim of a robbery than the average person. This trauma is rather different, perhaps, from the situation of a soldier in battle or a policeman at a horrific traffic accident. However, the bank clerk is probably in a more helpless and out-of-control situation, and may therefore be at equally great risk.

Generalisations about selection cannot confidently be made, but there is some evidence from unrelated work that selection can be effective at choosing people who are most suited for particularly stressful or dangerous jobs, as has been shown by the old work on bomb disposal officers in the UK. This work also suggested that candidates were effective at self-selection, with mostly suitable candidates applying. However, such self-selection procedures are rather less of a source of confidence when we remember that at least one study has indicated that volunteers for Vietnam were more likely to have PTSD than conscripts.

Preparing those who must be exposed

There appears to be an unco-ordinated but generally effective programme of preparing the general public for the consequences of traumatic events. The association of trauma and 'counselling' cannot have been unnoticed by many in the UK. While some do not accept it, the general assumption is that some form of intervention after trauma is expected and essential. This is the most obvious way in which the general public is prepared for the possible adverse effects of trauma. PTI is perhaps seen as rather more normal and acceptable than mental illness. Hopefully this means that people will be more likely to seek or at least accept treatment where necessary.

It seems unlikely that there could be any other formal plan to prepare the general public to cope with the effects of trauma and thus prevent PTI. However, various organisations have put effort into preparing their own staff in the hope of preventing PTI and its consequences. As previously hinted, the aims of the employers are not essentially altruistic but are mission orientated. They need their staff to be able to do their job. They need to avoid losing staff. More recently they need to avoid their staff suing them for personal injury because of the employer's failure to keep the employee safe at work.

Military preventive preparation

The military has always been seen as the principal example of training in anticipation to prevent problems and to aid the mission.

There has been long and carefully fostered dependence upon group cohesion and effective leadership in the army. In Britain, there has been a move away from the local regiments, in which a company came from a single town and a platoon from a single street or factory, since the First World War experience of whole male populations being wiped out in the fields of France in a single day. Nevertheless, group identification, and team membership down to section and even to two-man buddy level are greatly encouraged in the belief that members of such close-knit groups are collectively more able to cope with stress.

The Vietnam experience was one situation which did not really support this contention, however. As in Korea, the soldiers were individually drafted into theatre for fixed periods so that units were continuously rebuilt rather than moving en masse. Soldiers would travel individually to join strangers in Vietnam after their basic training. Despite this, in the early years of Vietnam the rate of psychiatric casualty evacuations was consistently low and less than 5% of the total evacuated (Jones, 1967; Jones and Johnson, 1975).

Armies have tended to give their men repeated practice in simulations of likely situations. The use of 'drill' is intended to drum procedures into people's heads over and over again until they become automatic. The expectation is that this automatic response will continue in the real-life situation and will be protective.

In armies there is a an overt and planned approach to teaching and training in the subject of possible PTI and battle shock. In the British army, it forms part of the annual training programme for all soldiers, having filtered down over the years from officer, to SNCO, to soldier level. The expressed aim is to normalise acute combat reactions and to teach soldiers to provide emotional first-aid in a buddy–buddy pattern in the same way as they provide physical first-aid. The importance of normalisation is that the emphasis is placed on the initial, normal reactions of those stressed in battle, along with the agreed response, which includes keeping the individual with the unit and in his role, and does not involve health care workers. This normalisation says that individuals will be acutely affected by stress at times but that they are not ill and can continue to do their work. Clearly the goal is mission orientated, but there is a presumption, although not totally supported by evidence, that this will also prevent long-term post traumatic illness.

Another way in which armies prepare their personnel for exposure to stress in the hope that they will not be disabled but will continue their mission is inoculation training. This will be discussed below, but is the implicit and explicit aim of such practices as soldiers being in positions in which live rounds fly past them or in which they are exposed to large concentrations of weapons and men moving and firing at the same time. It is hoped to inure them to the noise and chaos of a war situation.

Stress inoculation training

The idea that exposure to small doses of stressful situations will help the subject cope with the real thing has been used by armed and emergency forces for many years. A more formalised system of stress inoculation training which can be used in varying settings has been described in his book of the same name by Meichenbaum (1985). He sees it as being useful in those who can expect to be exposed in their work situation to stressful and traumatic situations. He uses a cognitive–behavioural approach and suggests that subjects should have 12 to 15 sessions of stress inoculation training followed by 'boosters' from time to time. He describes stages of:

> conceptualisation of the situation
> acquisition of skills and rehearsal
> application of skills and follow through.

One group who have been thought particularly at risk of PTI are those who have to handle bodies after disasters (McCarroll *et al.*, 1993; Fullerton *et al.*, 1993). For them, inoculation training is often used in various forms. For example, it is usual for such volunteers to see and handle dead bodies in a controlled environment before working in the field, they may be exposed to relevant film footage; and they may be exposed to the smell of burning human hair. There is no firm evidence of beneficial effect, but it is usual to teach them certain manoeuvres to reduce distress and involvement, such as breathing through the mouth to reduce the effect of smell, and avoiding direct eye-to-eye contact with dead victims.

Other employers' training

The Institute for Psychotrauma in Utrecht has produced secondary prevention packages for various organisations. Other bodies have also looked at such matters, including public and private sector organisations in the UK. Although there is not, as yet, a co-ordinated national strategy, each of the various fire and police authorities has a standard procedure for employees involved in stressful incidents, or at least for those who are recognised as having problems subsequently.

Another group of relevant employers is comprised of what used to be British Rail. For drivers in particular, there is a formal plan for intervention after an incident which usually includes a period of riding in the cab and driving accompanied before return to full duties.

The banking institutions present a good example of organisations with a formal plan for both primary and secondary intervention. The general public is mainly unaware of the frequency of robberies in banks. A number of the major companies have clearly defined strategies for the protection of staff.

As far as primary prevention is concerned, the banks obviously do all that they can to prevent incidents, with careful use of security. In addition staff are trained not only in security and prevention of robberies, but in how to respond in the case of an incident. Regular training programmes are reinforced by video presentations showing them how to behave. In addition, they are informed in advance of the post-robbery procedures, including procedures aimed at reducing time off work and PTI. One such procedure requires all staff to remain at work until the end of the working day, to be present the next working day at a counselling/debriefing session which includes all those present plus a professional who is a member of staff but from outside the branch. All staff are informed in writing and verbally of the procedures for seeking further help and of the possibility of tertiary referral if required. Sick absence after such incidents is carefully monitored.

Secondary prevention

This is the area most studied, particularly with reference to PTSD rather than other PTI. The basis of the prevention measure used is most commonly that of psychological debriefing. The usual methodology is to provide such intervention to all people identified as being victims or survivors of an incident plus potential secondary victims such as rescuers and family. In addition it is suggested that there is a need to provide psychological debriefing for those doing the debriefing, as few would deny that the process can be painful.

Psychological debriefing

The term was coined by Dyregrov, who was particularly talking about prevention of PTI in rescuers and emergency personnel. In his initial paper (Dyregrov, 1989), he refers to the original description of the method described by Mitchell (1983) and later called critical incident stress debriefing. Dyregrov talks of three principles in such debriefing:

- rapid outreach of services
- a focus on the present time
- mobilisation of existing resources internally and externally.

Although originally described and used for care workers and emergency workers, there has been a gradual and increasing spread of its use so that psychological debriefing is considered by many people to be a normal part of procedure for all survivors of traumatic events.

Critical incident stress debriefing

In many ways this is an extension of debriefing processes used for many years by uniformed services following missions in order to gain information. There are a number of ground rules in psychological debriefing which are explicit. Nobody is forced to speak. All communication is confidential. The debriefing is not a tactical critique of events.

Clearly these rules mean that any critical incident stress debriefing must be separate from a tactical debriefing and those in authority must respect and accept the separation so that participants can have faith in the process.

The debriefing may be done on an individual basis but, where possible, it is preferred to use a natural grouping of people who have shared the experience or the aftermath. As is the norm in group therapeutic processes, two debriefers should work together.

The identity of the debriefers is important, even more so when dealing with a group. The presence of an outsider is a problem. One of the ever-repeated cries of survivors is that those who were not there cannot possibly understand what they have gone through. Debriefers must be acceptable to the group. They must have some common ground, a common experience, and a common language. This is why many occupational debriefing schemes use internal staff or, for confidentiality and avoiding lines of management, those from other parts of the organisation. It is generally accepted that one of the most important and effective supportive forces is in the group itself.

It is generally recommended that debriefing should be soon after the incident, but after physical safety has been not only secured but also recognised by those involved. However, many workers carry out formal debriefing even months or years after the event if it has not been done previously.

The stages in critical incident stress debriefing are as follows.

1. *Introduction.* This includes explanation of the rules, identification of those conducting the debriefing, and explanation of the experience which entitles the debriefers to be present.
2. *Facts.* Members of the group are encouraged to recount the facts of events.
3. *Thoughts and sensory impressions.* Survivors then talk of what was going through their mind, of how they saw things.
4. *Emotional reactions.* Following the earlier stages, group members or individuals are now able to describe their emotional responses to the events described.
5. *Normalisation and anticipatory guidance.* After events, thoughts and emotions have been described and admitted, the debriefer helps normalise such responses, confirms that they are normal in an abnormal situation, and suggests ways to deal with future responses which can be anticipated.
6. *Future planning and coping.* With the debriefer the subjects consider how they will deal with issues in the future, their response to inevitable further situations, and strategies they can use to cope.
7. *Disengagement.* The purpose of the debriefing is to mobilise the resources and normalise the responses of the subjects rather than to engage them in formal treatment. Obviously dependence must not be encouraged, but internal and social supports should be. This must be overtly faced by the subjects as the debriefer raises the topic.

Multiple stress debriefing

Other variations in debriefing have been developed, again usually designed for those involved as rescuers or intervening agencies. One such has been used especially with those who are professional helpers and may have been involved in a range of different traumatic situations over time (Armstrong *et al.*, 1995). It has been used after hurricanes, earthquakes and fire-storms and has four phases:

1. description of factual events
2. expression of feelings and reactions
3. discussion and validation of coping strategies
4. termination.

Does psychological debriefing work?

The rise in popularity and acceptance of debriefing has been remarkable. One of the few things about psychological interventions which the general public can be expected to know is that people who survive trauma should be offered 'counselling'. However, psychological debriefing is definitely not an area of evidence-based medicine.

Much has been extrapolated from the results of early intervention in the later stages of the First World War and subsequent conflicts. However, such treatment strategies, which will be discussed below, were aimed not at survivors or carers, but at those seen to have been traumatised and to be in need of actual treatment.

At least two recent editorials have addressed the issue of the efficacy of psychological debriefing for PTSD. Bisson and Deahl (1994) posed the question 'Early interventions are intuitively appealing and a response to perceived need, but do they work?'.

The same sort of question has been raised by Raphael (Raphael, Meldrum and McFarlane, 1995) who finds that there is an enormous faith in debriefing but no evidence of its efficacy. She is one of those who have advocated controlled research and has asked the unpopular question as to whether there is any danger of such interventions doing harm.

Bisson and Deahl point out that most of the papers which advocate psychological debriefing either tacitly assume its efficacy as unarguable, or provide anecdotal or uncontrolled evidence (Armstrong, O'Callahan and Marmar, 1991).

Sloan's study (Sloan, 1988) of 30 survivors of a plane crash who received early psychological debriefing showed that their psychological distress reduced rapidly over eight weeks and then continued to fall more slowly. However, there were no controls and there was no evidence that the natural course would have been otherwise without intervention.

Robinson and Mitchell (1993) found that 60% of emergency workers thought psychological debriefing 'valuable', while nearly 70% of the assaulted psychiatric staff debriefed by Flannery found that after ten days they were 'regaining control'. Neither of these studies shows any actual preventive effect of psychological debriefing, but rather they help confirm its acceptance. Not everybody accepts psychological debriefing, and British general practitioners involved in emergency work in particular are reported as being one group who find it unacceptable (Doctors reject trauma help, 1991). They, like others, have reported that they will not accept counselling or debriefing from outside but provide all the help needed in an entirely unstructured way internally. Interestingly, a Norwegian study of fire-fighters (Hyton and Harle, 1989) found no difference in outcome between those who had psychological debriefing and those who reported that they had simply talked to colleagues at work. With an uncontrolled group of policemen after the Bradford football stadium fire (Duckworth, 1986), however, Duckworth showed that when those with higher immediate post-trauma GHQ scores were debriefed, their level of symptomatology fell. He is an advocate of debriefing for police personnel (Duckworth, 1991).

Some of the studies have been internally confusing. McFarlane's studies of 469 fire-fighters after the Ash Wednesday fires in Australia considered the presence and absence of psychological debriefing. In the early assessment, those who had been debriefed appeared to have had fewer acute stress reactions, but in the longer-term follow-up they had more psychopathology (McFarlane, 1988).

There have been a few controlled studies. One which showed a response to a crisis intervention scheme rather than simple debriefing was published in 1979 (Bordow and Porritt, 1979) and involved 70 victims of serious road traffic accidents who spent at least a week in hospital. The very small group of ten who had a brief 'review' assessment did better than those who had no intervention. Those who also had a programme of 'practical, social, and emotional support' did better still.

Brom *et al.* also studied road traffic accident victims (Brom, Kleber and Hofman, 1993). They offered a more complicated preventive package rather than psychological debriefing. It had no effect on actual mental health outcome but subjects felt it was helpful.

Deahl *et al.* (1994) carried out an opportunistic controlled trial of psychological debriefing after the Gulf War. The land war was over quickly, with few coalition casualties. Mental health workers were therefore not overloaded by working with vast numbers of combat stress reactions, and looked for those considered to be at most risk of PTI. They were aware that those working as body-handlers for war graves had a very traumatic experience, expressing severe but different stresses associated with handling a small number of British dead and a very much larger number of Iraqi bodies in varying degrees of decomposition. Some of the workers had done such duties before, some had volunteered and been trained in the UK, and some had volunteered and been trained in the Gulf. It was planned that they would all be offered prompt psychological debriefing, either in theatre or immediately on return to the UK. However, logistic mission factors meant that 20 of those followed up at nine months were not debriefed, while 42 were. PTI was common but there was no difference in 'caseness', GHQ score, or IES score, according to participation in psychological debriefing or otherwise. No protective effect at all was demonstrated. In addition it was found that neither previous experience nor longer training was protective, and the one identified predictive factor was a history of previous emotional problems.

That there was no benefit from psychological debriefing was surprising. The strength of the appeal of 'doing something' in response to need, perceived at least by the professional if not the subjects, is shown by a statement by the authors. They said that despite the results, they remained committed to psychological debriefing.

Following the Newcastle earthquake in Australia, another opportunistic experiment in debriefing of rescue personnel was carried out (Kenardy *et al.*, 1996). Sixty-two debriefed rescuers were compared with 133 who were not debriefed, on four occasions over two years. There was no evidence of a more rapid reintegration or of lower rates of psychopathology in the debriefed group.

No controlled studies or natural experiments have shown that psychological debriefing prevents PTSD. Recent, and as yet unpublished, work on psychological debriefing in situations other than war, body-handling, and road traffic accidents has also failed to demonstrate an effect, although it is generally well accepted and valued by subjects. At present the conclusion must be that there is no evidence that psychological debriefing is effective in the prevention of PTI. It is possible that it may have some effect, but it has not yet proven possible to demonstrate any such postulated effect.

This simple fact should be borne in mind by those planning responses to disasters and traumatic events, and also by those who allocate resources. On the one hand, the provision of widespread 'counselling' or debriefing to non-complaining survivors and potential secondary victims should be evidence based. On the other hand, there is also a real danger that those purchasing services may thankfully latch onto psychological debriefing as the appropriate response to PTI because it is clear that one or two session group interventions are much cheaper than formal treatment of PTSD and other PTI. The influx of squads of 'trained counsellors' does not provide an adequate replacement for formal mental health services.

Other generalised preventive responses

McFarlane (1989) considered preventive management after natural disasters. While he commented upon the methodological problems present in most studies, he agreed that 'despite the fact that counselling and an effective welfare relief programme had been provided by a specially instituted team of welfare workers who had contact with all the registered victims' of the Ash Wednesday fires, there was nevertheless a 50% excess of morbidity in those registered victims as measured by the GHQ. He comments upon the failure of this addition of social support as well as counselling to prevent morbidity. He also notes a lack of evidence that poor social support predicted poor outcome.

Singh and Raphael (1981) provided structured intervention for bereaved spouses with a possible beneficial effect, but a planned intervention after the Granville train disaster in Australia showed only 'tentative' evidence of a beneficial effect.

One of the events which has been quoted as an example of a psycho-therapeutic intervention after trauma is the Beverly Hills Club fire. However, it is difficult to draw any conclusions from this work. It has been reported that only 5% of those eligible accepted intervention. Of a group of 30 subjects who entered psychotherapy, (Lindy et al., 1983), the majority did not complete treatment as planned, and this was said to be predicted by therapist experience rather than by factors related to the fire.

Brom and the group from the Institute of Psychotrauma at Utrecht have written about the theory and practice of preventive programmes for PTI (Brom and Kleber, 1989). They describe a package which has been developed for a number of organisations including banks. Their account lists three main aims of early psychological intervention in subjects not identified as patients:

• the stimulation of healthy coping strategies
• the early recognition of disorders
• early psychotherapeutic treatment of recognised PTI.

In a later paper they described the use of the programme to prevent PTI after serious road traffic accidents (Brom, Kleber and Hofman, 1993). They emphasise the importance of fitting in with the needs and expectations of the victims and the superiority of internal over external groups.

They consider an occupational setting for intervention, and three factors which are specifically important therein. They say that there should be a standardised system that applies to all, that it should be agreed beforehand and officially sanctioned, and that it should take note of practical issues such as leave and redeployment where necessary.

The elements of the programme provided in this and other situations include:

1. practical help and information provision
2. psychological support

3.   reality testing of assumptions
4.   confrontation with the event
5.   several contacts over an extended period
6.   early formal treatment of recognised PTI.

One actual study which they published applied the elements of this programme to 68 victims of serious road traffic accident identified by police accident records, with 83 controls not having any intervention. When followed up at
six months, about 10% of both groups had been referred for formal treatment.
Although the intervention group felt that the programme had been helpful, it was
not possible to prove any beneficial effect and the rate of PTI was not reduced.

Stallard and Law (1993) carried out a small opportunistic study on later secondary prevention in a group of teenagers who had been in a minibus which
had crashed. About six months later one of the nine children sought mental
health help for PTI. Two sessions of psychological debriefing were arranged
and were attended by seven children and a teacher. Their questionnaire scores
were lower three months later but, even before the psychological debriefing
scores were lower than those after debriefing in teenagers who survived the
Jupiter sinking. None of the other teenagers sought help or was considered to
have PTI either before or after the delayed debriefing.

Early intervention

The authority most often quoted as the justification for the programmes of
psychological debriefing or other early intervention is the experience of mental
health professionals in a war situation, and the efficacy of the principles of
combat psychiatry as it has been called.

This has its origins again in the First World War. Before what was then called
shell shock and is now called acute stress disorder was recognised, those with
problems were evacuated to England and most did not recover. The establishment of treatment facilities in theatre led to many sufferers returning to duty.
This lesson has greatly influenced army psychiatry ever since. It probably
reached its pinnacle with the Israelis in the seventies and eighties.

Israeli experience in early treatment

The Israelis practise the principles of war psychiatry as explored in Chapter 8:

*   proximity
*   immediacy

- expectancy
- simplicity.

This was due partly to doctrine and partly to necessity. Unlike the Americans in Vietnam, they were fighting in their own back-yard rather than overseas. Those who were not treated in field medical units were inevitably in the next line of medical support, Israeli civilian hospitals. They had no real prospect of significant reinforcements and needed all the manpower available.

The four principles are logical in this situation. However, it is necessary to contrast the situation in a war zone with more normal medical practice. In the former the desired result is that the 'patient' picks up his rifle and goes back to fight. In the battle situation his chances of five-year survival are not immediately relevant. Proximity is important as it is hardly surprising that as victims get further from the point of injury their symptoms solidify and, at least unconsciously, they recognise that symptoms are necessary to prevent return. Immediacy is entirely logical. The sooner the problem is addressed, the less it will have crystallised. The expectation is that the victim will maintain a soldier role, will not become a patient in pyjamas, and will quickly return to duty. The treatment is simple because it may need to be applied to many and in poor conditions.

The elements of such initial treatment include: practical issues such as food, sleep and self-care; an opportunity for ventilation; maintenance of self-determination and role; re-establishment of the duty role; and especially normalisation. A major message is that what has happened happens to normal people in an abnormal situation and will normally go away.

Such treatment programmes have been shown to be effective in returning people to battle (Solomon and Benbenishty, 1986). They have also been shown to reduce the rate of PTSD to some extent on long-term follow-up. However, this must be put into perspective. Solomon and her colleagues have followed up combat stress reaction sufferers from both the Yom Kippur and Lebanon wars. For security reasons it is difficult to find the exact numbers of cases but they have followed groups in excess of 400. In one major study (Solomon *et al.*, 1987), they found that the rate of PTSD in veterans in general was 16% but in those who had been *successfully* treated for combat stress reaction it was 59%. Thus if a soldier had an acute stress reaction to trauma, immediate treatment was likely to render him fit to return to duty and finish the war but he still had a better than evens chance of developing chronic PTSD.

There are two main reasons why the war psychiatry research cannot be used as a justification for the use of psychological debriefing or other intervention in victims of disasters.

The first is that the proximity–immediacy–expectancy–simplicity model has never been provided to healthy soldier survivors, but only to those who 'broke down' and were defined as being disabled or ill at the time. It is quite unreasonable to extrapolate from this group to those who survive a natural disaster or witness sudden death or a near miss.

The second problem is the results. Even though defined cases may return to duties immediately, more than half of them seem to develop chronic illness anyway. This intervention has only been tried on what are probably the people with the worst prognosis.

Intervention for those with problems

While there is no firm evidence that the war psychiatry principles are applicable to survivors in general, they would seem to be appropriate for those who do develop an acute stress reaction. In this situation all the principles apply. It is probably appropriate for even those who recover to be followed up in the medium term given the Israeli experience.

It should be clearly recognised that intervention in such circumstances is not the same as psychological debriefing and that while psychological debriefing may be considered to be an appropriate element of the programme, it is not sufficient.

Summary and conclusions

It has to be accepted that there is, as of yet, no good evidence that any of the strategies used thus far is of value in preventing rather than treating PTI. The perceived need for planners and health professionals to do something should not result in the wholesale use of unproven interventions.

There is always a danger for those who are involved with people who are likely to be exposed to trauma or have been so exposed to follow the distorted logic:

> I must do something.
> This is something.
> I must do this !!!

- Employers and planners should obviously do all that they can to prevent people being exposed to trauma by increasing safety and security and perhaps by selection. They should avoid the unnecessary exposure of those not directly involved.

- There should be formal plans for action after trauma which take into account PTI, so that access to services is easy and is known by all. Plans should include, particularly for employers, some way of recognising or detecting problems over time.
- Those with appropriate responsibility should be aware of individuals or groups who, by reason of their role or other factors, are at most risk.
- There should be prior training, information passing, and inoculation.
- At this stage there is no evidence that psychological debriefing, counselling, or other intervention in those who are not diagnosed and do not see themselves as ill is of any value in preventing PTI or PTSD. This does not mean that it has no effect, and it may be that further research will find an effect or define alternative strategies which are protective. In the meantime, such interventions should not be seen as a substitute for services.
- Despite the above, some people find psychological debriefing somehow useful even if it does not prevent illness. It is often seen as supportive.
- There should be early intervention for those who present with symptoms.
- It should be recognised that quick recovery may still be followed by chronic symptoms.
- There is a very real need for empirical research into the question as to whether or not PTI can be prevented. Large-scale controlled trials are needed.
- In the meantime, Lundin's statement can be reasonably amended: 'It is not *at all* clear that it is possible to prevent PTSD *or other PTI*'.

References

Armstrong, K., Lund, P., McWright, L. and Tichenor, V. (1995). Multiple stressor debriefing and the American Red Cross: the East Bay Hills fire experience. *Social Work*, **40**, 1: 83–90.

Armstrong, K., O'Callahan, W. and Marmar, C.R. (1991). Debriefing Red Cross disaster personnel: the multiple stressor debriefing model. *Journal of Traumatic Stress*, **4**, 4: 581–93.

Bisson, J. and Deahl, M. (1994). Psychological debriefing and prevention of post-traumatic stress. More research is needed. [Editorial] *British Journal of Psychiatry*, **165**, 6: 717–20.

Bordow, S. and Porritt, D. (1979). An experimental evaluation of crisis intervention. *Psychology Bulletin*, **84**: 1189–217.

Brom, D. and Kleber, R.J. (1989). Prevention of post-traumatic stress disorders. *Journal of Traumatic Stress*, **2**, 3: 335–51.

Brom, D., Kleber, R.J. and Hofman, M.C. (1993). Victims of traffic accidents: Incidence and prevention of post-traumatic stress disorder. *Journal of Clinical Psychology*, **49**, 2: 131–40.

Deahl, M.P., Gillham, A.B., Thomas, J., Searle, M.M. and Srinivasan, M. (1994). Psychological sequelae following the Gulf War: Factors associated with subsequent morbidity and the effectiveness of psychological debriefing. *British Journal of Psychiatry*, **165**, 1: 60–65.

Doctors reject trauma help. (1991). *General Practitioner*, 4 May: 24.

Duckworth, D.H. (1986). Psychological problems arising from disaster work . *Stress Medicine*, **2**: 315–23.

Duckworth, D.H. (1991). Managing psychological trauma in the police service: from the Bradford fire to the Hillsborough crush disaster. *Journal of the Society of Occupational Medicine*, **41**, 4: 171–3.

Dyregrov, A. (1989). Caring for helpers in disaster situations: Psychological debriefing. *Disaster Management*, **2**, 1: 25–9.

Fullerton, C.S., Wright, K.M., Ursano, R.J. and McCarroll, J.E. (1993). Social support for disaster workers after a mass casualty disaster. Effects on the support provider. *Nordic Journal of Psychiatry*, **47**, 5: 315–24.

Hyton, K and Harle, A. (1989). Firefighters: A study of stress and coping. *Acta Psychiatrica Scandinavica*, **80**: 355.

Jones, F.D. (1967). Experiences of a division psychiatrist in Vietnam. *Military Medicine*, **132**, 12: 1003–8.

Jones, F.D. and Johnson, A.W. (1975). Medical and psychiatric treatment policy and practice in Vietnam. *Journal of Sociological Issues*, **31**, 4: 49–65.

Kenardy, J.A., Webster, R.A., Lewin, T.J., Hazell, P.L. and Carter, G.L. (1996). Stress debriefing, patterns of recovery following a natural disaster. *Journal of Traumatic Stress*, **9**, 1: 37–49.

Lindy, J.D., Green, B.L., Grace, M. and Titchener, J. (1983). Psychotherapy with survivors of the Beverly Hills Supper Club fire. *American Journal of Psychotherapy*, **37**, 4: 593–610.

Lundin, T. (1994). The treatment of acute trauma: Post-traumatic stress disorder prevention. *Psychiatric Clinics of North America*, **17**, 2: 385–91.

McCarroll, J.E., Ursano, R.J., Wright, K.M. and Fullerton, C.S. (1993). Handling bodies after violent death: strategies for coping. *American Journal of Orthopsychiatry*, **63**, 2: 209–14.

McFarlane, A.C. (1988). The longitudinal course of posttraumatic morbidity: The range of outcomes and their predictors. *Journal of Nervous and Mental Disease*, **176**, 1: 30–39.

McFarlane, A.C. (1989). The prevention and management of the psychiatric morbidity of natural disasters: an Australian experience. *Stress Medicine*, **5**, 1: 29–36.

Meichenbaum, D. 1985. *Stress Inoculation Training*. New York: Pergamon Press.

Mitchell, J.T. (1983). When disaster strikes. The critical incident stress debriefing process. *Journal of Emergency Medical Services*, **8**: 36–9.

Pugh, C. and Trimble, M.R. (1993). Psychiatric injury after Hillsborough. *British Journal of Psychiatry*, **163**: 425–9.

Raphael, B., Meldrum, L. and McFarlane, A.C. (1995). Does debriefing after psychological trauma work? *British Medical Journal*, **310**: 1479–80.

Richards, D. (1994). Traumatic stress at work: A public health model. *British Journal of Guidance and Counselling*, **22**, 1: 51–64.

Robinson, R.C. and Mitchell, J.T. (1993). Evaluation of psychological debriefings. *Journal of Traumatic Stress*, **6**: 367–82.

Rosenheck, R. and Nathan, P. (1985). Secondary traumatization in children of Vietnam veterans. *Hospital and Community Psychiatry*, **36**, 5: 538–9.

Singh, B. and Raphael, B. (1981). Post-disaster morbidity of the bereaved. A possible role for preventive psychiatry. *Journal of Nervous and Mental Disease*, **169**: 205–12.

Sloan, P. (1988). Post-traumatic stress in survivors of an airplane crash-landing: A clinical and exploratory research intervention. Special issue: Progress in traumatic stress research. *Journal of Traumatic Stress*, **1**, 2: 211–29.

Solomon, Z. and Benbenishty, R. (1986). The role of proximity, immediacy, and expectancy in frontline treatment of combat stress reaction among Israelis in the Lebanon War. *American Journal of Psychiatry*, **143**, 5: 613–17.

Solomon, Z., Weisenberg, M., Schwarzwald, J. and Mikulincer, M. (1987). Posttraumatic stress disorder among frontline soldiers with combat stress reaction: The 1982 Israeli experience. *American Journal of Psychiatry*, **144**, 4: 448–54.

Stallard, P. and Law, F.D. (1993). Screening and psychological debriefing of adolescent survivors of life-threatening events. *British Journal of Psychiatry*, **163**: 660–65.

Talbot, A. (1990). The importance of parallel process in debriefing crisis counsellors. *Journal of Traumatic Stress*, **3**: 265–77.

Tarrier, N. (1995). Psychological morbidity in adult burns patients: Prevalence and treatment. *Journal of Mental Health*, **4**, 1: 51–62.

CHAPTER 11

THE WAY AHEAD - WHITHER NOW?

Thus far this book has been intended to present the case for the importance and relevance of PTI in general and PTSD in particular. The aim of this chapter is to present some personal ideas and questions, and to try to consider the future direction of work on the psychological effects of trauma and the postulated physical effects in the brain of psychological trauma. It is unashamedly a personal view and is intentionally written without references, although hopefully the sources of most of the questions and problems have been detailed in the text thus far.

Trauma and mental illness are a subject which has inevitably preoccupied me over the years because of my employment. As a trainee psychiatrist in the army it seemed inevitable that I would be confronted with the history of battle shock and the future of combat stress in the anticipated battlefields of North West Europe. In the event the first case of PTI which I met was from one of the sad series of airline crashes which have come to be known by the name of the relevant city, or airfield, or flight number. What it taught me was the power of trauma and the intransigence of avoidance symptoms. A series of individual cases from Northern Ireland and from the Falklands taught me about PTI and then about PTSD. What they taught me was not so much the uniformity and the commonality of post-traumatic illnesses, but the variety of post-traumatic responses. What was interesting was not so much that some people got PTSD, as that not everybody did. Why was it that most people seemed not to get PTIs, some did but got better quickly, and a few seemed to stay disabled come what may?

Then as I began to study Falklands veterans and others, it became clear that not all of those who responded positively to questions about PTSD symptomatology seemed actually to be ill. It was not that they seemed to be telling lies, but that some of those who reported intrusive symptomatology in particular seemed quite unaffected by it, living their lives apparently successfully despite these reported symptoms. Many of them did not see themselves as ill.

Then there were the older patients, the ex Far East prisoners of war and other World War II veterans who came for assessments for pensions or seeking treatment. Some were presenting with what seemed to be PTSD but it was the first time that they had reported it, some 40 years after the event. It seemed not so much that they had simply ignored serious disability for 40 years, but that symptoms had not really been troublesome before and that some other event such as loss of work, of a supportive relationship, or of health, had led to their becoming ill.

Increasingly, through the eighties and early nineties I saw my role as championing the cause of PTI and PTSD. It seemed to be my job, along with my leaders, to have the concept and the consequences accepted as important by the medical services, the army management, and the population. This last was done for everyone most effectively by the media following Zeebrugge, Hillsborough, Lockerbie etc. etc. These events and experiences in Northern Ireland and elsewhere also influenced the army authorities, and it was considered appropriate that the opinions of psychiatrists including myself, were sought. The plans for the North West Europe scenario were extended and modified and the psychological effects of trauma became important, or at least recognised in standard procedure planning. Dealing with psychological injuries became part of the annual training objectives of all qualified soldiers.

With the recognition of the existence and significance of PTI came an acceptance of a number of other things, including the ubiquitous role of counselling. There was an implicit acceptance of debriefing and an open expression, in the army and elsewhere, of its value in prevention of PTI. Elsewhere, PTSD was being described after a wider and wider range of traumatic incidents. It seemed that anything and everything could cause PTSD, and that anyone and everyone not only could have, but did have, PTSD. It was an inevitable consequence of the media exposure.

Gradually doubt began to rise. Did all of these people really have PTSD? Did all of these events cause PTSD? Was PTSD the best explanation of all the problems that could follow trauma?

Much of the book has been devoted to a justification of the concept of PTI and of PTSD. However, there is some doubt. It is actually possible to construct arguments which bring into question many of the apparent facts and clear opinions about PTSD. Perhaps there is some value in a healthy cynicism.

First of all, trauma without physical injury is not only associated with PTSD. It has been associated with battle shock, which some equate with PTSD, but it has also been associated with conversion hysteria, with depression, with substance abuse, and with personality change, to name a few.

PTSD was only defined in 1980, which suggests that it is a new concept but an argument central to the concept, and the status of PTSD is that it is not new but has simply been renamed. Various ancient case histories are quoted, but inevitably none of them fulfills current diagnostic criteria. Is this because the right details were not recorded or are the conditions actually not coterminous? There are similarities between post-traumatic reactions over the centuries and that defined after Vietnam, but what is the justification for saying that they are the same? There are also differences. It has been suggested that PTSD is a new concept that has developed over the past hundred years or so, not because trauma is new, but because the way in which we remember things and the possession of memories are relatively new and newly developed concepts, not present previously. It is suggested that individually owned memories are an essential prerequisite of PTSD as it is seen now, but that such memories are a relatively recent development. Whatever the explanation, is there really any justification for saying that the problems experienced by the Swiss women trapped in an avalanche, by the World War I soldiers with hysterical paralyses and shell shock, by those with railway spine and soldier's heart, and those who are preoccupied with the content of their psychotic illness are fundamentally the same problems as that of the Vietnam veterans with their 'post-Vietnam syndrome'? Were Edmund Blunden and Siegfried Sassoon really the same as Rambo and the stars of The Deerhunter?

In the second half of the twentieth century and before Vietnam, there was some interest in post-traumatic neurosis and related problems, but it was often somewhat specialised. There was work into the state of the Holocaust survivors and their condition is really not that similar to that of Vietnam veterans after all. The other source of interest was rape victims and at the same time as there was a call for a post-Vietnam syndrome there was also a call for a rape trauma syndrome, this last with the three variants of typical, compounded or silent. Probably this was nearer to PTSD than the Holocaust response, with the silent variation being nearest to predominantly avoidant symptoms. Some of the work being done at this time, however, was perhaps less than mainstream, with published work like that investigating the effect of using psychedelic drugs to treat the psychological effects of industrial accidents.

It seems all the more surprising that the problems of the Vietnam veterans have led to the development of this apparently almost universal condition when one realises that the thrust of the whole Vietnam argument was that the Vietnam War was different from other wars and trauma, so that they had different problems and different needs. It was only when Congress accepted this difference that readily accessible services were provided for Vietnam veterans which had not been, and were not, provided for veterans of other wars. However, the next year PTSD was defined, explicitly emphasising the commonality of responses to varied trauma.

One of the curiosities of this 'different' war was that, unlike previous wars, there was an apparently very low rate of acute psychiatric illness during the war but then an apparently very high rate of chronic illness after the conflict was over. Bersoff studied the Rorschach ink blots of 1500 of those who actually were evacuated from Vietnam for psychological or psychiatric reasons and stated that only two of them had traumatic neuroses of war! This contrasts sharply with the First World War, which had troublingly high acute rates of illness followed by relatively high chronic rates.

While it is clear that there were some extremely good and very extensive studies of veterans, some of the initial work leading the way to them was less robust. A very frequently reported study by an influential writer seems to report a less than 10% response rate to a postal questionnaire and to base its conclusions on a far smaller subgroup numbering 39. Some of the papers suggested that many of the cases they reported had been diagnosed by others as having psychotic illnesses. This interests me as there does not appear to be a lot of more recent literature about significant numbers of cases of PTSD presenting as psychosis or being misdiagnosed as schizophrenia. It is interesting that schizophrenia is one of the few diagnoses not generally associated with PTSD as a comorbid or dual diagnosis.

One of the interesting but seldom quoted papers on veterans questioned the frequency with which post-Vietnam problems were detected and suggested that investigator priming might have had an effect. The study neatly demonstrated that if the investigators expected to find that subjects saw a negative effect of the war, that is what they got. If they expected a positive view of the experience the subjects would oblige.

One of the interesting things about PTSD and the Vietnam veterans, which is conveniently forgotten about when considering other causes of PTSD, is the forensic implication. Rightly or wrongly, one of the most prevalent perceptions of the Vietnam veteran with PTSD was of violent behaviour, with or without law-breaking. Nobody has suggested an increase in violent crime in victims of road traffic accidents, in the survivors of natural disasters, or in the 46% of people with a recent psychotic illness who are said to have PTSD.

In a lecture I once, jokingly, compared PTSD with a unicorn. It is a mythical beast. It would be nice if it existed and it certainly should exist. It is a bit hard to work out what it is in such a way that it is easily recognised as being different from horse, giraffe and rhinoceros. It would be extremely helpful if there was a more practical way of finding it than having a virgin sit in a clearing in the forest and wait for it to put its head in her lap!

In truth, PTSD is a condition in which certain stressors produce certain symptoms in certain people. The problem is that there is still doubt about which stressors produce which symptoms in which people. Can we answer these questions?

The criterion which describes the stressor has not been too stable since the definition of PTSD. Interestingly, the historical examples purporting to be cases of PTSD have always been from fairly impressive natural and man-made disasters like being trapped under the snow for days, or in the trenches of the First World War, or in the Great Fire of London. DSM-III initially considered PTSD to be a sequel of catastrophic experiences and focused on the universality of the effect, talking about events which would be likely to cause great distress in almost anyone. However, there was an almost immediate interest in small numbers of people who apparently had similar symptomatology following less catastrophic events. DSM-IIIR then talked of events outside the range of usual human experience.

Even if you do research into catastrophic experiences it rapidly becomes clear that there is no universal catastrophic-type event. If you look at a group of people involved in the same incident, it becomes clear even before you start to look at meaning and interpretation that not everybody has had the same experience. If you look at several hundred victims of a major fire, some will have nearly been killed, some will have lost relatives, some will have lost their belongings, some will have been temporarily inconvenienced. When soldiers go into battle some will be wounded, some will kill at close range, some will have near misses, some will have days and weeks of fear and boredom. There is almost inevitably a range of experience, even in a single incident.

When we then go on to take into account the individual's perception, it becomes even more complicated. If three men are in an armoured vehicle and the vehicle next to them bursts into flames, one may feel that witnessing the probable death of close peers is terrible. A second may see this as an indicator that they too will inevitably be killed, heightening his fear. The third may see it as a lucky escape and proof of personal invulnerability.

Given that there appears at first glance to be some difficulty with recognising definitive PTSD-generating trauma, it is hardly surprising that a wider and wider range of stimuli came to be promoted. Indeed there has, of course, been a mildly vociferous argument about the possibility of disposing of the stressor criterion as a hurdle altogether. Thus, if people had intrusive, avoidant and arousal symptoms and some degree of disability for more than a month after anything happened, then they would have post 'whatever it was' disorder.

In fact, as we know, the DSM-IV committee steered a middle course and defined the stressor hurdle as requiring some form of 'exposure' to real or potential harm to someone, plus intense fear or horror. However, this does seem to be a really rather wide goal-mouth. The increasing list of trauma-producing events seems to move further and further away from the initial triumvirate of combat exposure, rape, and concentration camp experience. Is it really only me that finds it a little odd that things like near-miss car crashes are seen to be in the same league? Are people sitting at home who work for ferry companies and hear that a ferry belonging to another company has sunk with many lives lost, really in the same position as the Vietnam veterans? Does the apparently normal process of childbirth have the same meaning? Can the distress caused by suffering a psychotic illness, or the pressure of a bullying line manager really have the same effect as being in a concentration camp?

It seems to me that there are still many questions to be asked about the nature and meaning of the stressor criterion. Can these things all be equivalent? Is there any significance to the fact that some types of stressful events can have the same effect on disparate communities as regards conditions such as depression, but widely differing effects as regards PTSD? What is the importance of who the individual is and what their previous life experience has been?

There are occasions when we seem to shoot ourselves in the foot in the search to have the importance of psychological effects of traumatic incidents recognised. For example, a paper extolling the value of including mental health professionals in disaster response teams stated: 'the less serious the accident, or the closer the near-miss, the more likely the worker will develop neurotic symptoms'. Is this really what is meant, that the less the stress the more likely the psychological response? I hope not. If it were true it would suggest that there was a directly opposite effect in accidents from that seen in combat. It is a matter of some concern that it is really only in combat that exposure has been consistently shown to account for much of the variance of PTSD, and then only for about 35%. We really do not know what dictates who will get PTSD. If 35% of the variance is accounted for by the trauma, then presumably the rest is accounted for by things like previous trauma history, previous illness, family history, personality, experience, support networks, and subsequent experience. Nevertheless, people have thus far failed to come near explaining the whole, or nearly the whole, of the variance. We do not really know why some people get PTSD and some do not. All of the features mentioned have some bearing but you cannot predict or explain it.

Having decided that it is very difficult to come to any firm decisions about which stressors can cause PTSD because apparently nearly everything can, we now look at the symptom profile. Here we are on steadier ground. DSM-III, DSM-IIIR and DSM-IV have changed the symptoms somewhat but have essentially consolidated the idea that there are three groups of symptoms, intrusive, avoidant and arousal. There is even some statistical analytic support for these three groups of symptoms, at least in Vietnam veterans. It seems a pity that the World Health Organisation has decided effectively to call the intrusive symptoms essential and the others common but not necessary. This is particularly disappointing if one looks at the influential work by Horowitz and the effectively confirmatory recent opinions supporting the theory of a phasic nature of the condition, with intrusive symptoms intermittently predominating or intruding against a background of avoidance.

Unfortunately none of the symptoms is pathognomonic. However, this is not that surprising as there is a limited number of possible psychiatric symptoms. The most specific seem to be the intrusive symptoms, but even if they do not appear specifically in other diagnostic criteria sets, most of them do occur elsewhere.

DSM, of course, unlike the ICD, is quite specific about the number of symptoms required to make the diagnosis. Various investigators have gone further and used the total number or the frequency and severity of symptoms as a specific measure of the severity of disease. However, are either of these sets of assumptions justified?

Why does DSM require one symptom from one group, two from another, and three from a third? The empirical basis for this distribution has not been widely demonstrated. What the criteria mean is that if a person has all but one of the necessary symptoms they do not fulfill diagnostic criteria for PTSD. It does not matter which one of the required six is missing. Logically this suggests that the various symptoms must be free from overlap both within the three groups and across the groups. They must all be distinct and valid if they carry equivalent weight in the diagnostic process. However, simple study of the various symptoms does not really support the contention that they are actually 17 separate entities.

- If you get intrusive memories which cause distress, are you not likely to become distressed if exposed to reminders?

- Do not frequent distressing dreams result in sleep disturbance?
- Is avoidance of thoughts and feelings really separate from and distinguishable from avoiding reminders?
- Can many patients reliably differentiate between feelings of detachment or estrangement and a restricted range of affect with inability to have loving feelings?

While the idea of the three separate groups of symptoms does seem to have validity as noted above, the same is not proven for each of the symptoms. They do not necessarily separate within the groups and there is some overlap across groups. Indeed, some of the symptoms may not necessarily always be symptoms. Is an inability to remember an important element of the incident necessarily a symptom of PTSD?

Anyway, even if some of the symptoms do seem to overlap to some degree, at least it is clear that PTSD is a distinct stand-alone illness which is separate from other illnesses, or at least it should be.

One of the strange things about PTSD is how often there is another co-morbid condition. It is clear that the Epidemiological Catchment Areas have shown that the presence of almost any one psychiatric disorder seems to predispose to the concurrent presence of a wide range of others. However, at least in those presenting for any form of treatment, the rate of comorbidity in patients with PTSD is enormous, perhaps 80%. This seems a difficult finding to assimilate into a concept of PTSD as a distinct, identifiable illness. Surely the majority of cases should be in a pure form. Of course, because most of the PTSD symptoms are also found in other conditions, they can generally be 'used' more than once, so that the same individual symptoms are seen as fulfilling the diagnostic criteria for more than one condition. The absence of the hierarchical approach means that all possible diagnoses are applied and none is considered paramount. It is certainly possible that in some cases there can be doubt about what the diagnosis of PTSD adds to the management of the case, for example if the other diagnosis is of specific phobia of driving.

The symptoms of PTSD may not be such that PTSD can be easily separated from other disorders on clinical criteria on all occasions, and the stressors can be variable. It seems appropriate to consider how many people get PTSD and whether there is anything specific about which people do and do not get the disorder.

The suggestion that the findings for rates of PTSD are surprisingly consistent despite significant differences in methodology is surprising when one considers that two of the biggest studies have shown current rates with a sevenfold difference, and lifetime rates with a twofold difference. Even more surprising, both of these studies were looking at the same group, Vietnam veterans. For various other classes of stressors rates have varied from 0% to 90%, from 4% to 81%, from 1% to 38% etc. The contention that the prevalence rates are surprisingly congruent only applies if you provide explanations which exclude the ones which do not fit. The rates are all the same except for those which are different, and they are wrong!

The reason why rates vary from stressor to stressor is presumably because stressors do not all have the same effect in producing PTI. The reasons why rates vary within the same class of stressor may be about a differential effect of different subclasses or severities of stressor, but may also be about both individual variation and the diagnostic method.

There has been a lot of interest in the failure of people to report their symptomatology, even when asked to do so. It is generally held that this shows the importance of persistent enquiry. However, it may also show that many cope well despite some symptoms. If they do not complain of their problems, appear to function well, do not see the need of help, and do not want to speak to psychiatrists, is it not possible that they are actually generally healthy? Surely there is some inherent danger in investigators labelling people as ill if they do not see themselves as ill and do not act as if ill. There may also be some danger inherent in labelling them as cases of PTSD when this may not be the most appropriate explanation of the situation.

It is a less popular area of study but there has also been some over-reporting of PTSD. Apart from the individual cases of people misguidedly thinking that PTSD explains their problems, or hopefully seeking medical or financial input by claiming that it does, there have been a few fascinating legal cases of apparent fabrication. Obviously there is no suggestion that these particularly infamous cases are representative, but they do highlight the fact that dissimulation is possible. While the use of questionnaires and psychometric instruments will improve diagnostic reliability, most of them presume that the subject will report honestly. Questionnaires simply ask questions that could be put in interview. They contain no internal magic ingredient for diagnosis. Some of the more complicated instruments have been tested in 'staged' dissimulation, but until there is some independent way to diagnose PTSD it is impossible to know how good any of the measures are at detecting faking.

What is needed is a simple and reliable objective test for PTSD, like a blood test. There is little doubt that the most hopeful at present concerns physiological response to exposure *in vivo* or *in vitro*. While there is good evidence of biochemical and neurochemical changes in the brain in certain cases of PTSD, the testing is not yet at a stage where it could be used for actual diagnosis in individual cases. The work on physiological changes seems relatively further advanced and nearer to application in diagnosis. However, I have two concerns about this. The theoretical one is that this seems, at first glance, to tap only one aspect of PTSD, the arousal symptomatology. We would need to be quite sure that it was not possible to get, say, avoidance without arousal, or distressing intrusive symptoms without arousal, before we could be sure that the test was diagnostic. My more practical concern is that this has really only been investigated to any significant extent on one group of sufferers thus far. We have already seen that the assumption that there is complete homogeneity across stressors and patient groups is based more on belief than upon evidence. It has been shown that Vietnam veterans can be differentiated from other veterans with and without other psychiatric disorders by physiological response. However, apart from a little work in road traffic accidents, there is no evidence yet that these results are universal. This seems necessary if physiological response is to be seen as a method of specific diagnosis.

If we were able somehow to come across a single diagnostic test, then we would effectively redefine, at least temporarily, PTSD as that condition which resulted in a positive test. We could then examine the disparate presentations of PTSD in different groups at different times. Do the acutely distressed patients whose lives are disrupted by distressing reminders of a robbery, who avoid travelling, and who are in a constant state of arousal six months on have the same fundamental condition as the embittered and distrusting veteran ten years on who, far from avoiding reminders, is almost totally preoccupied with his experiences and with his grievances? I am not suggesting that either is not suffering, but it does seem to take quite an effort of will to suggest that they have the same problem. If they do have the same condition, how does the veteran get to that position when, on the balance of probabilities, the robbery victim will return to normal function, affected by the incident, but no longer disabled? It seems to me that we have to find some common substrate other than the simple idea of a 'major stressor' if they are to be the same.

Alternatively, perhaps they are not the same. Perhaps we have worked too hard over the past 20 years to push everyone into the same pigeon-hole. People are beginning to question this. ICD-10 has given us the concept of an enduring change in personality and, while I have concerns about this idea, it does suggest that all that glitters is not PTSD. The proposed DSM disorder of DESNOS (disorders of extreme stress not otherwise specified) was not accepted, but reflects a perception that there is more to specific post-traumatic illness than PTSD. People like Marmar have suggested that there is a concept of uncomplicated as opposed to complicated PTSD, that there is more than one predictable course, and therefore perhaps more than one entity. It seems that there is a growing perception that not all specific post-traumatic illness is PTSD, that there are variations on a theme. There is a need to start trying to separate out these variations and to look at who gets them, and after which traumata.

Identifying variants of PTSD or other PTI may help us to allocate treatment logically. There is no doubt that certain types of treatment have a positive effect: behavioural treatments, antidepressants, probably psychotherapeutic treatments. The perception is that the condition generally has a good prognosis and ICD-10, at least, states this openly. However, the published trials of treatment, while recognising some response, are far less positive. They show problems in the very definition of improvement, with differences between patient, therapist, and observer perception. They show a tendency for symptom levels to return to a pre-treatment baseline after treatment whether intervention is initially followed by improvement or deterioration. Certainly for established and chronic cases there is a high relapse rate. It is difficult to find any definite empirical evidence, but a perception is that combat veterans do rather worse than many other victims, particularly those who have been exposed to brief, even if catastrophic, trauma. Perhaps response to treatment will help us to sort out variants of PTSD. The treatment studies carried out thus far have been surprisingly small. We need more, and collaborative, probably multicentre, studies.

While further examining the treatment response in PTSD, there is also a very urgent need for further examination of the concept of prevention of ongoing disability after the traumatic event. There has been a general acceptance that the influx of 'specially trained counsellors' after any traumatic event is both necessary and inevitable. A few communities have anecdotally complained about the intrusion, but nevertheless there has grown a whole industry of counselling or debriefing. Thankfully, in recent years important players such as Raphael have started to point out that for all its blind acceptance, there is no substantiated evidence at all that debriefing in its various forms prevents PTSD. What evidence there is suggests no significant effect of debriefing, even though many victims are supportive of it. In addition, we cannot simply assume that such intervention is necessarily harmless. There has certainly been some suggestion that some intervention in PTI or PTSD can actually aggravate matters. There is a real need, not only for the larger-scale studies of treatment of PTSD, but also for such studies of the much-vaunted prevention measures and early interventions.

Summary

So what is the purpose of this clumsy attempt apparently to dismantle the carefully constructed concept of PTSD?

I am not, in any sense, attempting to suggest that post-traumatic illnesses do not occur. They clearly do, and one of the major successes of the PTSD story is that this is a concept almost universally accepted today, so that post-traumatic problems are accepted by health services and those who plan and pay for them, as well as by employers, by courts, and by the public. However, it seems to me that PTSD is almost a victim of its own success. There is some degree of a backlash as a wider and wider range of people claim greater and greater sums of compensation following an apparently spreading degree of involvement in an increasing variety of traumatic incidents. Not only does this cause some resentment and suggestion that people are perhaps no longer able to sustain the normal stresses and vicissitudes of life, but as the syndrome spreads it must surely be diluted and more heterogeneous, so that investigation becomes more difficult and more speculative. There is a need to step back and look dispassionately at the arena of post-traumatic problems. Does the concept have the same value if it applies to almost anyone after almost anything? We need to compare like with like. If the effects of everyday normal stresses of life initially specifically excluded from definitions of PTSD are the same as the effects of catastrophe, then PTSD needs to be rethought and perhaps renamed. If not, then we need to examine its boundaries further. What is really needed, if unlikely to be possible, is a really large-scale prospective study of a group of young people, looking at what traumata they experience, what else their world and history contains, and what their responses to the traumata and subsequent treatment and experience turn out to be.

An attempt to summarise the conclusions and the unsolved problems which come to mind would be as follows.

- Mental health problems can follow a wide range of stressful events and situations.
- There have probably always been responses to stresses but the confident assertion that they have remained unchanged in character and detail over hundreds of years is not really proven and is probably incorrect. Life is changing.
- The response to stresses is not always uniform and does not always constitute an illness.
- The idea that responses to various stresses is uniform, or that stresses can readily be equated on the basis of severity, is less than proven.

- When an illness is present the diagnosis is often a 'standard' one.
- There is some objective evidence of particular symptom clusters after certain forms of trauma which seem to correspond to PTSD symptomatology. However, not all of the individual symptoms have been demonstrated to be independent of each other or of equivalent importance. None of them is pathognomonic of PTSD.
- We need an objective measure which can be used to diagnose PTSD and does not rely upon response to questions in whatever form. At present comparison of diagnoses is necessarily theoretically based. There is a circular relationship between diagnosis and definition which could only be broken if there were a pathological test.
- There is a need for more knowledge about course and about response to treatment. There is an urgent need for more knowledge about the effect of debriefing and early intervention.
- PTSD is a useful concept, but we still need a healthy scepticism and some more research. If you do not need 'abnormal' or 'unusual' or 'extreme' or 'catastrophic' stresses to cause PTSD then perhaps some redefinition and new description are required. In the meantime, we need to keep trying to find out which stresses cause which symptoms in which people, and what happens then.

INDEX